THIS BOOK BELONGS TO

_____

This educational resource is being provided to you by
Otsuka America Pharmaceutical, Inc.

 Otsuka America Pharmaceutical, Inc.

ATLAS OF VASCULAR DISEASE

SECOND EDITION

ATLAS OF VASCULAR DISEASE

SECOND EDITION

EDITOR
MARK A. CREAGER, MD

Associate Professor
Department of Medicine
Harvard Medical School
Cardiovascular Division
Simon C. Fireman Scholar in Cardiovascular Medicine
Director, Vascular Center
Brigham and Women's Hospital
Boston, Massachusetts

SERIES EDITOR
EUGENE BRAUNWALD, MD, MD (HON), ScD (HON)

Distinguished Hersey Professor of Medicine
Faculty Dean for Academic Programs at Brigham and Women's
  Hospital and Massachusetts General Hospital
Harvard Medical School
Vice President for Academic Programs
Partners HealthCare System
Boston, Massachusetts

With 19 contributors

Developed by Current Medicine, Inc.

Philadelphia

CURRENT MEDICINE, INC.

400 Market Street, Suite 700 • Philadelphia, PA 19106

Developmental Editor . . . .*Teresa M. Giuliana*
Commissioning Supervisor . . . .*Annmarie D'Ortona*
Cover Design . . . .*Jennifer Knight*
Design and Layout . . . .*William C. Whitman, Jr.*
Illustrators . . . .*Wieslawa Langenfeld and Maureen Looney*
Assistant Production Manager . . . .*Margaret LaMare*
Index . . . .*Dorothy Hoffman*

Library of Congress Cataloging-in-Publication Data

Atlas of vascular disease / editor, Mark A. Creager.-- 2nd ed.
    p. ; cm.
  Rev. ed. of: Vascular disease / volume editor, Mark A. Creager. c1996.
  Includes bibliographical references and index.
  ISBN 1-57340-191-9 (hardcover : alk. paper)
   1. Blood-vessels--Diseases--Atlases. I. Title: Vascular disease. II. Creager, Mark A.
  [DNLM: 1. Vascular Diseases--Atlases. WG 17 A884683 2002]
 RC682 .A825 2002
 616.1'3--dc21

                               2002067395

ISBN 1-57340-191-9

Printed in Thailand by Imago Productions (FE) Ltd.

10 9 8 7 6 5 4 3 2 1
For more information please call 1 (800) 427-1796 or (215) 574-2266
or e-mail us at inquiry@phl.cursci.com

www.current-science-group.com

PREFACE

Vascular diseases constitute the most common causes of disability and death in Western society. Atherosclerosis, thrombosis, hypertension, and their clinical sequelae, including myocardial infarction, disabling claudication, limb loss, and stroke, occur far too frequently. Indeed, vascular pathology in one form or another is responsible for over one hundred billion dollars of costs annually in the United States for medical expenses and lost productivity.

There have been rapid advancements in vascular biology, pharmacology, and technology for vascular disease. Basic science discoveries have led to our recognition of the human vasculature as not simply a passive conduit, but as a complex organ that responds to both intrinsic and extrinsic stimuli with definable pathologic processes. In addition, technologic advances have redefined the role of imaging modalities. The enhanced resolution of techniques such as ultrasonography, computed tomography, and magnetic resonance angiography has enabled the clinician to accurately diagnose vascular diseases noninvasively, thereby avoiding the risks inherent to invasive procedures. As diagnostic modalities have become less invasive, therapeutic options have moved from the purely surgical arena. Innovations in endovascular intervention have provided less invasive therapeutic strategies for patients affected by clinically significant atherosclerosis of peripheral and renal arteries. Endovascular placement of stented grafts is now employed for selected patients with aortic aneurysms. Advances in surgical techniques coupled with perioperative cardiac risk assessment and management have yielded lower operative mortality and morbidity rates and consequently improved the outcome for patients with arterial aneurysms, ischemic extremities, and cerebrovascular disease.

This second edition of the *Atlas of Vascular Disease* reviews a number of important vascular disorders that are encountered in clinical practice, including aortic aneurysms and dissection, peripheral arterial occlusive disease, renovascular hypertension, cerebrovascular disease, vasospasm, venous thromboembolism, venous insufficiency, and lymphedema. For each major vascular condition, the pathophysiology, clinical presentation, associated conditions (*eg*, atherosclerosis, hypertension, and vasculitis), contemporary diagnostic testing (*eg*, vascular ultrasonography, magnetic resonance imaging, and angiography), and therapeutic strategies are discussed. One of the most perplexing issues to face the clinician is how to manage the patient undergoing vascular surgery, since many of these patients have coexisting coronary artery disease. Therefore, we have devoted a chapter to preoperative risk assessment, decision analysis, and medical management.

The chapter on vascular neoplasms logically categorizes and beautifully illustrates the pathology of these blood vessel tumors. We have also dedicated a chapter to Kawasaki disease, an important infectious disease that affects blood vessels, particularly in children, and one that is of growing interest to clinicians.

Our understanding of vascular biology is increasing rapidly and our ability to favorably influence outcome in patients with vascular disease has never been greater. This atlas is designed to provide the physician with a practical and informative framework, illustrating the clinical options in a logical and algorithmic fashion. In addition, it will serve as a useful teaching aid for those who educate medical students, house staff, fellows, and colleagues. It is hoped that this atlas will enable the readers to deal effectively with a broad range of vascular diseases that are encountered in practice.

MARK A. CREAGER, MD

CONTRIBUTORS

ANDREW W. BRADBURY, BSC, MBCHB (HCUS), MD, FRCSED
Professor
Department of Surgery
University of Birmingham
Birmingham Heartlands Hospital
Birmingham, United Kingdom

MARK A. CREAGER, MD
Associate Professor
Department of Medicine
Harvard Medical School
Cardiovascular Division
Simon C. Fireman Scholar in
  Cardiovascular Medicine
Director, Vascular Center
Brigham and Women's Hospital
Boston, Massachusetts

MAGRUDER C. DONALDSON, MD
Associate Professor
Department of Surgery
Harvard Medical School
Brigham and Women's Hospital
Boston, Massachusetts

SAMUEL Z. GOLDHABER, MD
Associate Professor
Department of Medicine
Harvard Medical School
Staff Cardiologist
Director, Venous Thromboembolism
  Research Group
Director, Anticoagulation Service
Brigham and Women's Hospital
Boston, Massachusetts

MARDI GOMBERG-MAITLAND, MD, MSC
Mount Sinai School of Medicine
New York, New York

SCOTT R. GRANTER, MD
Associate Professor
Department of Pathology
Harvard Medical School
Associate Pathologist
Brigham and Women's Hospital
Boston, Massachusetts

JONATHAN L. HALPERIN, MD
Professor
Department of Cardiology
Mount Sinai School of Medicine
Director, Cardiology Clinical Service
The Zena and Michael A. Wiener
  Cardiovascular Institute
Mount Sinai Medical Center
New York, New York

MARIE GERHARD-HERMAN, MD
Assistant Professor
Department of Medicine
Cardiovascular Division
Medical Director, Vascular Diagnostic Laboratory
Brigham and Women's Hospital
Boston, Massachusetts

ALAN T. HIRSCH, MD
Associate Professor
Departments of Medicine and Radiology
Director, Vascular Medicine Program
University of Minnesota Medical School
Minneapolis, Minnesota

ERIC M. ISSELBACHER, MD
Assistant Professor
Department of Medicine
Harvard Medical School
Medical Director, Thoracic Aortic Center
Massachusetts General Hospital
Boston, Massachusetts

FRANCES E. JENSEN, MD
Director, Cardiovascular Division
Brigham and Women's Hospital
Boston, Massachusetts

ALEXANDER J. F. LAZAR, MD, PHD
Clinical Fellow
Department of Pathology
Harvard Medical School
Brigham and Women's Hospital
Boston, Massachusetts

JANE W. NEWBURGER, MD, MPH
Professor
Department of Pediatrics
Harvard Medical School
Associate Cardiologist-in-Chief
Children's Hospital of Boston
Boston, Massachusetts

JEFFREY W. OLIN, DO
Director, Vascular Medicine Program
The Zena and Michael A. Wiener
  Cardiovascular Institute
Mount Sinai School of Medicine
New York, New York

JOSEPH F. POLAK, MD, MPH
Associate Professor
Department of Radiology
Harvard Medical School
Director of Noninvasive Vascular Imaging
Brigham and Women's Hospital
Boston, Massachusetts

KHETHER E. RABY, MD
Assistant Clinical Professor
Department of Medicine
Boston University School of Medicine
Boston, Massachusetts

STANLEY ROCKSON, MD
Associate Professor
Division of Cardiovascular Medicine
Stanford University School of Medicine
Chief, Consultative Cardiology
Stanford University Medical Center
Stanford, California

C.VAUGHAN RUCKLEY, MB, CHM, FRCSE, FRCPE
Professor Emeritus
Department of Vascular Surgery
The University of Edinburgh
Edinburgh Royal Infirmary
Edinburgh, Scotland

KATHRYN A. TAUBERT, PHD
Professor
Department of Physiology
University of Texas Southwestern Medical School
Vice President, Science and Medicine
American Heart Association
National Center
Dallas, Texas

CONTENTS

1

CHAPTER

AORTIC AND ARTERIAL ANEURYSMS

Mardi Gomberg-Maitland, Jonathan L. Halperin, and Mark A. Creager

The aorta is the body's major conductance vessel, through which all oxygenated blood passes. As an elastic artery, the aortic wall consists of three layers: intima, media, and adventitia. The arteries arising along its course give rise to the vasa vasorum, which supply a capillary network to the adventitia and media of the thoracic aorta; however, vasa vasorum do not supply the media of the abdominal aorta. Systolic ejection of blood from the left ventricle creates a pressure wave that traverses the aorta producing radial expansion and contraction and transfer of energy to the aortic wall. During diastole, the aortic wall recoils, transforming potential to kinetic energy and driving blood into the peripheral vessels.

The term aneurysm originates from the Greek *aneurysma*, for dilation. The pathologic concept is distinct from ectasia, the modest generalized arterial dilation that normally accompanies aging. Aneurysms may be classified anatomically or etiologically; true aneurysms may be either fusiform or saccular. The limited orifice of a saccular aneurysm may protect the thin wall from aortic pressure, thereby reducing the risk of rupture, while the entire circumference of a fusiform aneurysm is exposed to distending forces. Infrarenal aortic aneurysms, the most common type, are almost exclusively fusiform. Aneurysms are classified according to the segment of aorta affected, since clinical features depend largely on location. Aneurysms of more peripheral arteries carry a lower risk of rupture than those of the aorta, but a greater propensity to thromboembolic complications. A pseudoaneurysm, or false aneurysm, is essentially a contained arterial rupture, in which the wall of the aneurysm is composed of thrombotic material; the relatively narrow communication between the sac and main lumen may resemble a saccular true aneurysm.

Dilatation of the aorta may occur as a consequence of aging, as well as of atherosclerosis, infection, inflammation, trauma, congenital anomalies, and medial degeneration. The pathologic changes that accompany these conditions cause the aorta to thicken, thin, bulge, tear, rupture, stenose or dissect, or be altered by combinations of these conditions. Atherosclerotic lesions occur more extensively in the abdominal aorta than in any part of the arterial tree and initially affect only the intima, but fibrocalcific degeneration leads to secondary atrophy of the medial layer. The ascending aorta is generally spared by atherosclerosis until the most advanced stages, and aneurysmal disease of the ascending aorta is more often nonatherosclerotic. Cystic medial necrosis, with elastic fiber degeneration, necrosis of muscle cells, and cystic spaces filled with mucoid material, is most frequent in the ascending aorta but may be seen in the remainder of the aorta as well, particularly in Marfan syndrome.

In addition to the etiology and location of aortic aneurysms, the risk of rupture of aortic aneurysms correlates with diameter, accounting for at least 30% of deaths. Aneurysms typically produce no symptoms prior to rupture, but a variety of symptom complexes may arise depending on size and location. Diagnosis of an abdominal aortic aneurysm may be suggested by prominent widening of the epigastric pulsation. Epigastric bruit is a nonspecific finding, and other findings on physical examination reflect co-existing atherosclerosis. Plain roentgenograms may reveal calcification in the opposing walls, and ultrasonography helps confirm its size and demonstrate thrombus formation on the intimal surface extending into the lumen. Computed tomography accurately outlines the configuration, especially when enhanced by the intravenous injection of contrast material. Magnetic resonance imaging is a sensitive tool for early detection of dissection. Contrast aortography is reserved for preoperative definition of the relationship of the aneurysm to adjacent vascular structures in patients with concomitant arterial occlusive disease.

The surgical technique for repair of aortic aneurysms has evolved over the past 50 years since the first resection of an abdominal aortic aneurysm was reported in 1952 [1]. Today, most surgeons use a modification of the method advanced by Crawford and Coselli. Following dissection just beyond the proximal and distal margins of the aneurysm, heparin is administered and the aorta is cross-clamped. The aorta is incised, and a woven Dacron (Dupont, Wilmington, DE) graft is inserted within the aneurysmal sac and anastomosed to the less diseased portions. After the anastomoses are complete, the clamps are released and the wall of the aneurysm is then wrapped around the outside of the prosthetic graft.

Operative repair of thoraco-abdominal aneurysms still carries a high mortality rate; major complications include paraplegia, renal insufficiency, and myocardial infarction. The outlook for repair of abdominal aortic aneurysms is considerably better, with in-hospital mortality rates around 1%. There have been several controlled trials comparing surgical and nonsurgical management of patients with abdominal aortic aneurysms of 4.0 to 5.5 cm. There is no survival advantage of early elective repair of small aneurysms compared with careful surveillance when surgical repair is deferred until aneurysm size exceeds 5.5 cm or expands at a rate of 1 cm or more per year.

The 5-year survival rate in patients with untreated aneurysms larger than 5 cm in diameter ranges between 5% and 10%, while the survival rate for such patients after surgery is over 50%. After recovery from surgical repair, long-term survival is limited principally by concomitant coronary or cerebrovascular disease [9]. It is hoped that the introduction of intraluminal stent graft repair will reduce the operative mortality of aortic aneurysm correction, but the relative durability of this approach compared with conventional open aneurysmorrhaphy must be established.

Evaluation and management of patients with aneurysmal disease of the aorta and peripheral arteries requires appreciation of the various factors that bear upon prognosis and careful balancing of the complexity of surgical intervention against alternative measures to reduce the risk of rupture. Control of hypertension, medications that reduce the rate of rise of arterial pressure during systole, and general steps to prevent thromboembolic complications and retard progression of atherosclerotic disease seem of diminishing value as the expansion of an aneurysm threatens cardiovascular catastrophe. A successful outcome depends upon close serial evaluation by means of appropriate noninvasive imaging methodology and timely, judicious intervention.

Evaluation and management of patients with aneurysmal disease of the aorta and peripheral arteries require an appreciation of the factors that influence prognosis and careful balancing of the risk of surgical intervention against the limited nonoperative measures available to reduce the chance of rupture. Control of hypertension, medications that reduce aneurysmal wall stress, and measures to prevent thromboembolic conditions and retard progression of atherosclerotic disease diminish in value as the expansion of an aneurysm threatens cardiovascular catastrophe. A successful outcome depends on close serial evaluation by means of appropriate noninvasive imaging methodology and timely, judicious intervention.

THE NORMAL AORTA

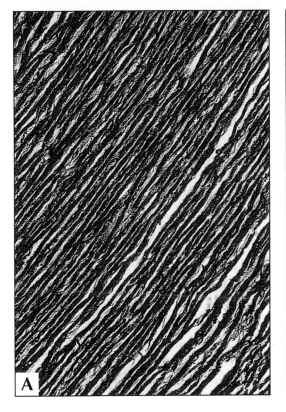

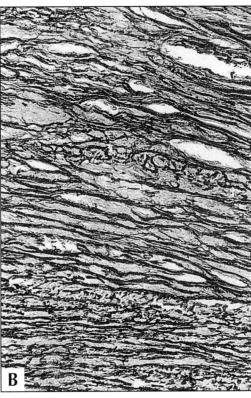

FIGURE 1-1. Histology of the normal aorta. Compare the composition of elastin in the aortic wall of a child (**A**) with that in an elderly adult (**B**). Each component of the aortic wall changes with age: elastic fibers fragment, collagen becomes more prominent at the expense of smooth muscle cells, and acid mucopolysaccharide ground substance accumulates progressively. The wall weakens, leading to dilation of the lumen and elongation and uncoiling of the aortic arch. The process of ectasia that accompanies aging is distinct from the pathologic changes that produce aneurysm formation. (Orcein and Giesen stain; magnification, ×414.) (*From* Nichols and O'Rourke [2]; with permission.)

CLASSIFICATION OF AORTIC ANEURYSMS

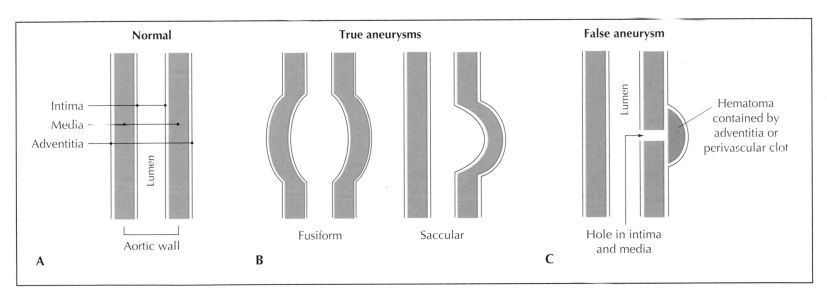

FIGURE 1-2. Classification of aortic aneurysms. **A,** The normal aortic lumen is lined by intimal endothelium, a muscular medial layer, and a surrounding fibrous adventitia. **B,** True aneurysms are localized dilatations involving all three layers. Circumferential or fusiform aneurysms are distinguished from saccular aneurysms because of differences in etiology and natural history. **C,** A false aneurysm, or pseudoaneurysm, is essentially a hematoma formed when a perforation of the intima and media is contained by a thin layer of adventitia or perivascular thrombus. (*Adapted from* Diminick *et al.* [3].)

Thoracic aortic aneurysms
  Ascending aorta
  Aortic arch
  Descending thoracic aorta
Thoraco-abdominal aortic aneurysms
Abdominal aortic aneurysms
  Aneurysms involving the origins of the renal arteries
  Infrarenal aneurysms
Visceral artery aneurysms
Iliac artery aneurysms
Femoropopliteal aneurysms
Carotid artery aneurysms
Aneurysms of other arteries of the extremities

FIGURE 1-3. Anatomic classification of aortic aneurysms, in which thoracic and abdominal portions are distinguished and the thoracic aorta is subdivided into ascending, transverse (arch), and descending segments. Normally, the ascending aorta has a maximum diameter of 3 cm, the aortic arch 2.5 to 3.5 cm (depending on body size and age), and approximately 20 cm from the arch the diameter of the thoracic aorta tapers to about 2 cm. The abdominal aorta descends in front of the vertebral column approximately 15 cm and then divides into the two iliac arteries. Along this course, its diameter narrows further, averaging 1.7 to 1.9 cm and about 2 mm larger in males than in females.

AORTIC ANEURYSMAL DISEASE: ETIOLOGIC AND ASSOCIATED CONDITIONS

Atherosclerosis	Infectious aortitis
Cystic medial necrosis	Congenital
Vasculitis	Traumatic

FIGURE 1-4. Etiologic and associated conditions of aortic aneurysmal disease. Dilatation of the aorta may occur as a consequence of aging, as well as of atherosclerosis, infection, inflammation, trauma, congenital anomalies, or medial degeneration. The principal consequences of atherosclerosis in the aorta are aneurysmal dilatation and stenotic obstruction. The former process is more generalized, potentially affecting the entire length of the aorta, while obstruction is limited mainly to the abdominal portion. The proximal thoracic aorta is rarely a site of atherosclerotic formation unless there is independent disease of the media. When the arch and descending portions are aneurysmal, there is usually involvement of the abdominal aorta as well, since the abdomen is the most common site of aneurysm formation.

Congenital aneurysms are often associated with other congenital cardiac defects such as bicuspid aortic valve or coarctation, and sometimes involve cystic medial necrosis. Following chest trauma, aneurysms most often develop in the descending thoracic aorta just beyond the origin of the left subclavian artery. Aortic aneurysms resulting from sudden horizontal deceleration injury usually involve the mobile subclavian isthmus at the ligamentum arteriosus. Vertical deceleration injuries commonly produce aneurysms of the ascending aorta. Because of the unpredictable risk of rupture, surgical repair is usually advised for traumatic aneurysms, even when they are remote from the inciting injury. Other etiologic subtypes of aortic aneurysms are discussed in Figures 1-5 through 1-9.

CYSTIC MEDIAL NECROSIS AND THE MARFAN SYNDROME

CAUSES OF CYSTIC MEDIAL NECROSIS OF THE AORTA

Primary
Marfan syndrome
Ehlers-Danlos syndrome

FIGURE 1-5. Causes of cystic medial necrosis of the aorta. Histologic evidence of severe elastic fiber degeneration, necrosis of muscle cells, and cystic spaces filled with mucoid material (*see also* Fig. 1-6) are most often encountered in the ascending aorta from the region of the valve to the brachiocephalic artery, although similar changes may occur in the remainder of the aorta as well. Aneurysms in these cases are almost invariably fusiform. Aortic regurgitation may occur as a consequence of dilatation of the aortic root even though the valve leaflets themselves are unaffected histologically.

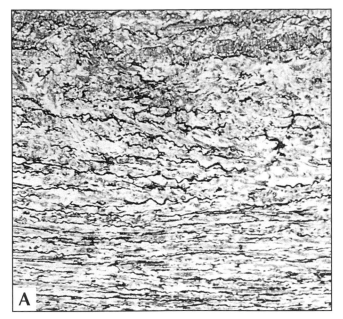

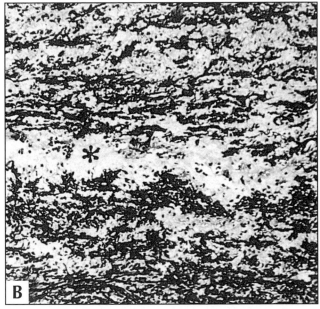

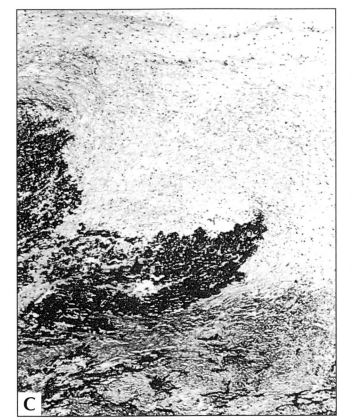

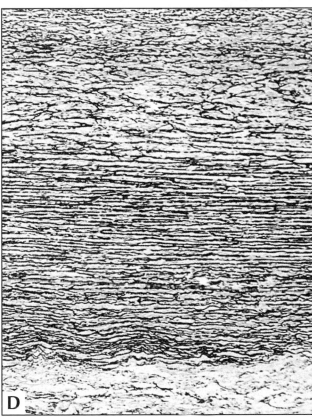

FIGURE 1-6.
Histologic changes of medial degeneration progressing to cystic medial necrosis of the aorta. **A,** Mild elastic tissue fragmentation in a patient with Marfan syndrome. **B,** Higher-power photomicrograph of a section of the aortic wall from another patient demonstrating cyst formation (*asterisk*), with depletion of elastic tissue, focal loss of medial smooth muscle cells, and mucopolysaccharide accumulation. **C,** Advanced cystic medial necrosis, with gross deficiency of elastic tissue. **D,** Normal aorta, for comparison. All sections were prepared with a stain in which elastic tissue appears black. (*From* Schoen [4]; with permission.)

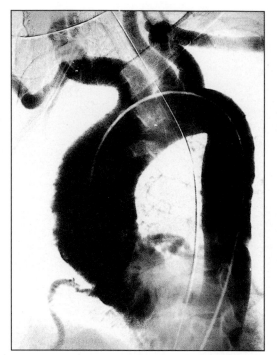

FIGURE 1-7. The aorta in Marfan syndrome. This syndrome is an inherited disorder characterized by arachnodactyly, redundant ligaments, ectopia lentis, ascending aortic dilatation, and incompetency of the aortic and/or mitral valves. Aneurysms in this disorder are characterized by annulo-aortic ectasia involving the sinuses of Valsalva and the tubular portion of the aorta, and are produced by degeneration of elastic fibers and accumulation of mucoid material within the medial layer of the aortic wall, grossly resembling cystic medial necrosis. Dissection is relatively frequent and may involve the entire length of the aorta, with or without other histologic features of the syndrome or aortic valvular incompetence. True dissection tends not to develop in cases in which fusiform aneurysm formation is present in patients with Marfan syndrome, such that there are two patterns of presentation: dissection and aneurysmal degeneration. (*From* Creager *et al.* [5]; with permission.)

MISCELLANEOUS CAUSES OF AORTIC ANEURYSMAL DISEASE

VASCULITIS SYNDROMES ASSOCIATED WITH AORTIC ANEURYSM FORMATION

Takayasu's arteritis
Giant cell arteritis
Ankylosing spondylitis
Rheumatoid arthritis
Reiter's syndrome
Relapsing polychondritis

FIGURE 1-8. Vasculitis syndromes associated with aortic aneurysm formation. Takayasu's arteritis, also designated "pulseless disease" or "idiopathic medial aortopathy," is a chronic vasculitis of unknown etiology, with a predilection for the aorta and its primary branches. Aneurysms may be associated with thromboembolic phenomena, but rupture is uncommon. Giant cell arteritis, typically occurring in individuals over 55 years of age, affects more distal arteries of the upper half of the body than arteritis of the Takayasu type; aneurysmal complications are less frequent in the aorta. Among the seronegative spondyloarthropathies, ankylosing spondylitis is associated with several cardio-aortic anomalies, including aortic regurgitation, dilatation, and dissection. Abnormalities of the proximal aorta associated with ankylosing spondylitis include dilatation of the valve annulus, fibrous thickening and focal inflammation of the valve cusps (which may prolapse into the left ventricular cavity), dilatation of the sinuses of Valsalva, and degeneration of the medial layer of the aortic wall. Rheumatoid arthritis, relapsing polychondritis, and Reiter's syndrome have each been associated with dilatation of the aorta, sometimes accompanied by valvular aortic regurgitation.

INFECTIOUS CAUSES OF AORTIC ANEURYSMAL DISEASE

Syphilitic aortopathy
Tuberculous aortopathy
Mycotic aneurysms
  Staphylococcus
  Streptococcus
  Salmonella
  Pseudomonas species

FIGURE 1-9. Infectious causes of aortic aneurysmal disease. Syphilitic aneurysms are typically saccular, and involve the ascending aorta whether or not the transverse and descending portions are also affected. Rupture is the major complication, but the enlarging aneurysm may also compress or erode adjacent structures of the mediastinum. Since the inflammatory process tends to interrupt the medial layer by transverse scars, dissection is uncommon. Linear calcification of the wall of the ascending aorta may appear on roentgenography of the chest, a finding not typically encountered in other types of aneurysmal disease of the ascending aorta. Tuberculous aneurysms result usually from direct extension of infection from hilar lymph nodes and subsequent granulomatous destruction of the medial layer leading to loss of aortic wall elasticity. The posterior or posterolateral aortic wall is usually the site of saccular aneurysm formation in such cases. Primary mycotic aneurysms may arise as complications of infective endocarditis or arterial catheterization. An intrinsically abnormal aorta, however, may become infected as a consequence of bacteremia from any cause, producing suppurative aortitis leading to weakness of a portion of the aortic wall. In these cases aneurysms are typically saccular, with a comparatively high propensity to rupture.

AORTIC IMAGING METHODS

FIGURE 1-10. Diagnostic methods for imaging of the aorta. Plain roentgenography frequently suggests the diagnosis in asymptomatic patients. Anteroposterior or "across-table" lateral views may reveal calcification in the opposing walls of an aortic aneurysm. Two-dimensional echocardiography may be employed to assess the proximal ascending aorta. Ultrasound examination provides accurate estimates of the diameter of the abdominal aorta and may demonstrate thrombus formation on the intimal surface extending into the lumen. Contrast-enhanced computed tomography is both sensitive and specific for assessment of aneurysms of the thoracic aorta and is particularly useful for outlining the length as well as the diameter and shape of thoraco-abdominal aortic aneurysms. Magnetic resonance imaging, which avoids nephrotoxic contrast agents, increasingly is favored as a noninvasive method for diagnosis of aortic aneurysms. Contrast aortography is the principal diagnostic test for confirming an aneurysm of the thoracic aorta and for determining morphology. Although noninvasive diagnostic procedures may establish the diagnosis, aortography often is performed preoperatively to address the length of the aneurysm and involvement of branch vessels prior to operative correction of thoraco-abdominal aneurysms.

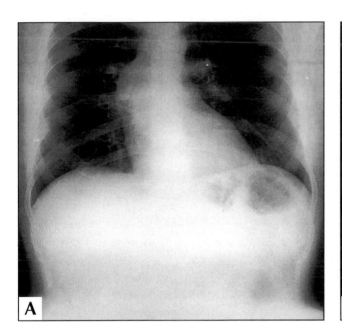
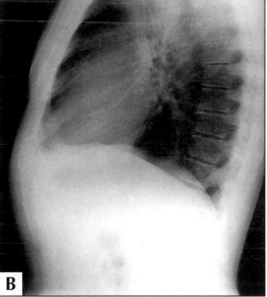

FIGURE 1-11. Chest roentgenograms in the posteroanterior (**A**) and left lateral (**B**) projections of a 43-year-old man with asymptomatic aneurysmal dilation of the ascending aorta. Increasingly recognized is the association of proximal aortic dilation with congenital bicuspid aortic valve, with or without hemodynamically significant valvular stenosis or regurgitation. Whether this is mediated by cystic medial necrosis of the aorta in all or some cases is not yet clear.

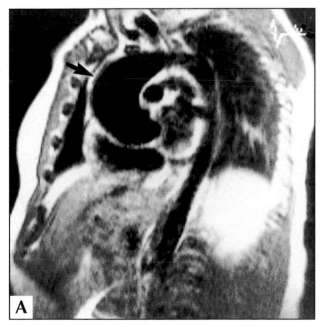
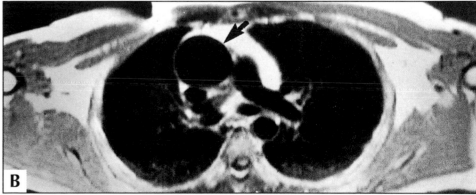

FIGURE 1-12. Magnetic resonance imaging scans of the thorax of the patient in Figures 1-11 and 1-13 demonstrate 5-cm diameter fusiform dilatation of the ascending aorta in the sagittal (**A**) and transverse (**B**) planes. The aorta narrows to normal diameter at the level of the arch. *Arrows* designate the dilated ascending aortic segment.

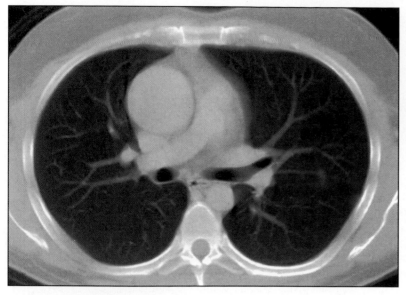

FIGURE 1-13. Contrast-enhanced computed tomography scan of the thorax of the patient in Figures 1-11 and 1-12, illustrating dilatation of the proximal portion of the ascending aorta without dissection.

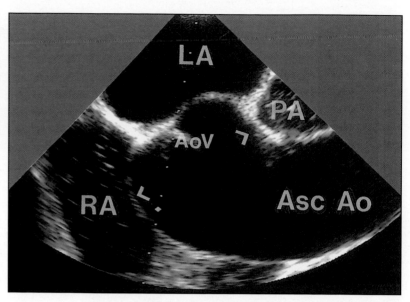

FIGURE 1-14. Aneurysm of the ascending aorta (Asc Ao), measuring 4.8 cm in diameter at the level of the sinuses of Valsalva, imaged by transesophageal echocardiography. The relative accuracy of the various vascular imaging modalities for measurement of the aortic diameter and identification of early markers of rupture or dissection is controversial. *Brackets* mark the ends of the line of measurement. AoV—aortic valve; LA—left atrium; PA—pulmonary artery; RA—right atrium.

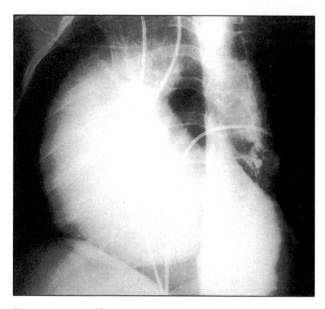

FIGURE 1-15. Chest roentgenogram of a patient with annulo-aortic ectasia involving the transverse arch. (*From* Cooley [6]; with permission.)

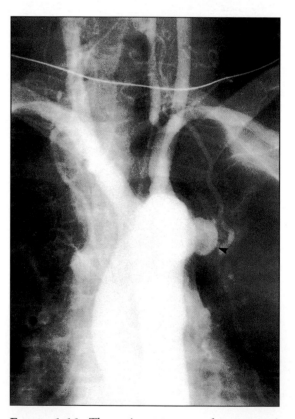

FIGURE 1-16. Thoracic aortogram demonstrating a saccular aneurysm (*arrowhead*) involving the aortic arch. (*From* Creager *et al.* [5]; with permission.)

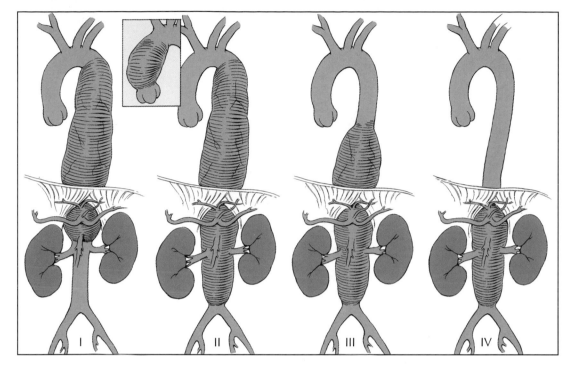

FIGURE 1-17. Classification of thoraco-abdominal aortic aneurysms. Type I aneurysms involve most of the descending aorta from near the origin of the left subclavian artery to the abdominal vessels, but the renal arteries are not involved. Type II aneurysms also begin near the origin of the left subclavian artery, but extend below the origins of the renal arteries in the abdomen. Type III aneurysms arise more distally and involve less of the descending thoracic aorta but often involve more of the abdominal aorta than type I and II aneurysms. Type IV aneurysms arise at the level of the diaphragm and typically extend to a point below the origins of the renal arteries. (*Adapted from* Crawford and Coselli [7].)

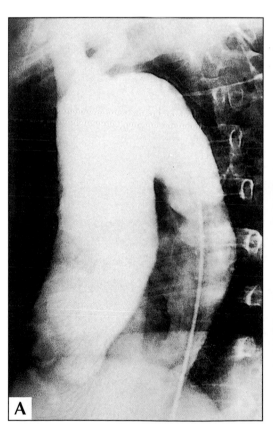

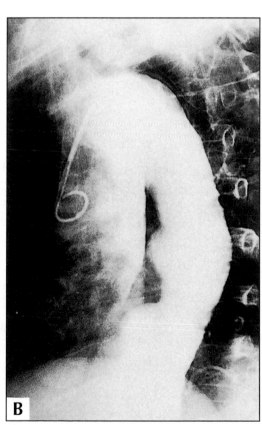

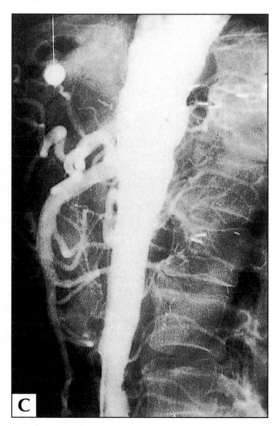

FIGURE 1-18. Aortograms demonstrating an extensive thoraco-abdominal aortic aneurysm. **A,** Ascending thoracic aorta. **B,** Descending thoracic aorta. **C,** Abdominal aorta. (*From* Creager *et al.* [5]; with permission.)

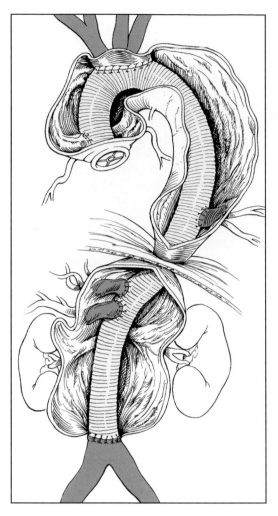

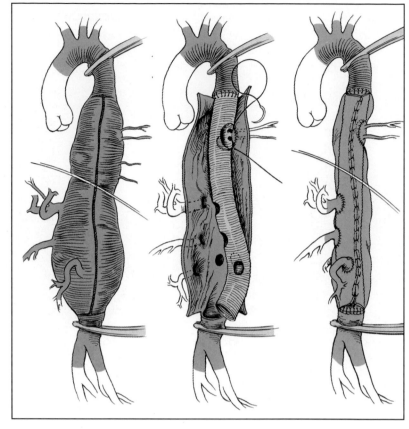

FIGURE 1-19. General technique for endoaneurysmorrhaphy for repair of aortic aneurysms. Emphasis is on repair and restoration of circulatory continuity rather than on excision. (*Adapted from* Cooley [6].)

FIGURE 1-20. Repair of thoraco-abdominal aortic aneurysm using the graft inclusion technique, with anastomosis of intercostal and visceral vessels. The procedure involves a thoraco-abdominal incision, cross-clamping of the thoracic aorta, and replacement of the aneurysmal segment of the aorta. Here the lateral aspect of the aorta is incised (*left*), and an intraluminal graft is incorporated within the opened aneurysmal sac (*center*), incorporating intercostal and visceral arterial ostia. The completed graft is then surrounded by the collapsed walls of the aneurysm (*right*). Cardiac afterload is reduced pharmacologically during the procedure, and renal perfusion with a chilled crystalloid solution may be employed. (*Adapted from* Whittemore and Mannick [8].)

ABDOMINAL AORTIC ANEURYSMS

FIGURE 1-21. Epidemiology of abdominal aortic aneurysms. (*Adapted from* Ernst [9].)

EPIDEMIOLOGY OF ABDOMINAL AORTIC ANEURYSMS

Incidence	12/100,000 population in 1950 → 36/100,000 in 1980
Mortality	15,000/y among population >55 years of age
Gender ratio	2:1 male predilection
Race differential	4.2% incidence in white males vs 1.5% in black males
Comorbidity	Occur in 5% of patients with coronary disease and 10% of those with atherosclerotic peripheral arterial disease
Surgery	40,000 operations for repair/y
Cost of rupture	2000 deaths/y; $50 million spent in medical costs over elective repair

A. PREVALENCE OF ABDOMINAL AORTIC ANEURYSM, BY SIZE	
DIAMETER, *CM*	PREVALENCE, %
≥ 3.0	4.2
≥ 4.0	1.3
≥ 5.0	0.5
≥ 6.0	0.2
≥ 7.0	0.1
≥ 8.0	0.03

B. PREVALENCE OF ABDOMINAL AORTIC ANEURYSM, BY SEX		
	PERCENTAGE WITH AAA	
AGE, *y*	MEN	WOMEN
65	5.9	0
65–70	5.9	1.0
71–75	9.0	1.8
76–80	9.2	1.6
Total	7.6	1.3

FIGURE 1-22. Prevalence of abdominal aortic aneurysm (AAA). **A**, Prevalence of AAA by diameter in the Veterans Administration Cooperative Study of 126,196 men between 50 and 79 years of age with no history of documented AAA who underwent ultrasound screening [10]. Age, smoking, family history of AAA, and atherosclerotic diseases remained the principal positive associations.

B, Prevalence of AAA in 9342 women and 6433 men between the ages of 65 and 80 years in Chichester, United Kingdom. The prevalence of AAA in women was six times lower than that in men for all age groups; the overall prevalence was 1.3% in women compared with 7.6% in men [11].

A. VARIABLES ASSOCIATED WITH ANEURYSM RUPTURE		
BASELINE VARIABLE*	HAZARD RATIO (95TH CI)	*P*
Age, *y*	1.02 (0.93–1.13)	0.67
Female sex	4.50 (1.98–10.2)	0.0
AAA diameter, *cm*	2.51 (1.08–5.80)	0.032
Current smoker†	2.11 (0.95–4.67)	0.066
Mean BP, *mm Hg*	1.04 (1.02–1.07)	0.002

*Cox regression analysis; all baseline variables adjusted for one another.
†People who never smoked and ex-smokers were combined and compared with current smokers.

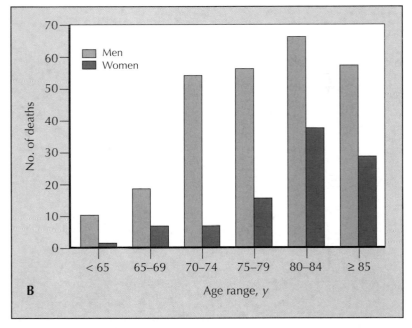

FIGURE 1-23. Variables associated with abdominal aortic aneurysm (AAA) rupture. **A**, In addition to initial AAA diameter in the United Kingdom Small Aneurysm Trial of 2257 patients, estimated hazard ratios identified female gender, higher mean arterial blood pressure (BP), and current smoking, as factors associated with increased risk of aneurysm rupture. The cohort included patients whose AAA diameter never exceeded 4.0 cm or who were unfit for or refused surgery. When the analysis was limited to a more homogenous group of 1090 otherwise healthy patients with AAAs 4.0 to 5.5 cm in diameter (with 25 that ruptured), current smoking had borderline significance, while initial AAA diameter, female gender, and higher mean BP were independently and significantly associated with rupture [12]. **B**, Mortality from ruptured AAAs. Women in

whom AAAs 3 cm in diameter or larger were detected in the study by Scott *et al.* [11] were followed with repeat ultrasonography at intervals depending on the diameter of the aneurysm. Surgical repair was considered when the aortic diameter measured 6 cm or more, the diameter increased by 1 cm or more annually, or symptoms developed. The number of deaths from aneurysm rupture in the unscreened local population is shown by age and gender. More than half the deaths from ruptured aneurysms in men occurred before age 80 years, while the majority of women (70%) died from rupture after age 80 years [11].

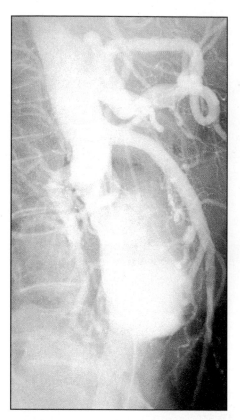

FIGURE 1-24. Abdominal aortogram demonstrating an infrarenal fusiform abdominal aortic aneurysm. In over 90% of cases, the superior margins of abdominal aortic aneurysms are below the level of the renal arteries. The average rate of expansion was 0.21 cm/y in one series, and 24% expanded faster than 0.4 cm/y. In 24,000 consecutive autopsies performed over a 23-year period there were 591 cases of abdominal aortic aneurysm. One hundred eighteen had ruptured. Of these, 9.5% were smaller than 4 cm in diameter; 25% were 4 to 7 cm in diameter; 45% were 7 to 10 cm; and 60% were larger than 10 cm. (*From* Creager *et al.* [5]; with permission.)

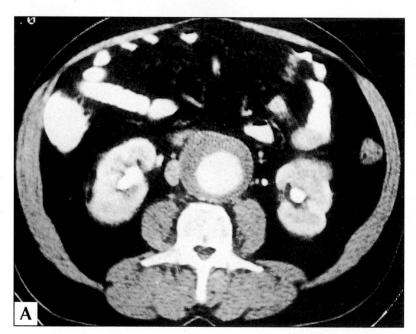

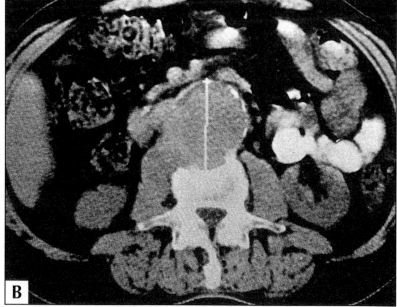

FIGURE 1-25. Computed tomographic images of patients showing abdominal aortic aneurysms located immediately anterior to the vertebral column. **A,** The aortic lumen is highlighted by an intravenous contrast agent, and can be distinguished from the surrounding mural thrombus. **B,** Another case imaged without intravenous contrast in which an adjacent vertebral body has been eroded. (*From* Creager *et al.* [5]; with permission.)

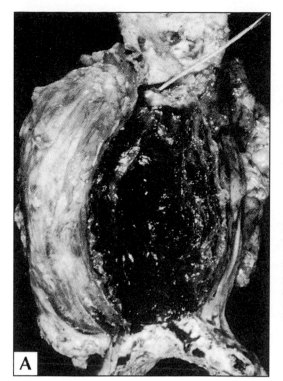
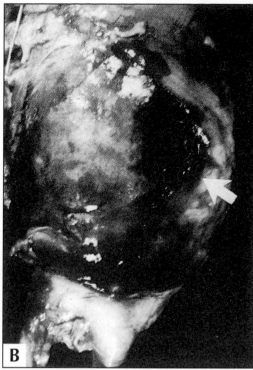

FIGURE 1-26. Autopsy specimen of an atherosclerotic abdominal aortic aneurysm following fatal rupture. **A,** Open view, demonstrating extensive intraluminal thrombosis. **B,** Closed anterior view. The site of rupture appears as a dark crescent-shaped patch on the anterolateral surface (*arrow*). (*From* Schoen [4]; with permission.)

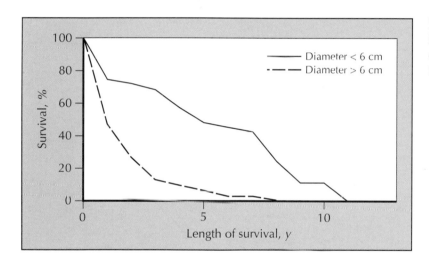

FIGURE 1-27. Comparative survival data for patients with abdominal aortic aneurysms without surgery. Three-year survival based on an aneurysmal diameter greater than ($n = 61$) or less than ($n = 44$) 6 cm.

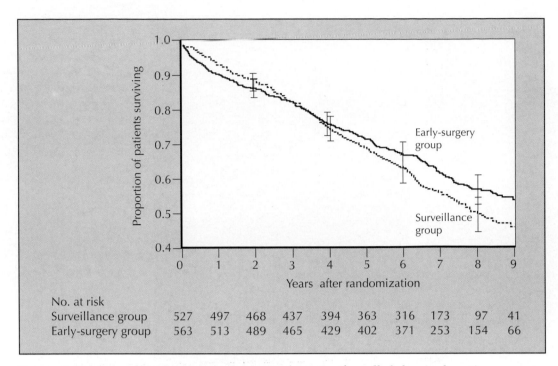

FIGURE 1-28. Surveillance versus early surgical repair of small abdominal aortic aneurysms (AAAs). The risk of rupture seems low for AAAs smaller than 5 cm in diameter. The United Kingdom Small Aneurysm Trial [14] and a Veterans Administration Cooperative Study [15] addressed whether early elective surgery would reduce mortality. In the United Kingdom study, 1090 patients 60 to 76 years of age with asymptomatic AAAs 4.0 to 5.5 cm in diameter were randomized to early elective open surgery ($n = 563$) or ultrasonographic surveillance ($n = 527$) and were followed for a mean of 8 years, with surgical repair recommended if the diameter of aneurysms in the surveillance group exceeded 5.5 cm. There was a survival disadvantage for patients in the elective surgery group early in the follow-up period, balanced by a higher rate of aneurysm rupture in the surveillance group. Mortality did not differ significantly between groups at 8 years, though women had a higher risk of aneurysm rupture than men. Ultrasonographic surveillance for small AAAs was a safe initial strategy [14]. Findings in the Veterans Administration Cooperative Trial were similar [15].

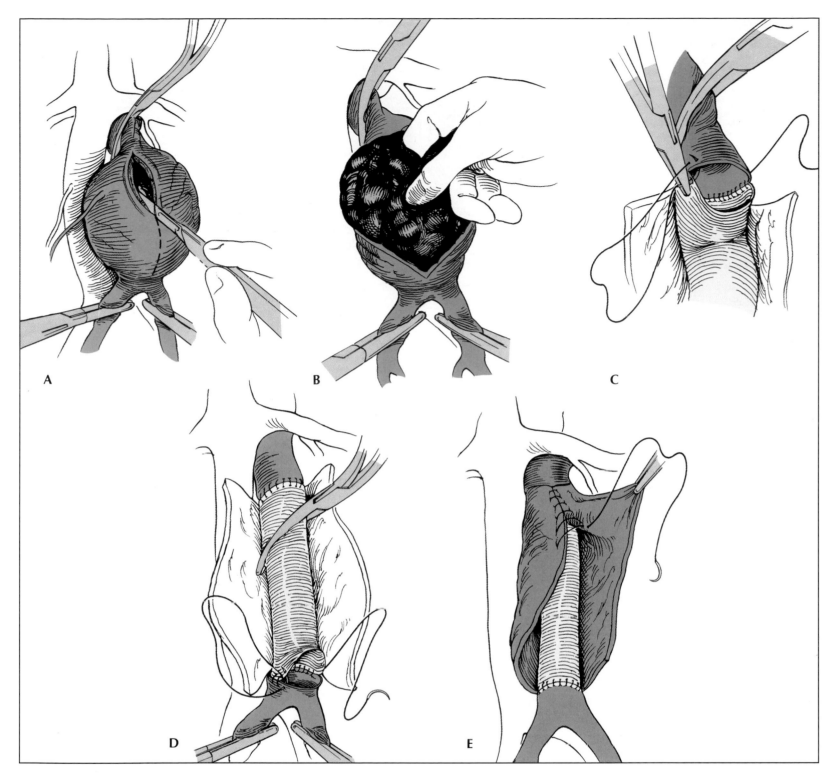

Figure 1-29. Surgical technique for repair of infrarenal abdominal aortic aneurysm. **A,** Following retroperitoneal exposure, the aneurysm is isolated between occluding cross-clamps and the sac is incised longitudinally. **B,** Intraluminal thrombus is evacuated and backbleeding lumbar vessels are oversewn. **C,** The proximal anasto-mosis is formed by continuously suturing the graft end-to-end to the neck of the aneurysm. **D,** The distal anastomosis is completed at the aortic bifurcation, also using monofilament suture. **E,** After flow is restored, the wall of the aneurysm is reapproximated over the graft to protect adjacent viscera. (*Adapted from* Greenhalgh [16].)

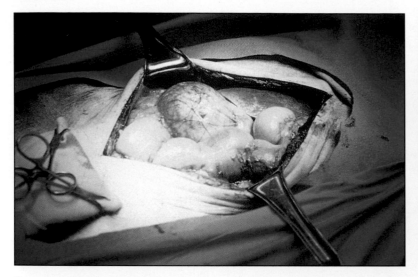

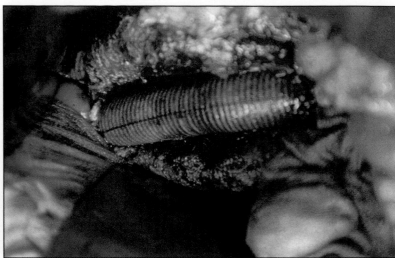

FIGURE 1-30. Intraoperative photograph showing retroperitoneal exposure for repair of an abdominal aortic aneurysm.

FIGURE 1-31. Intraoperative photograph showing a tubular polyethylene terephthalate (Dacron; Dupont, Wilmington, DE) aortic graft in place following repair of abdominal aortic aneurysm.

FIGURE 1-32. Outcome of surgery for repair of intact abdominal aortic aneurysm. (*Adapted from* Ernst [9].)

RESULTS OF SURGERY FOR NONRUPTURED ABDOMINAL AORTIC ANEURYSMS

STUDY	STUDY PERIOD	PATIENTS, *n*	DEATHS, *n*	MORTALITY, %
Crawford *et al.* [17]	1955–1980	860	41	4.8
McCabe *et al.* [18]	1972–1977	364	9	2.5
Diehl *et al.* [19]	1974–1978	350	18	5.1
Hertzer *et al.* [20]	1978–1981	840	55	6.5
Donaldson *et al.* [21]	1972–1983	476	24	5.0
Reigel *et al.* [22]	1980–1985	499	14	2.8
Green *et al.* [23]	1983–1987	379	8	2.1
Johnston [24]	1986	666	32	4.8
Leather *et al.* [25]	Not stated	299	11	3.7
Sicard *et al.* [26]	1983–1988	213	3	1.4
Golden *et al.* [27]	1973–1989	500	8	1.6
AbuRahma *et al.* [28]	1983–1987	332	12	3.6
Ernst [9]	1980–1989	710	25	3.5
Total	—	6488	260	4.0

RESULTS OF SURGERY FOR RUPTURED ABDOMINAL AORTIC ANEURYSM

STUDY	STUDY PERIOD	PATIENTS, n	DEATHS, n	MORTALITY, %
Crawford et al. [17]	1955–1980	60	14	23
McCabe et al. [18]	1972–1977	73	38	52
Wakefield et al. [29]	1964–1980	116	60	52
Hoffman et al. [30]	1975–1979	152	58	38
Donaldson et al. [21]	1972–1983	81	35	43
Meyer et al. [31]	Not stated	97	45	46
Shackleton et al. [32]	1975–1985	106	43	41
Chang et al. [33]	1983–1989	63	16	25
Ouriel et al. [34]	1979–1988	243	133	55
Sullivan et al. [35]	1978–1989	69	24	35
AbuRahma et al. [36]	1983–1987	73	45	62
Harris et al. [37]	1980–1989	113	72	64
Johansen et al. [38]	1980–1989	180	124	69
Gloviczki et al. [39]	1980–1989	214	97	45
Ernst [9]	1980–1989	91	41	45
Total	—	1731	845	49

FIGURE 1-33. Outcome of surgery for ruptured abdominal aortic aneurysm. (*Adapted from* Ernst [9].)

LATE SURVIVAL AFTER REPAIR OF AN ABDOMINAL AORTIC ANEURYSM

STUDY	STUDY PERIOD	PATIENTS, n	SURVIVAL RATE, %		
			1-YEAR	5-YEAR	10-YEAR
Crawford et al. [17]*	1955–1980	860	95	62	38
Hollier et al. [40]*	1970–1975	1066	91	68	41
Reigel et al. [22]	1980–1985	499	95	74	—
Ernst [9]	1980–1989	801	87	64	—
Total†	—	3226	92	67	40

*Ruptured aneurysms were included in this study.
†Survival rates shown are averages for the four studies.

FIGURE 1-34. Late survival after repair of abdominal aortic aneurysm. (*Adapted from* Ernst [9].)

INDICATIONS FOR SURGERY OF AORTIC ANEURYSMS

ASCENDING THORACIC AORTA	ABDOMINAL AORTA
Marfan syndrome	5 cm maximal diameter
5 cm maximal diameter	Enlargement faster than 1 cm annually
All patients	Symptomatic compression of surrounding structures
6 cm maximal diameter	Aortic wall tenderness
Enlargement >1 cm annually	Intestinal ischemia
Symptoms resulting from compression of surrounding tissues	Distal atheroembolism

FIGURE 1-35. Indications for surgery of aortic aneurysms.

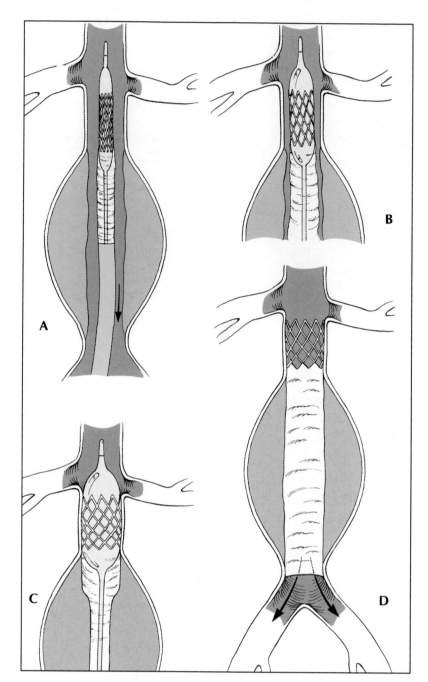

FIGURE 1-36. Treatment of infrarenal abdominal aortic aneurysm with a percutaneous intraluminal stent graft. The compressed stent is introduced transfemorally on a deployment catheter (**A**) and positioned with its proximal end above the point of aneurysmal dilatation (**B**). The stent is deployed over an expandable balloon (**C**) and then extruded distally within the lumen, terminating above the iliac bifurcation (**D**). (*Adapted from* Parodi *et al.* [41].)

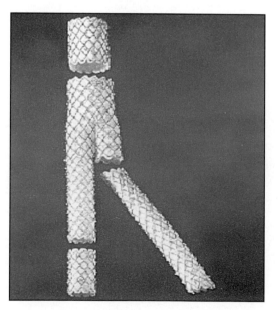

FIGURE 1-37. Example of a commercially available aortic stent-graft system. The modular stent graft components consist of a thin-walled, woven polyester graft supported by a nickel-titanium alloy. The modular components are a main bifurcated segment and contralateral iliac limb. Modular proximal (aortic) and distal (iliac) extender cuffs allow adjustment of length [42].

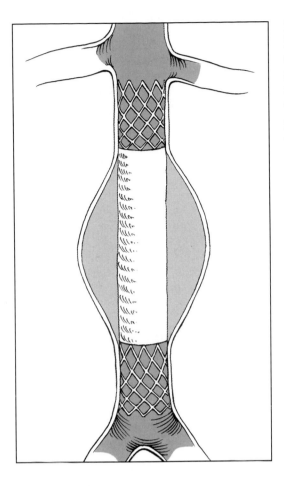

FIGURE 1-38. Diagram showing an intraluminal stent graft in place in an infrarenal aneurysm of the abdominal aorta. (*Adapted from* Parodi *et al.* [41].)

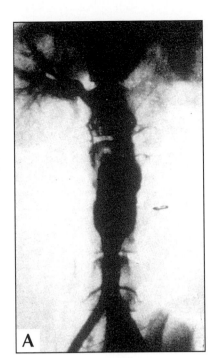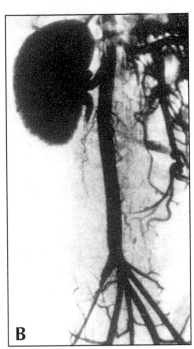

FIGURE 1-39. Abdominal aortograms obtained before (**A**) and after (**B**) percutaneous placement of an intraluminal stent graft. (*From* Parodi *et al.* [41]; with permission.)

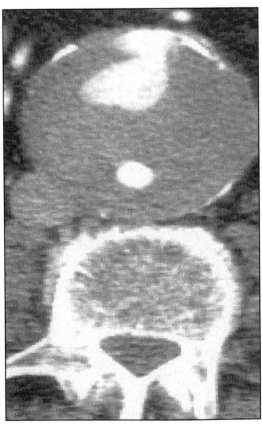

FIGURE 1-40. Computed tomography scan of a leak from an intraluminal stent graft into the aneurysm sac (endoleak) that occurred following stent grafting of an abdominal aortic aneurysm. (*Courtesy of* Michael L. Marin, MD.)

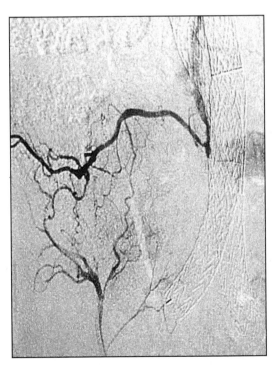

FIGURE 1-41. Digital subtraction angiogram demonstrating retrograde flow in lumbar, accessory renal, and inferior mesenteric arteries resulting from an endoleak following stent-graft repair of an abdominal aortic aneurysm. The optimum method for detection of endoleaks and the approach to clinical management remain controversial. Some advocate early postoperative computed tomographic imaging and open surgical repair, while others recommend an expectant observational approach without intervention in the absence of symptoms or hemodynamic compromise. (*Courtesy of* Michael L. Marin, MD.)

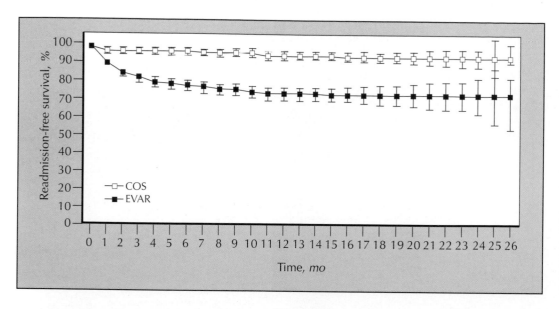

FIGURE 1-42. Durability of endovascular versus open surgical repair of abdominal aortic aneurysms (AAAs). In a nonrandomized study of 337 patients undergoing repair of AAAs, the conventional open surgical technique was used on 163 cases and endovascular repair was performed on 174 patients using a variety of devices. Endovascular repair resulted in less initial morbidity and shorter length of hospital stay compared with conventional surgery (5 vs 8 days; $P = 0.009$). Each year, 5% of patients were readmitted to the hospital after open repair compared with 29% of those undergoing endovascular repair ($P < .001$). The most common reason for readmission was endoleak occurring within the first few months following repair [43].

PERIPHERAL ARTERIAL ANEURYSMS

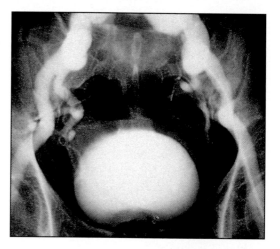

FIGURE 1-43. Abdominal angiogram demonstrating bilateral iliac aneurysms. (*From* Creager *et al.* [5]; with permission.)

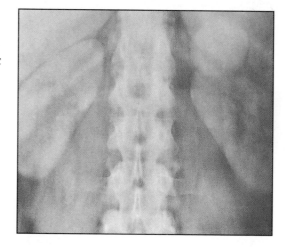

FIGURE 1-44. Nephrographic tomogram of the abdomen in a patient with hypertension. The round density in the left upper quadrant was later found at angiography to represent a splenic artery aneurysm. (*From* Joyce [44]; with permission.)

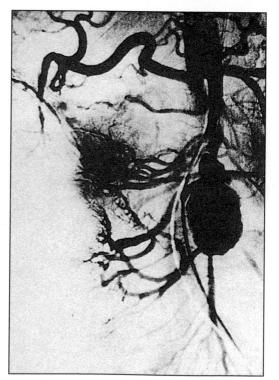

FIGURE 1-45. Mycotic aneurysm of the superior mesenteric artery that was subsequently excised; arterial reconstruction was achieved using autologous saphenous vein grafts. (*From* Whittemore and Mannick [8]; with permission.)

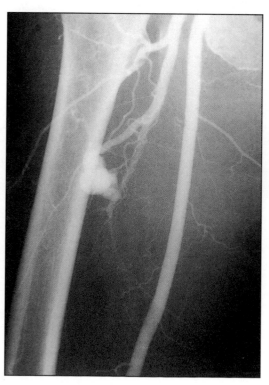

FIGURE 1-46. Right transfemoral angiogram demonstrating leaking pseudo-aneurysm of the profunda femoris artery that developed following blunt limb trauma in a patient with insufficiency of the aortic valve. (*From* Squire *et al.* [45]; with permission.)

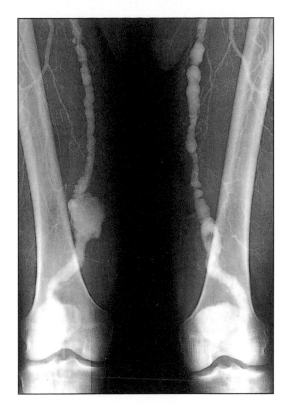

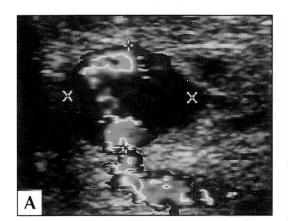

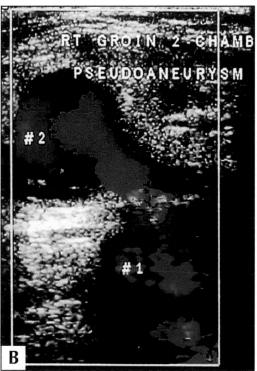

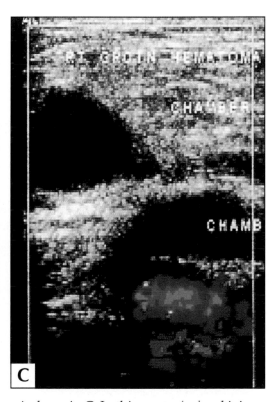

FIGURE 1-48. Femoral artery pseudoaneurysm. **A**, Color-enhanced duplex ultrasonogram of a femoral artery pseudoaneurysm. Femoral artery pseudoaneurysm is a frequent complication of diagnostic or therapeutic catheterization. Diagnosis may be suggested by detection of a systolic bruit over the groin in a patient with a large hematoma, and confirmed by color-enhanced duplex ultrasonography. **B**, Obliteration using thrombin injection. Femoral arterial pseudoaneurysms may thrombose spontaneously or require closure by ultrasound-guided compression, thrombin injection, or surgical repair. **C**, In this example, local injection of 0.5 to 1 mL of a 2000 U/mL solution of activated thrombin into the neck of the pseudoaneurysm under ultrasound visualization was used to induce thrombosis [46].

REFERENCES

1. Dubost C: Resection of an aneurysm of the abdominal aorta: re-establishment of the continuity by a preserved human arterial graft with results after 5 months. *Arch Surg* 1952, 64:405–408.

2. Nichols WW, O'Rourke MF: Aging, high blood pressure and disease in humans. In *McDonald's Blood Flow in Arteries: Theoretic, Experimental and Clinical Principles,* edn 3. Edited by Nichols WW, O'Rourke MF. Philadelphia: Lea & Febiger; 1990:398–420.

3. Diminick K, Kaplan S, Salmeron J: Peripheral vascular disease. In *Pathophysiology of Heart Disease: A Collaborative Project of Medical Students and Faculty.* Edited by Lilly LS. Philadelphia: Lea & Febiger; 1993:239–254.

4. Schoen FJ: *Interventional and Surgical Cardiovascular Pathology.* Philadelphia: WB Saunders Co.; 1989.

5. Creager MA, Halperin JL, Whittemore AD: Aneurysmal disease of the aorta and its branches. In *Vascular Medicine: A Textbook of Vascular Biology and Diseases.* Edited by Loscalzo J, Creager MA, Dzau VJ. Boston: Little, Brown & Co.; 1992:903–930.

6. Cooley DA: Experience with hypothermic circulatory arrest and the treatment of aneurysms of the ascending aorta. *Semin Thorac Cardiovasc Surg* 1991, 3:166–170.

7. Crawford ES, Coselli JS: Thoracoabdominal aortic aneurysms. *Semin Thorac Cardiovasc Surg* 1991, 3:300–322.

8. Whittemore AD, Mannick JA: Principles of vascular surgery. In *Vascular Medicine: A Textbook of Vascular Biology and Diseases.* Edited by Locscalzo J, Creager MA, Dzau VJ. Boston: Little, Brown & Co.; 1992:683–713.

9. Ernst CB: Abdominal aortic aneurysm. *N Engl J Med* 1993, 328:1167–1172.

10. Lederle FA, Johnson GR, Wilson SE, *et al.*: The aneurysm detection and management study screening program: validation cohort and final results. *Arch Intern Med* 2000, 160:1425–1430.

11. Scott RA, Bridgewater SG, Ashton HA: Randomized clinical trial of screening for abdominal aortic aneurysm in women. *Br J Surg* 2002, 89:283–285.

12. Brown LC, Powell JT: Risk factors for aneurysm rupture in patients kept under ultrasound surveillance. *Ann Surg* 1999, 230:289–296.

13. Szilagyi DE, Smith RF, DeRusso FJ, *et al.*: Contribution of abdominal aortic aneurysmectomy to prolongation of life. *Ann Surg* 1966, 164:678–699.

14. Long-term outcomes of immediate repair compared with surveillance of small abdominal aortic aneurysms. *N Engl J Med* 2002, 346:1445–1452.

15. Lederle FA, Wilson SE, Johnson GR, *et al.*: Immediate repair compared with surveillance of small abdominal aortic aneurysms. *N Engl J Med* 2002, 346: 1437–1444.

16. Greenhalgh RM: *Vascular Surgical Techniques: An Atlas.* Philadelphia: WB Saunders Co.; 1989.

17. Crawford ES, Saleh SA, Babb JW III, *et al.*: Infrarenal abdominal aortic aneurysm: factors influencing survival after operation performed over a 25-year period. *Ann Surg* 1981, 193:699–709.

18. McCabe CJ, Coleman WS, Brewster DC: The advantage of early operation for abdominal aortic aneurysm. *Arch Surg* 1981, 116:1025–1029.

19. Diehl JT, Cali RF, Hertzer NR, *et al.*: Complications of abdominal aortic reconstruction: an analysis of perioperative risk factors in 557 patients. *Ann Surg* 1983, 197:49–56.

20. Hertzer NR, Avellone JC, Farrell CJ, *et al.*: The risk of vascular surgery in a metropolitan community: with observations on surgeon experience and hospital size. *J Vasc Surg* 1984, 1:13–21.

21. Donaldson MC, Rosenberg JM, Bucknam CA: Factors affecting survival after ruptured abdominal aortic aneurysm. *J Vasc Surg* 1985, 2:564–570.

22. Reigel MM, Hollier LH, Kazmier FJ, *et al.*: Late survival in abdominal aortic aneurysm patients: the role of selective myocardial revascularization on the basis of clinical symptoms. *J Vasc Surg* 1987, 5:222–227.

23. Green RM, Ricotta JJ, Ouriel K, DeWeese JA: Results of supraceliac aortic clamping in the difficult elective resection of infrarenal abdominal aortic aneurysm. *J Vasc Surg* 1989, 9:124–134.

24. Johnston KW: Multicenter prospective study of nonruptured abdominal aortic aneurysms: II. Variables predicting morbidity and mortality. *J Vasc Surg* 1989, 9:437–447.

25. Leather RP, Shah DM, Kaufman JL, *et al.*: Comparative analysis of retroperitoneal and transperitoneal aortic replacement for aneurysm. *Surg Gynecol Obstet* 1989, 168:387–393.

26. Sicard GA, Allen BT, Munn JS, *et al.*: Retroperitoneal versus transperitoneal approach for repair of abdominal aortic aneurysms. *Surg Clin North Am* 1989, 69:795–806.

27. Golden MA, Whittemore AD, Donaldson MC, *et al.*: Selective evaluation and management of coronary artery disease in patients undergoing repair of abdominal aortic aneurysms: a 16-year experience. *Ann Surg* 1990, 212:415–423.

28. AbuRahma AF, Robinson PA, Boland JP, *et al.*: Elective resection of 332 abdominal aortic aneurysms in a southern West Virginia community during a recent five-year period. *Surgery* 1991, 109:244–251.

29. Wakefield TW, Whitehouse WM Jr, Wu SC, *et al.*: Abdominal aortic aneurysm rupture: statistical analysis of factors affecting outcome of surgical treatment. *Surgery* 1982, 91:586–596.

30. Hoffman M, Avellone JC, Plecha FR, *et al.*: Operation for ruptured abdominal aortic aneurysms: a community-wide experience. *Surgery* 1982, 91:597–602.

31. Meyer AA, Ahlquist RE Jr, Trunkey DD: Mortality from ruptured abdominal aortic aneurysms: a comparison of two series. *Am J Surg* 1986, 152:27–33.

32. Shackleton CR, Schechter MT, Bianco R, *et al.*: Preoperative predictors of mortality risk in ruptured abdominal aortic aneurysm. *J Vasc Surg* 1987, 6:583–589.

33. Chang BB, Shah DM, Paty PSK, *et al.*: Can the retroperitoneal approach be used for ruptured abdominal aortic aneurysms? *J Vasc Surg* 1990, 11:326–330.

34. Ouriel K, Geary K, Green RM, *et al.*: Factors determining survival after ruptured aortic aneurysm: the hospital, the surgeon and the patient. *J Vasc Surg* 1990, 11:493–496.

35. Sullivan CA, Rohrer MJ, Cutler BS: Clinical management of the symptomatic but unruptured abdominal aortic aneurysm. *J Vasc Surg* 1990, 11:799–803.

36. AbuRahma AF, Woodruff BA, Lucente FC, *et al.*: Factors affecting survival of patients with ruptured abdominal aortic aneurysm in a West Virginia community. *Surg Gynecol Obstet* 1991, 172:377–382.

37. Harris LM, Faggioli GL, Fiedler R, *et al.*: Ruptured abdominal aortic aneurysms: factors affecting mortality rates. *J Vasc Surg* 1991, 14:812–820.

38. Johansen K, Kohler TR, Nicholls SC, *et al.*: Ruptured abdominal aortic aneurysm: the Harborview experience. *J Vasc Surg* 1991, 13:240–247.

39. Gloviczki P, Pairolero PC, Mucha P Jr, *et al.*: Ruptured abdominal aortic aneurysms: repair should not be denied. *J Vasc Surg* 1992, 15:851–859.

40. Hollier LH, Plate G, O'Brien PC, *et al.*: Late survival after abdominal aortic aneurysm repair: influence of coronary artery disease. *J Vasc Surg* 1984, 1:290–299.

41. Parodi JC, Palmaz JC, Barone HD: Transfemoral intraluminal graft implantation for abdominal aortic aneurysms. *Ann Vasc Surg* 1991, 5:491–499.

42. Zarins CK, White RA, Schwarten D, *et al.*: AneuRx stent graft versus open surgical repair of abdominal aortic aneurysms: multicenter prospective clinical trial. *J Vasc Surg* 1999, 29:292–308.

43. Carpenter JP, Baum RA, Barker CF, *et al.*: Durability of benefits of endovascular versus conventional abdominal aortic aneurysm repair. *J Vasc Surg* 2002, 35:222–228.

44. Joyce JW: Aneurysmal disease. In *Cardiovascular Clinics: Clinical Vascular Disease*. Edited by Spittell JA. Philadelphia: F.A. Davis; 1983:89–101.

45. Squire A, Miller CM, Horowitz SF, *et al.*: Femoral pseudoaneurysm following nonpenetrating trauma in a patient with aortic insufficiency. *Am J Med* 1985, 78:719–720.

46. Hughes MJ, McCall JM, Nott DM, Padley SP: Treatment of iatrogenic femoral artery pseudoaneurysms using ultrasound-guided injection of thrombin. *Clin Radiol* 2000, 55:749–751.

CHAPTER 2

AORTIC DISSECTION

Eric M. Isselbacher

Aortic dissection, also known as dissecting aortic aneurysm, is a life-threatening condition with an early mortality as high as 1% per hour [1]. However, with prompt diagnosis and the institution of appropriate medical or surgical therapy, a patient's chance of early survival can be as high as 74% to 92% [2]. While most cases of aortic dissection present with classic symptoms, such as severe "sharp" or "stabbing" chest pain, other cases present with much less specific signs or symptoms, making diagnosis a challenge. Therefore, vigilance for any risk factors, symptoms, or physical findings consistent with aortic dissection is essential if a timely diagnosis is to be made.

Once aortic dissection is suspected clinically, its presence or absence must be determined with an imaging study. Options include computed tomography, magnetic resonance imaging, transesophageal echocardiography, and aortography. Knowledge of the relative advantages and disadvantages, diagnostic performance, and practical utility of each of these imaging modalities is essential when selecting among them.

When an aortic dissection is suspected clinically, medical therapy should still be instituted immediately and continued until a conclusive diagnosis has been established. If the presence of an aortic dissection is confirmed, definitive treatment is initiated with either medical therapy or direct surgical repair, based on the location of the dissection (proximal or distal) as well as several other factors. Even with successful "definitive" in-hospital treatment of aortic dissection, patients remain at considerable risk for late complications such as recurrence or extension of the aortic dissection as well as aortic aneurysm formation and rupture. These patients should be managed indefinitely with β-blockers and antihypertensive therapy, and should undergo serial imaging with either computed tomography or magnetic resonance imaging at least annually for life.

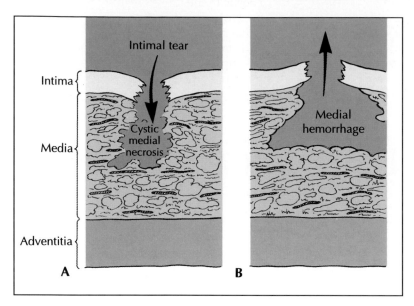

FIGURE 2-1. The mechanism of intimal tearing in aortic dissection. This illustration shows the two possible mechanisms for the pathogenesis of aortic dissection. **A,** In this mechanism of intimal tear, which is believed to be the more likely one, there is a primary intimal tear followed by dissection of blood from the aorta into the media. Propagation usually occurs antegrade, driven by the natural forward pressure of blood flow in the aorta, but retrograde propagation may occur as well. The presence of an intimal tear allows the transmission of aortic pressure into the disrupted media, causing progressive separation of the tissue planes and propagation of the dissection. **B,** In this mechanism, the primary event is rupture of the vasa vasorum with hemorrhage in the aortic media and then through the intima into the aortic lumen. When such medial hemorrhage occurs without intimal rupture, it produces a variant of aortic dissection called intramural hematoma (*see* Fig. 2-46). (*Adapted from* Eagle *et al.* [3].)

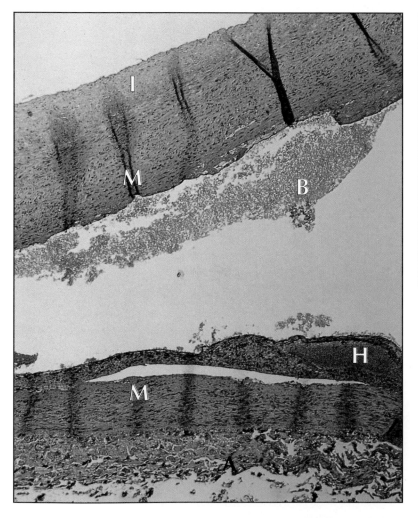

FIGURE 2-2. Histologic section demonstrating medial hemorrhage. This specimen is from the aorta of a patient who suffered an aortic dissection. Note the presence of blood (B), which has cleaved the laminar planes of the media (M) and thus dissected the aortic wall. Also evident is a small hematoma (H) within the media. A—adventitia; I—intima.

ETIOLOGY OF AORTIC DISSECTION: PREDISPOSING FACTORS

Advanced age (mean age, 63 years)
Male gender (65%)
History of hypertension (72%)
Known aortic aneurysm (16%)
Marfan's syndrome (5%)
Bicuspid aortic valve (5%)
Peripartum period of pregnancy (1%)
Cardiac catheterization (2%)
Prior cardiac surgery (18%)

FIGURE 2-3. Etiology of aortic dissection in 464 patients in the International Registry of Aortic Dissection. Other uncommon but important predisposing factors include cocaine abuse and blunt trauma. Any disease process or other condition that undermines the integrity of the aortic media (either its elastic or muscular component) may predispose to aortic dissection. Cystic medial necrosis is the common denominator in nontraumatic cases. Elderly patients with a history of hypertension are the most typical population presenting with aortic dissection. Patients with Marfan syndrome are at particularly high risk for aortic dissection, as well as recurrent dissections, and therefore often require a more aggressive diagnostic and therapeutic approach.

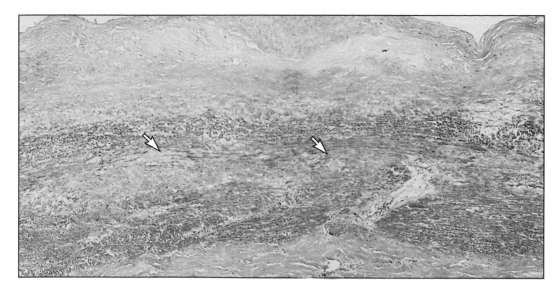

FIGURE 2-4. Histologic specimen of cystic medial necrosis. This section is from a patient with Marfan syndrome and a prior healed aortic dissection showing a portion of aortic tissue uninvolved by the dissection. Note the extensive areas of cystic medial necrosis (*arrows*) in which the usual elastic lamellar appearance of the media is disrupted. Cystic medial necrosis is found in many but not all patients who suffer aortic dissection.

CLASSIFICATION

CLASSIFICATION OF AORTIC DISSECTION BY ITS DURATION	
TYPE	TIME ELAPSED SINCE ONSET OF SYMPTOMS
Acute	< 2 weeks
Chronic	> 2 weeks

FIGURE 2-5. Classification of aortic dissection by its duration. The early mortality and risk of progression of aortic dissection are greatly influenced by the age of the dissection, with risk decreasing over time. Accordingly, therapeutic strategies may be quite different for a dissection that presents acutely versus one that has become chronic. Two weeks or more is defined as the age at which an aortic dissection is considered "chronic," because it is at about this time that the mortality curve for untreated aortic dissection begins to level off.

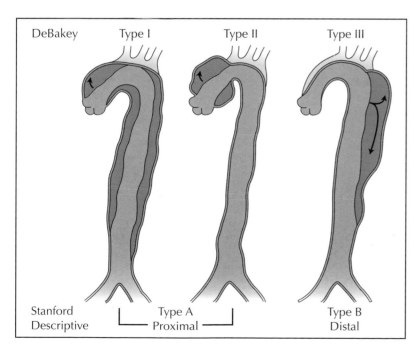

FIGURE 2-6. Classification of aortic dissection by the extent of aortic involvement. This diagrammatic representation of aortic dissection shows the anatomy of the three most common types. The intimal tear is represented by the arrows, which cross from the true lumen out into the false lumen (represented here by the darker red). Three classification systems are commonly used to describe aortic dissections. These three systems share the same basic principle of distinguishing dissections that involve the ascending aorta from those that do not, because involvement of the ascending aorta has important prognostic and therapeutic implications. Most would consider involvement of the ascending aorta an indication for surgery, while a lack of involvement would favor medical therapy. Since management of DeBakey types I and II is usually similar, the other classification systems have combined these two types into a single group, called *type A* or *proximal*. Type A aortic dissections outnumber type B aortic dissections by approximately 2 to 1. (*Adapted from* Eagle *et al*. [3].)

RELATIVE FREQUENCY OF SITES OF INTIMAL TEAR IN AORTIC DISSECTION	
SITE OF INTIMAL TEAR	PERCENT
Ascending aorta	61
Aortic arch	9
Descending aorta	29
Abdominal aorta	1

FIGURE 2-7. The relative frequency of sites of intimal tear in aortic dissection. The large majority of aortic dissections originate from an intimal tear in either the proximal ascending aorta within several centimeters of the aortic valve or in the descending aorta just distal to the origin of the left subclavian artery. In addition to the multiple sites of origin, aortic dissections may also differ with respect to the extent of the aorta (proximal and/or distal to the site of intimal tear) involved by the dissection. (*Adapted from* Richartz *et al.* [4].)

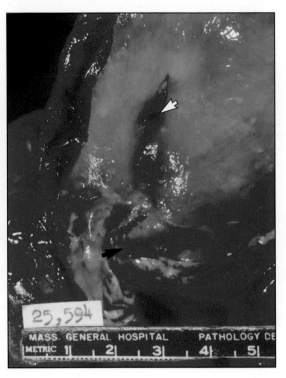

FIGURE 2-8. Pathologic specimen showing an intimal tear. Shown is a specimen of the aortic root from a patient with a proximal aortic dissection demonstrating a discrete intimal tear (*white arrow*) just distal to the sinus of Valsalva (*black arrow*). Proximal aortic dissections most commonly originate within a few centimeters of the aortic valve.

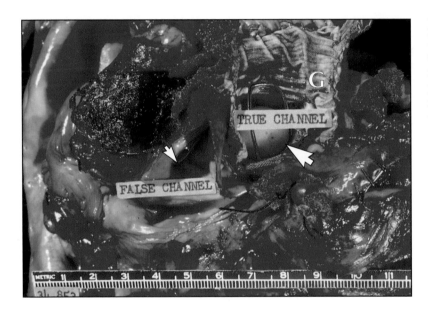

FIGURE 2-9. Pathologic specimen showing the true and false lumina. Shown is a specimen of the aortic root from a patient with a proximal aortic dissection who underwent an attempted aortic repair using a composite aortic root graft (G) with a Starr-Edward prosthetic valve (*large arrow*). The true and false lumina are identified, with the aortic graft positioned within the true lumen. The tip of a probe (*small arrow*) can be seen within the false lumen.

TYPICAL PRESENTING SYMPTOMS IN 464 PATIENTS WITH AORTIC DISSECTION

	TYPE OF AORTIC DISSECTION		
SYMPTOM	ALL (N = 464), %	TYPE A (N = 289), %	TYPE B (N = 175), %
Pain	96	94	98
Chest	73	79	63
Anterior	61	71	44
Posterior	36	33	41
Back	53	47	64
Abdominal	30	22	43
Abrupt onset	89	85	84
Severe	91	90	90
Sharp	64	62	68
Tearing	51	49	52
Syncope	9	13	4

FIGURE 2-10. Presenting symptoms in 464 patients with aortic dissection [2]. The majority of patients with acute aortic dissection present with severe thoracic pain, either anterior or interscapular, or both. The pain may be migratory and its location often, but not always, correlates with the segments of the aorta involved. The pain is typically of sudden onset, is most severe at its start, and is most often described as "sharp," "stabbing," or "tearing" in quality. The pain is often distinguished from the pain of angina or myocardial infarction by its sudden onset, in contrast to the typical crescendo nature of the pain of coronary ischemia. (*Adapted from* Hagan *et al.* [2].)

PERTINENT PHYSICAL FINDINGS IN 464 PATIENTS WITH AORTIC DISSECTION

	TYPE OF AORTIC DISSECTION		
PHYSICAL FINDING	ALL (N – 464), %	TYPE A (N = 289), %	TYPE B (N = 175), %
Hypertension (SBP ≥ 150 mm Hg)	49	36	70
Normotensive (SBP 100–149 mm Hg)	35	40	26
Hypotensive (SPB 80–99 mm Hg)	8	12	2
Shock (SBP < 80 mm Hg)	8	13	2
Auscultated murmur of AI	32	44	12
Pulse deficit	15	19	9
Cerebrovascular accident	5	6	2
Congestive heart failure	7	9	3

FIGURE 2-11. Pertinent physical findings in 464 patients presenting with aortic dissection. Hypertension is seen in 70% of patients with type B aortic dissection, whereas hypotension and shock occur more commonly with type A aortic dissection. The associated findings of pulse deficits (or unequal blood pressures), the murmur of aortic insufficiency, and cerebrovascular accidents occur much more often with type A than with type B aortic dissection. AI—aortic insufficiency; SBP—systolic blood pressure. (*Adapted from* Hagan *et al.* [2].)

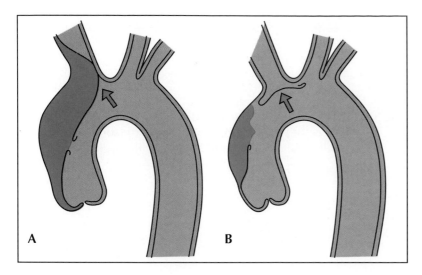

FIGURE 2-12. The mechanisms by which aortic dissection may cause loss of pulses. **A,** The intimal flap and false lumen extend into the right innominate artery to narrow or occlude the lumen. **B,** A mobile portion of the intimal flap has folded over the orifice of the right innominate artery, obstructing blood flow. (*Adapted from* Eagle *et al.* [3].)

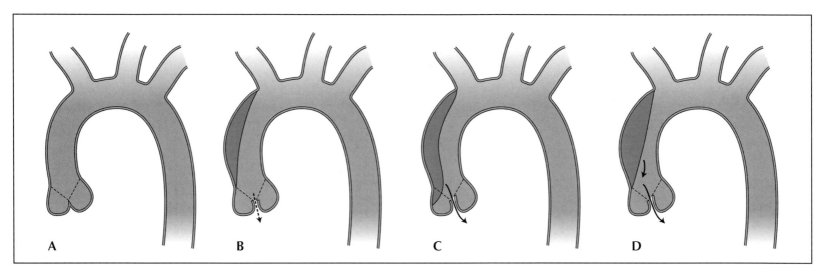

FIGURE 2-13. The mechanisms by which aortic dissection may induce aortic regurgitation. **A,** Normal aortic valve anatomy, with the leaflets suspended (*dotted lines*) from the sinotubular junction. **B,** A type A dissection dilates the ascending aorta, in turn widening the sinotubular junction from which the aortic leaflets hang so that the leaflets are unable to coapt properly in diastole (incomplete closure). Aortic regurgitation (*arrow*) results.

C, A type A dissection extends into the aortic root and detaches an aortic leaflet from its commissural attachment to the sinotubular junction, resulting in diastolic leaflet prolapse. **D,** In the setting of an extensive or circumferential intimal tear, the unsupported intimal flap may prolapse across the aortic valve and into the left ventricular outflow tract, preventing normal leaflet coaptation. (*Adapted from* Isselbacher [5].)

ROENTGENOGRAPHIC FINDINGS IN PATIENTS WITH AORTIC DISSECTION

FINDING	PERCENT
Widened superior mediastinum	62
Abnormal aortic contour	50
Displacement of intimal calcium	14
Pleural effusion (typically on left)	19
Normal chest radiograph	12

FIGURE 2-14. Roentgenographic findings in patients with aortic dissection. While the radiographic findings associated with aortic dissection may be helpful in raising or supporting one's clinical suspicion for the presence of dissection, they remain nevertheless quite nonspecific. Sometimes these radiographic changes are subtle and are only recognized when the film is compared with a prior radiograph (*see* Fig. 2-17). Some patients with aortic dissection will have one or more of these radiographic findings, while in other cases of dissection the chest radiograph may be entirely unremarkable. It must therefore be understood that a normal chest radiograph cannot serve to rule out aortic dissection (*see* Fig. 2-15). (*Adapted from* Hagan *et al.* [2].)

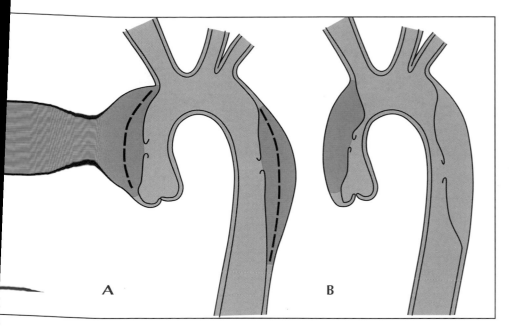

FIGURE 2-15. A dissecting hematoma may variably affect aortic size and contour on a chest radiograph or aortogram. **A,** The proximal and distal false lumina have expanded outward, producing an enlarged aortic silhouette with an abnormal bulging contour, while the diameter of the true lumen is narrowed minimally. **B,** The false lumen has expanded inward, causing marked narrowing of the true lumen, but this results in little or no change in the silhouette of the ascending or descending aorta. An unremarkable chest radiograph might be seen in this case. (*Adapted from* O'Gara and DeSanctis [6].)

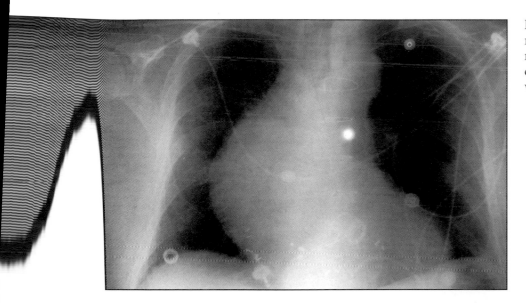

FIGURE 2-16. Chest radiograph suggestive of aortic dissection. This radiograph in a patient with a proximal aortic dissection shows marked widening of the mediastinum and an abnormal aortic contour. This patient was found to have a type A aortic dissection with an ascending aortic aneurysm measuring 12 cm in diameter.

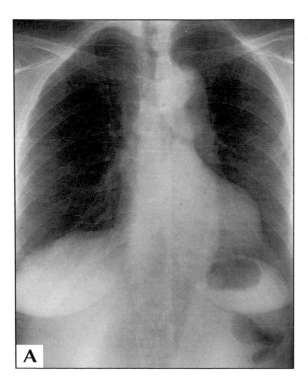
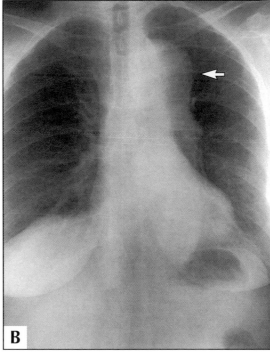

FIGURE 2-17. Chest radiographs showing a change from a patient's baseline study. While the chest radiograph of a patient presenting with suspected aortic dissection may at first appear unremarkable, a comparison with a previous examination from the same patient often reveals an interval change in the appearance of the aorta or mediastinum, which may suggest the presence of an aortic dissection. **A,** This patient's normal baseline chest radiograph 3 years prior to presentation. **B,** The same patient's chest radiograph at the time of presentation, which is remarkable for the interval enlargement of the aortic knob (*arrow*). The patient was found to have a type A aortic dissection.

DIAGNOSTIC TECHNIQUES

DIAGNOSTIC MODALITIES FOR EVALUATING PATIENTS WITH SUSPECTED AORTIC DISSECTION

Aortography
Contrast-enhanced computed tomography
Magnetic resonance imaging
Transesophageal echocardiography

FIGURE 2-18. Diagnostic mo
patients with suspected aort
has particular advantages a
nostic accuracy, convenience
nique is appropriate for all p
caring for a patient with sus
fore be familiar with both the
imaging modality in order to
study for a given patient situ
such as local availability or o
also factor significantly in the

DIAGNOSTIC INFORMATION SOUGHT IN PATIENTS WITH SUSPECTED AORTIC DISSECTION

Presence or absence of aortic dissection

Involvement of the ascending aorta

Extent of dissection

Sites of entry and re-entry

Thrombus in the false lumen

Branch vessel involvement by dissection

Aortic insufficiency

Pericardial effusion

Coronary artery involvement by intimal flap

FIGURE 2-19. Diagnostic infor
suspected aortic dissection. W
define all of the above anatom
aortic dissection, no single dia
information. Instead, on a cas
cion, together with considerati
should determine which diag
patient management. In fact, i
diagnostic study may be requi
an aortic dissection adequately

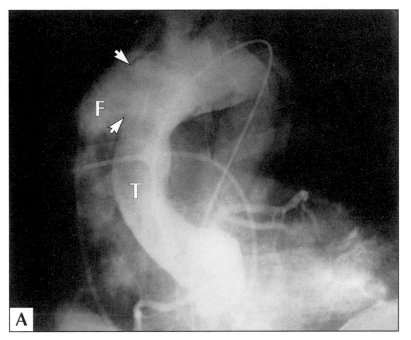

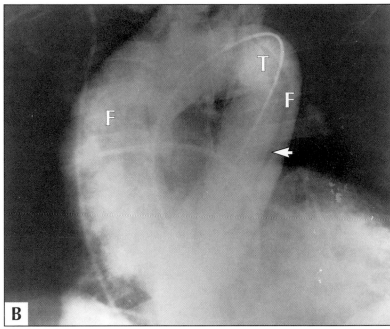

FIGURE 2-20. Anteroposterior aortograms demonstrating the presence of a type A aortic dissection. **A,** The well-opacified true lumen (T) and the poorly opacified false lumen (F) are separated by an intimal flap, which is visible on the ascending aorta as a thin radiolucent line within the aorta (*arrows*). Additionally, the prox- imal portions of both coronary arteries are well visualized. **B,** In a subsequent aortographic exposure, the false lumen has filled in late and the intimal flap is now clearly visible (*arrow*) as it courses distally down the descending aorta. (*Panel A from* Cigarroa *et al.* [7]; with permission.)

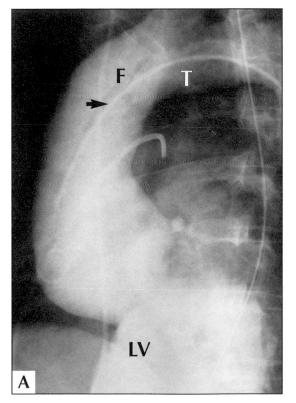

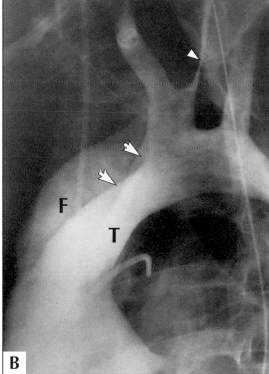

FIGURE 2-21. Left anterior oblique aortograms demonstrating a type A aortic dissection and its associated cardiovascular complications. **A,** The aortic root is dilated. The true lumen (T) and false lumen (F) are separated by a faintly visible radiolucent line (following the contour of the pigtail catheter), which is the intimal flap (*arrow*). The abundance of contrast in the left ventricle (LV) is indicative of significant aortic insufficiency (*see* Fig. 2-13). **B,** The true lumen is better opacified than the false lumen, and two planes of the intimal flap can now be distinguished (*arrows*). Additionally, the branch vessels are opacified and the marked narrowing of the right carotid artery (*arrowhead*) suggests that it is compromised by the dissection (*see* Fig. 2-12). (*Panel A from* Cigarroa *et al.* [7]; with permission.)

ANGIOGRAPHIC FINDINGS IN 52 CASES OF AORTIC DISSECTION

DIAGNOSTIC FINDING	PATIENTS, %
Opacification of false lumen	87
Deformity of true lumen	85
Visualization of intimal flap	70
Intimal tear defined	56
False lumen not opacified	13

FIGURE 2-22. Angiographic findings in 52 cases of aortic dissection. The various angiographic findings are used collectively by the radiologist to diagnose the presence or absence of aortic dissection. False lumen opacification is the most common finding. The site of intimal tear is defined in just over half of the cases. (*Adapted from* Earnest *et al.* [8].)

DIAGNOSTIC ACCURACY OF AORTOGRAPHY IN 126 CASES OF SUSPECTED AORTIC DISSECTION

Sensitivity	88%
Specificity	94%

FIGURE 2-23. Diagnostic accuracy of aortography in 126 cases of suspected aortic dissection. Aortography was for many years considered the gold standard for diagnosing aortic dissection. However, with the more recent introduction of alternative imaging techniques (including computed tomography, magnetic resonance imaging, and transesophageal echocardiography) for evaluating suspected aortic dissection, the limited sensitivity of aortography (88%) has become apparent. Moreover, when the definition of aortic dissection is broadened to include intramural hematoma, the sensitivity of aortography is only 77% [9]. (*Adapted from* Erbel *et al.* [10].)

ADVANTAGES AND DISADVANTAGES OF AORTOGRAPHY IN THE EVALUATION OF SUSPECTED AORTIC DISSECTION

ADVANTAGES

Well established—radiologists, cardiologists, and surgeons are comfortable with its use

Shows presence of aortic insufficiency

Shows extent of dissection

Often shows site of intimal tear

Reveals presence of branch vessel involvement

Often reveals patency of coronary arteries

DISADVANTAGES

Risk of invasive procedure

Risk of contrast

Time lag in obtaining study

Duration of the study

Unstable patients must travel to angiography suite

FIGURE 2-24. Advantages and disadvantages of aortography in the evaluation of suspected aortic dissection. Defining the presence or absence of branch vessel involvement remains one of the major strengths of aortography compared with the other available imaging modalities. The aortic arch and arch vessels are especially difficult to define adequately with computed tomography or transesophageal echocardiography, but are well delineated by aortographic examination. Aortography is also very effective in demonstrating the full extent of the aorta involved by the dissection, and is especially useful in cases when the dissection extends from the thoracic and into the abdominal aorta, where assessment of the origin of the branch vessels and the iliac arteries can be readily accomplished.

COMPUTED TOMOGRAPHY

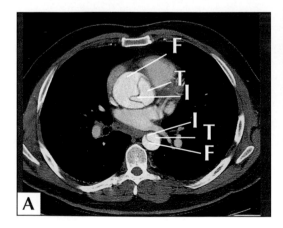

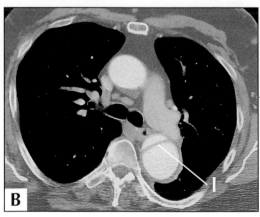

FIGURE 2-25. Computed tomography (CT) for diagnosing aortic dissection. **A**, A contrast-enhanced spiral CT scan of the chest at the level of the pulmonary artery showing an intimal flap (I) in the both the ascending thoracic aorta (above) and descending thoracic aorta (below) separating the true (T) and false (F) lumina in a type A aortic dissection. **B**, A contrast-enhanced spiral CT scan of the chest at the level of the pulmonary artery showing an intimal flap (I) in the descending thoracic aorta separating the two lumens in a type B aortic dissection.

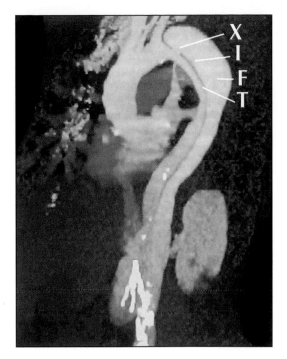

FIGURE 2-26. Advanced computed tomography (CT) of aortic dissection. Newer techniques in CT scanning can produce images that provide better anatomical resolution than conventional axial CT imaging, and are particularly useful in diagnosing and defining the extent of aortic dissection. Shown is a CT scan of the same patient shown in Figure 2-25B. A 3-dimensional reconstruction technique produces a tomographic image of the entire thoracic aorta in the left anterior oblique plane. The type B aortic dissection is easily identified. The intimal flap (I) originates just distal to the left subclavian artery and extends distally into the abdominal aorta. The intimal tear (X) is identified. The true lumen (T) is smaller than the false lumen (F), as is often the case in aortic dissection.

DIAGNOSTIC ACCURACY OF SPIRAL CONTRAST-ENHANCED CT SCANNING IN 81 CASES OF SUSPECTED AORTIC DISSECTION

Sensitivity	96%
Specificity	96%

FIGURE 2-27. Diagnostic accuracy of spiral contrast-enhanced computed tomography (CT) in 81 cases of suspected aortic dissection. In the past, conventional CT was used routinely, but its sensitivity and specificity for aortic dissection were lower. The introduction of spiral (helical) CT scanning has significantly improved the accuracy of the technique and the anatomical resolution of its images. (*Adapted from* Small *et al.* [11].)

ADVANTAGES AND DISADVANTAGES OF CONTRAST-ENHANCED CT IN THE EVALUATION OF SUSPECTED AORTIC DISSECTION

ADVANTAGES

Noninvasive

Quickly obtained

Identifies causes of aortic widening other than aortic dissection, *eg*, abnormal layers of fat or periaortic hematoma

May distinguish intraluminal thrombus from blood

Identifies presence of pericardial effusion

DISADVANTAGES

Risk of intravenous contrast

Cannot reliably identify the presence of aortic insufficiency or involvement of the coronary arteries

FIGURE 2-28. Advantages and disadvantages of contrast-enhanced computed tomography (CT) in the evaluation of suspected aortic dissection. The fact that CT scanners are present and quickly accessible in most hospital emergency rooms makes this technique attractive as a screening study for aortic dissection. However, if the presence of aortic dissection is confirmed, the lack of diagnostic information regarding the presence of aortic insufficiency may necessitate the performance of additional diagnostic studies.

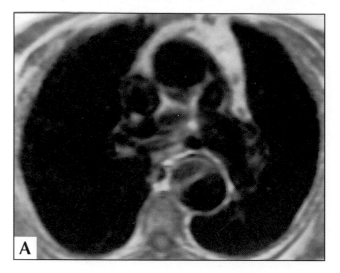

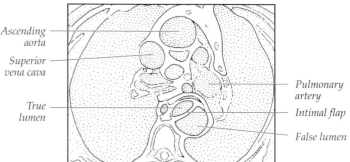

Ascending aorta
Superior vena cava
True lumen
Pulmonary artery
Intimal flap
False lumen

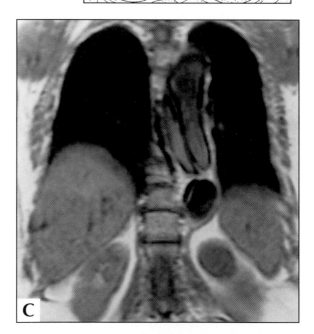

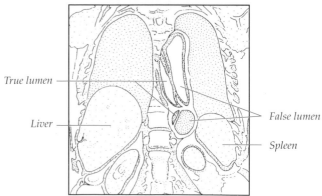

True lumen
Liver
False lumen
Spleen

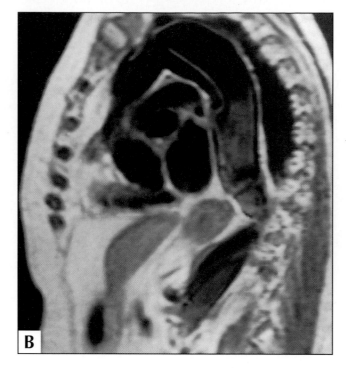

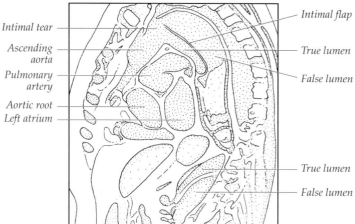

Intimal tear
Ascending aorta
Pulmonary artery
Aortic root
Left atrium
Intimal flap
True lumen
False lumen
True lumen
False lumen

FIGURE 2-29. Magnetic resonance images using the black-blood technique in three planes in a patient with a type B aortic dissection. **A,** This image in the transverse plane through the upper thorax at the level of the pulmonary artery shows an intact ascending aorta, but in the descending aorta it reveals an intimal flap separating the true lumen and false lumen. Also seen are the pulmonary artery at its bifurcation and the superior vena cava.

B, This image in the sagittal plane of the aorta shows the site of intimal tear together with the intimal flap, which begins just distal to the take-off of the left subclavian artery and spirals distally along the descending aorta. The true lumen and false lumen are identified in both the descending thoracic aorta above as well as in the abdominal aorta below. The aortic root and ascending aorta are uninvolved by the dissection. Also seen here are the left atrium and the pulmonary artery at its bifurcation.

C, This image in the coronal plane posteriorly reveals the dissected descending aorta with its true lumen and false lumen separated by the intimal flap. The descending aorta is cut in the long axis above and then in the short axis below as its turns anteriorly to enter the abdomen. Other landmarks include the liver and spleen. Note in all three views of this patient's aorta that the false lumen originates posteriorly and is wider than the true lumen. This pattern is quite typical in type B aortic dissections.

ACCURACY OF MRI IN 105 PATIENTS WITH SUSPECTED AORTIC DISSECTION

DIAGNOSTIC FINDING	SENSITIVITY, %	SPECIFICITY, %
Aortic dissection	98	98
Site of entry	88	100
Thrombus	98	99
Pericardial effusion	100	100

FIGURE 2-30. Accuracy of magnetic resonance imaging (MRI) in 105 patients with suspected aortic dissection. In addition to its remarkably high sensitivity and specificity for diagnosing the presence or absence of aortic dissection, MRI is also extremely accurate in defining many of the associated pathologic findings, such as site of intimal tear and the presence of thrombus in the false lumen. (*Adapted from* Nienaber *et al.* [12].)

ADVANTAGES AND DISADVANTAGES OF MRI IN THE EVALUATION OF SUSPECTED AORTIC DISSECTION

ADVANTAGES

Noninvasive

No intravenous contrast

No ionizing radiation

High-quality detailed images in multiple planes—transverse, sagittal, coronal, oblique

Useful in patients with pre-existing complicated aortic disease

DISADVANTAGES

May not be readily available

May not be suitable for unstable patients

Lengthy study (30–60 min)

Contraindicated in patients with pacemakers or implantable defibrillators

Contraindicated in patients with certain metallic prosthetic valves* or certain vascular clips

Limits presence of many monitoring and support devices in the imaging suite, and limits patient accessibility during scanning

Provides limited information about arch vessel and coronary artery involvement

May not always identify presence of aortic insufficiency

*While some of the older model prosthetic heart valves are considered a contraindication to MR imaging, patients with most current model prostheses can be scanned safely.

FIGURE 2-31. Advantages and disadvantages of magnetic resonance imaging (MRI) in the evaluation of suspected aortic dissection. MRI provides images in multiple planes through the body and thereby facilitates a 3-dimensional appreciation of the aorta and its intimal flap. It is particularly helpful in evaluating patients with pre-existing aortic disease. This modality has the additional appeal of being noninvasive and requiring no radiation or contrast exposure. Still, an important limitation is that magnetic resonance scanners are not present or readily available in many hospitals and, when available, may not allow for adequate monitoring and management of unstable patients during the lengthy procedure.

TRANSTHORACIC ECHOCARDIOGRAPHY

DIAGNOSTIC ACCURACY OF TTE

DIAGNOSTIC FINDING	SENSITIVITY, %	SPECIFICITY, %
Presence of aortic dissection	59–85	63–96
Identifying involvement of the		
Ascending aorta	78–100	—
Descending aorta	10–55	—

FIGURE 2-32. Diagnostic accuracy of transthoracic echocardiography (TTE). In comparison with the other available imaging modalities discussed here, TTE is of limited utility in the evaluation of suspected aortic dissection. On transthoracic imaging the ascending aorta is usually more clearly and more extensively visualized than is the descending aorta, accounting for the greater sensitivity in detecting dissections involving the ascending aorta. Still, even when considering proximal dissections alone, both the sensitivity and specificity of TTE remain relatively low. (*Adapted from* Cigarroa *et al.* [7].)

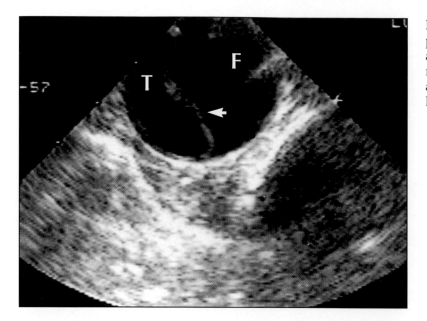

FIGURE 2-33. Transesophageal echocardiogram in the transverse plane through the descending aorta in a patient with a type A aortic dissection. Easily identified is an intimal flap (*arrow*) separating the true (T) and false (F) lumina. Note that the intimal flap appears to have peeled away from the aortic wall in the false lumen but still lines the wall of the true lumen.

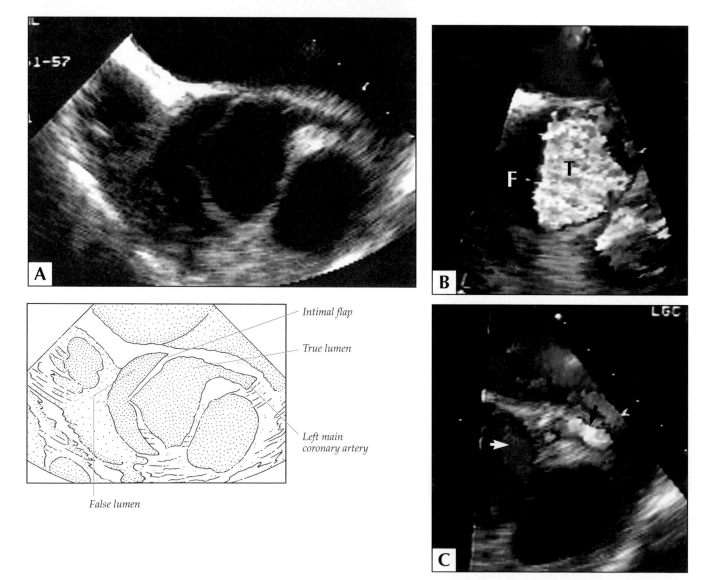

FIGURE 2-34. Transesophageal echocardiogram in the transverse plane through the aortic root in a patient with a type A aortic dissection. The imaging plane is just above (distal to) the level of the aortic valve, allowing visualization of the left main coronary artery. **A,** An intimal flap separates the true and the false lumina. The proximal segment of the left main coronary artery is visualized well in this view. **B,** The addition of color flow Doppler demonstrates that there is significant blood flow in the true lumen (T) with minimal flow in the false lumen (F), thereby confirming the presence of two lumina and the diagnosis of aortic dissection. **C,** Blood flow is also seen in the left main coronary artery (*black arrow*), confirming that it originates from the true lumen (*white arrow*) and that it appears uninvolved by the dissection.

DIAGNOSTIC ACCURACY OF TEE IN THE EVALUATION OF SUSPECTED AORTIC DISSECTION

Sensitivity	97%
Specificity	95%

FIGURE 2-35. Diagnostic accuracy of transesophageal echocardiography (TEE) in the evaluation of suspected aortic dissection. In addition to its excellent sensitivity for the detection of aortic dissection, TEE can locate the site of intimal tear in 75% of cases, and detect all cases of aortic insufficiency (which is essential data for a surgeon planning a repair). (*Adapted from* Isselbacher [5].)

ADVANTAGES AND DISADVANTAGES OF TEE IN THE EVALUATION OF SUSPECTED AORTIC DISSECTION

ADVANTAGES

Readily available

Quickly completed (5–15 min)

Performed at the bedside

Relatively noninvasive

No intravenous contrast

No ionizing radiation

Detects the presence of aortic insufficiency

Allows assessment of left ventricular wall motion abnormalities

May detect coronary artery involvement by the intimal flap

DISADVANTAGES

Contraindicated in some patients (*eg*, those with known esophageal disease: varices, strictures, tumors, *etc.*)

Rare complications, occurring in less than 1% (*eg*, bradycardia, atrioventricular block, hypertension, bronchospasm, esophageal perforation)

FIGURE 2-36. Advantages and disadvantages of transesophageal echocardiography (TEE) in the evaluation of suspected aortic dissection. In addition to its high sensitivity for detecting aortic dissections, TEE has the distinct advantages that it is readily accessible, can be completed quickly, and can be performed at bedside for unstable patients. TEE also provides a host of other information about aortic anatomy and cardiac function. In the case that a suspected aortic dissection is excluded, TEE can identify unsuspected cardiac pathology, which may facilitate a diagnosis or alter further management [13].

DIAGNOSTIC PERFORMANCE OF IMAGING MODALITIES IN THE EVALUATION OF SUSPECTED AORTIC DISSECTION

DIAGNOSTIC PERFORMANCE	ANGIOGRAPHY	CT	MRI	TEE
Sensitivity	++	+++	+++	+++
Specificity	+++	+++	+++	+++
Site of intimal tear	++	+	+++	++
Presence of aortic insufficiency	+++	-	+	+++
Pericardial effusion	-	+++	++	+++
Branch vessel involvement	+++	++	++	+
Coronary artery involvement	++	-	-	++

+++ — Excellent; ++ — good; + — fair; - — not detected.

FIGURE 2-37. Summary of the diagnostic performance of the four imaging modalities in the evaluation of suspected aortic dissection. The sensitivities of computed tomography (CT), magnetic resonance imaging (MRI), and transesophageal echocardiography (TEE) are all equally high, so no one technique is considered the preferred modality. In most cases, CT and TEE are the modalities used for the evaluation of patients in the acute setting, whereas MRI is often reserved for patients with chronic aortic dissections. Given its lower sensitivity, aortography is now generally reserved for cases in which branch vessel involvement is suspected and definition is required (ie, in the arch or abdominal aorta). (*Adapted from* Isselbacher [5].)

PRACTICAL ASSESSMENT OF IMAGING MODALITIES IN THE EVALUATION OF SUSPECTED AORTIC DISSECTION

ADVANTAGES	ANGIOGRAPHY	CT	MRI	TEE
Readily obtained	+	+++	+	++
Quickly performed	+	+++	+	++
Performed at bedside	-	-	-	+++
Noninvasive	-	+++	+++	++
No intravenous contrast	-	-	+++	+++
Cost	-	++	+	++

+++ — Very favorable; ++ — favorable; + — fair; — unfavorable.

FIGURE 2-38. Practical assessment of the four imaging modalities in the evaluation of suspected aortic dissection. While the accuracy of each diagnostic modality remains extremely important, when evaluating an acute (and possibly unstable) patient with aortic dissection several practical issues must be considered as well, including the emergency availability of the procedure, how speedily it can be performed, and any risks involved. In this regard, computed tomography (CT) and transesophageal echocardiography (TEE) are favored overall. Computed tomography typically is the most readily available modality in the emergency department, and TEE is the preferred modality for evaluating unstable patients presenting with suspected aortic dissection. MRI—magnetic resonance imaging. (*Adapted from* Isselbacher [5].)

STEPS IN THE EARLY MEDICAL MANAGEMENT OF A PATIENT PRESENTING WITH SUSPECTED ACUTE AORTIC DISSECTION

1. Immediate monitoring and stabilization of vital signs
2. Quick assessment: directed history, physical examination, chest radiograph, ECG, labwork
3. Reduce dP/dT with intravenous β-blockers: propranolol, labetalol, metoprolol, or esmolol
4. Treat hypertension to reduce dP/dT: intravenous nitroprusside (use in the presence of a β-blocker since alone it may increase dP/dT); goal is to reduce systolic blood pressure to 100–120 mm Hg or the lowest level possible while still maintaining cerebral and vital organ perfusion
5. If β-blockers are absolutely contraindicated, consider using intravenous calcium channel blockers or enalaprilat
6. Pain control with morphine as needed
7. Select and proceed promptly to a diagnostic study
8. Decide on medical vs surgical therapy (and determine surgical candidacy as well)

FIGURE 2-39. Steps in the early medical management of a patient presenting with suspected acute aortic dissection. The risk of complications from aortic dissection is highest within the first hours after onset, with a mortality rate for those untreated as high as 1% per hour. It is therefore essential to institute appropriate therapy as soon as the diagnosis of dissection is reasonably suspected, rather than waiting for the diagnosis to be confirmed. Specific management goals include: 1) comprehensively examining the patient for evidence of aortic dissection and the associated complications; 2) stabilizing the patient as necessary, and treating the patient pharmacologically to minimize the risk of progression or rupture of the dissection by reducing the slope of increasing pressure (dP/dT); and 3) selecting and obtaining a diagnostic imaging study as promptly as possible, and deciding between medical and surgical therapy if the diagnosis of dissection is confirmed. ECG—electrocardiogram.

INDICATIONS FOR DEFINITIVE SURGERY IN AORTIC DISSECTION

Treatment of choice for acute type A aortic dissection
Treatment of choice for chronic type A aortic dissection complicated by
  Significant aortic regurgitation
  Development of a large thoracic aortic aneurysm
Treatment of choice for acute or chronic type B aortic dissection complicated by
  Compromise of blood flow to vital organs or extremities
  Development of a large thoracic or abdominal aortic aneurysm
  Leaking or rupture of the aorta
  Retrograde extension into the ascending aorta

FIGURE 2-40. Indications for definitive surgery in aortic dissection. As a general rule, aortic repair is indicated for the management of acute type A aortic dissection, since survival in this group is improved when compared with medical management [14,15]. For acute and uncomplicated type B aortic dissection, however, aortic repair does not provide a survival advantage over medical therapy [16], so in such cases medical therapy is preferred. Nevertheless, if an acute distal dissection leads to complications, surgery may well be indicated. In the setting of chronic aortic dissection, surgery is indicated when there is evidence of significant aortic aneurysm formation. (*Adapted from* Isselbacher [5].)

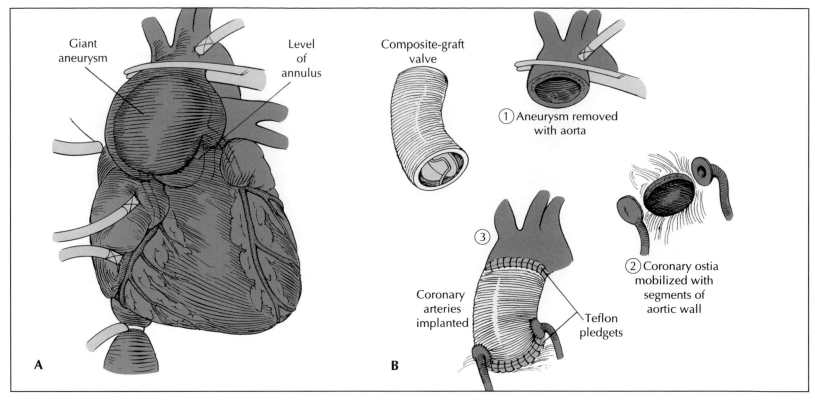

FIGURE 2-41. Repair of a proximal aortic dissection with a composite graft and reimplantation of the coronary arteries. **A,** A large dissecting ascending aortic aneurysm that involves the sinuses of Valsalva and has produced aortic insufficiency. **B,** After the patient is placed on full cardiopulmonary bypass, the aortic aneurysm is resected with the native aortic valve (1), and the coronary ostia are mobilized by excising them with a small button of the native aortic wall (2). A composite woven Dacron (C. D. Bard, Billerica, MA) graft, which includes a prosthetic aortic valve previously attached to one end, is sewn into place and Teflon (DuPont, Wilmington, DE) felt strips are used to reinforce the suture lines along the friable aorta (3). The ostia of the coronary arteries are then reimplanted into the composite graft. (*Adapted from* Eagle and DeSanctis [17].)

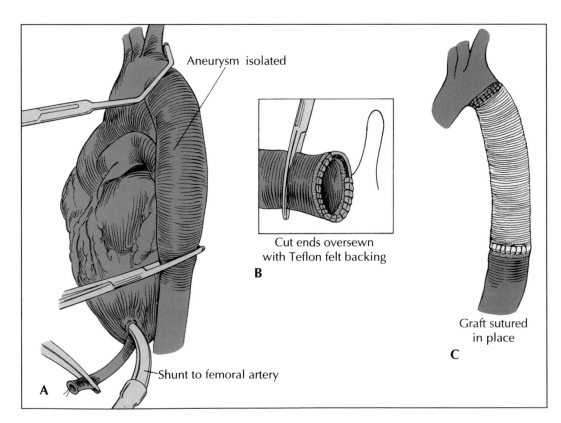

FIGURE 2-42. Repair of a type B aortic dissection. **A,** The involved segment of the descending aorta is cross-clamped and isolated and a shunt is placed from the apex of the left ventricle to the femoral artery to bypass the isolated portion of the aorta and maintain distal circulation during the surgical repair. The diseased segment of the aorta is then resected. **B,** The severed ends of the remaining aorta are oversewn with Teflon (DuPont, Wilmington, DE) felt strips to strengthen any friable aortic tissue. **C,** A woven Dacron (C.D. Bard, Billerica, MA) graft is then interposed to complete the repair of the descending aorta. (*Adapted from* Eagle et al. [3].)

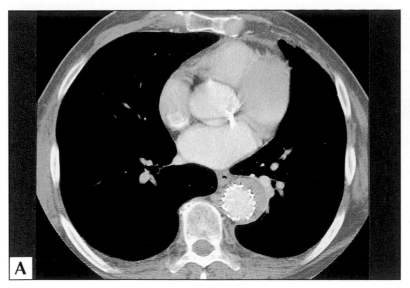 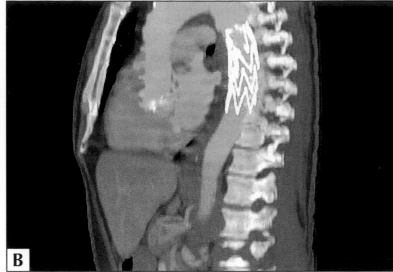

FIGURE 2-43. Endovascular aortic stent-grafts for nonsurgical management of type B dissection. Stent-grafts can be placed percutaneously via the transfemoral catheter technique. The purpose of the stent-graft is to close of the site of entry into the false lumen (*ie*, the intimal tear), thus decompressing the distended false lumen and promoting its thrombosis. For those with acute vascular complications, this should in turn relieve any obstruction of branch arteries. Such stent-grafts can only be placed in the descending aorta (*ie*, to treat distal dissections) since they cannot be passed through the aortic arch to reach the ascending aorta. In a study of 19 patients with acute dissection and a patent false lumen by Dake *et al.* [18], this technique produced complete thrombosis of false lumen in 79%, partial thrombosis in 21%, and restoration of flow to ischemic arteries with relief of corresponding symptoms in 76%. Larger studies with more patients and longer follow-up will be needed, however, before stent-graft therapy becomes a standard therapy for distal aortic dissection. **A**, A contrast-enhanced computed tomographic (CT) scan of the chest demonstrating a stent-graft in the descending aorta of a patient who presented with a type B aortic dissection. Note that there is flow in the true lumen (within the stent) but the false lumen (outside the stent) has thrombosed. **B**, A 3-dimensional reconstruction in the left anterior oblique view of the contrast-enhanced CT scan of the same patient demonstrating the position of the stent-graft within the descending thoracic aorta.

INDICATIONS FOR MEDICAL THERAPY IN AORTIC DISSECTION

1. Treatment of uncomplicated acute proximal aortic dissection if there is a specific contraindication to surgery (*eg*, stroke, severe debility, severe renal failure)
2. Treatment of chronic proximal aortic dissection, which is uncomplicated and without any other independent indication for surgery (*eg*, severe aortic insufficiency, localized aortic aneurysm)
3. Treatment of uncomplicated acute or chronic distal aortic dissection and without any other independent indication for surgery

FIGURE 2-44. Indications for medical therapy in aortic dissection. As discussed in Fig. 2-40, medical therapy is the treatment of choice in uncomplicated acute type B dissections and most uncomplicated chronic dissections. Long-term medical therapy involves both treating hypertension and reducing the slope of increasing pressure (dP/dT) in an effort to limit progression of the dissection. β-blockers are the mainstay of medical therapy and should be instituted in all cases unless specific contraindications exist [19]. Angiotensin-coverting enzyme inhibitors, added to the β-blocker therapy, have been used with increasing frequency to manage hypertension. (*Adapted from* Isselbacher [5].)

OTHER ACUTE AORTIC SYNDROMES

ACUTE AORTIC SYNDROMES

Aortic dissection

Intramural hematoma

Penetrating artherosclerotic ulcer

Focal aortic tear/contained rupture

Rapidly expanding thoracic aortic aneurysm

Traumatic aortic transection

FIGURE 2-45. Acute aortic syndromes that may present with symptoms and/or physical findings suggestive of acute aortic dissection. Intramural hematoma (*see* Fig. 2-46) is considered a variant of classic aortic dissection and occurs in a population with similar risk factors. A penetrating atherosclerotic ulcer (*see* Fig. 2-47) is typically a more localized process than aortic dissection and tends to occur in an older population with severe aortic atherosclerosis. A focal aortic tear or contained rupture may produce the same chest symptoms as aortic dissection, but its focal nature and lack of an intimal flap can make detecting it on computed tomography, magnetic resonance imaging, and transesophageal echocardiogram challenging. A rapidly expanding thoracic aortic aneurysm, typically one that involves the descending aorta, may produce significant pain, but its gradual onset and lesser severity usually distinguish it from aortic dissection. Deceleration injuries and blunt trauma to the aorta are more likely to cause aortic transsection rather than dissection; transsection is a full thickness tear through the aortic wall which, if not fatal, results in a pseudoaneurysm at the site of tear.

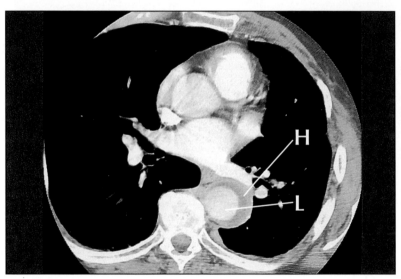

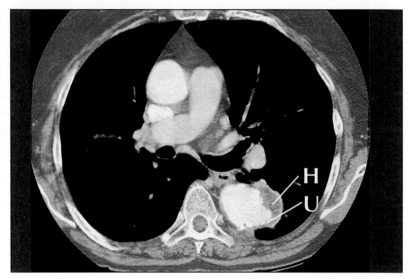

FIGURE 2-46. Intramural hematoma of the aorta. Unlike classic aortic dissection, intramural hematoma is not caused by a tear in the intima but by the rupture of the vasa vasorum within the aortic media, producing a hematoma within the wall (*see* Fig. 2-1). Since there is no intimal tear, there is no communication with the aortic lumen and thus no flow within the aortic wall hematoma. Consequently, intramural hematoma has a distinctly different— and less obvious—appearance on aortic imaging studies. Intramural hematoma is identified most readily on contrast-enhanced computed tomography (CT). The natural history of intramural hematoma is similar to that of classic aortic dissection, so its classification and its management strategies are essentially the same as for aortic dissection. Shown is a contrast-enhanced CT scan of the chest at the level of the pulmonary artery showing an intramural hematoma of the descending aorta. The hematoma (H) appears as a crescentic thickening of the aortic wall. Unlike what is seen on CT in a classic aortic dissection, with intramural hematoma there is no false lumen since there is no flow within the hematoma, there is no intimal flap, and the true lumen (L) maintains its normal shape and caliber.

FIGURE 2-47. Contrast-enhanced computed tomographic scan of a penetrating atherosclerotic ulcer of the descending thoracic aorta. The penetrating atherosclerotic ulcer appears as a contrast-filled outpouching (U) of the aorta (in the absence of an intimal flap or false lumen) with thickening of the aortic wall (H) similar to an intramural hematoma. A penetrating atherosclerotic ulcer begins as an ulceration of an atherosclerotic lesion of the aorta that penetrates into the media of the aorta, and then often produces a hematoma within the aortic wall that is either localized or extends several centimeters in length. On occasion, it can progress to classic aortic dissection. Penetrating atherosclerotic ulcerations occur almost exclusively in the descending thoracic aorta. Patients tend to be elderly with hypertension and evidence of atherosclerotic disease elsewhere. Presenting symptoms include chest and back pain similar to that of aortic dissection. The natural history of penetrating atherosclerotic ulcer is unclear, but at present management strategies are essentially the same as for classic aortic dissection.

LATE COMPLICATIONS OF AORTIC DISSECTION AND FOLLOW-UP EVALUATION

Late complications
  Recurrent dissection or progression of dissection
  Progressive aortic insufficiency requiring aortic valve replacement (in patients not initially having undergone aortic valve replacement)
  Aneurysm formation—may lead to aortic rupture
Patients at particularly high risk
  Those with Marfan syndrome—very high risk of recurrent dissection or of aneurysm formation with rupture
  Those with a patent false lumen—increased incidence of late complications and death
Imaging modalities frequently used to follow patients long-term
  Chest radiography
  Computed tomography
  Magnetic resonance imaging
  Transesophageal echocardiography

FIGURE 2-48. Late complications of aortic dissection and follow-up evaluation. While mortality is greatest following the acute phase of aortic dissection, even if the patient survives hospitalization, long-term morbidity and mortality may still result from late complications [20]. Close patient surveillance by the physician, thorough physical examinations, and follow-up imaging studies [21] performed at regular intervals (*ie*, annually) are essential to detect evidence of progression of a chronic dissection. All patients, whether treated initially with medical or surgical therapy, merit such careful follow-up.

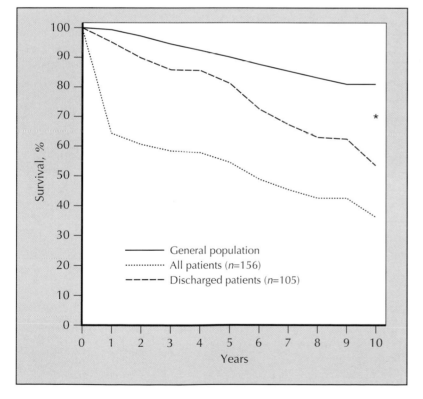

FIGURE 2-49. Ten-year actuarial survival in 156 patients with aortic dissection who received in-hospital treatment, either medical or surgical as indicated clinically. Depicted are actuarial survival curves for all 156 patients with aortic dissection, those 105 patients who were discharged from the hospital, and the general population matched for age and sex. The *asterisk* indicates a statistically significant difference in survival between the general population and the two aortic dissection groups. (*Adapted from* Doroghazi *et al.* [22].)

REFERENCES

1. Hirst AE Jr, Johns VJ Jr, Kime SW Jr: Dissecting aneurysm of the aorta: a review of 505 cases. *Medicine* 1958, 37:217–279.

2. Hagan PG, Nienaber CA, Isselbacher EM, *et al.*: The International Registry of Acute Aortic Dissection (IRAD): new insights into an old disease. *JAMA* 2000, 283:897–903.

3. Eagle KA, Doroghazi RM, DeSanctis RW, Austen GW: Aortic dissection. In *The Practice of Cardiology,* 2nd ed. Edited by Eagle KA, Haber E, DeSanctis RW, Austen WG. Boston: Little Brown; 1989:1369–1392.

4. Richartz BM, Smith DE, Cooper JV, *et al.*: New classifications of aortic dissection with improved impact on prognosis. *J Am Coll Cardiol* 2002, 39:264A.

5. Isselbacher EM: Diseases of the aorta. In *Heart Disease: a Textbook of Cardiovascular Medicine*, 6th ed. Edited by Braunwald E, Zipes DP, Libby P. Philadelphia: WB Saunders; 2001:422–456.

6. O'Gara PT, DeSanctis RW: Aortic dissection. In *Vascular Medicine.* Edited by Loscalzo J, Creager MA, Dzau VJ. Boston: Little Brown; 1992:931–956.

7. Cigarroa JA, Isselbacher EM, DeSanctis RW, Eagle KA: Diagnostic imaging in the evaluation of suspected aortic dissection: old standards and new directions. *N Engl J Med* 1993, 328:35–43.

8. Earnest F, Muhm JR, Sheedy PF: Roentgenographic findings in thoracic aortic dissection. *Mayo Clin Proc* 1979, 54:43–50.

9. Bansal RC, Chandrasekaran K, Ayala K, Smith D: Frequency and explanation of false negative diagnosis of aortic dissection by aortography and transesophageal echocardiography. *J Am Coll Cardiol* 1995, 25:1393–1401.

10. Erbel R, Daniel W, Visser C, *et al.*: Echocardiography in diagnosis of aortic dissection. *Lancet* 1989, 1:457–460.

11. Small JH, Dixon AK, Coulden RA, *et al.*: Fast CT for aortic dissection. *Br J Radiol* 1996, 69:900–905.

12. Nienaber CA, von Kodolitsch Y, Nicolas V, *et al.*: Definitive diagnosis of thoracic aortic dissection: the emerging role of noninvasive imaging modalities. *N Engl J Med* 1993, 328:1–9.

13. Chan KL: Usefulness of transesophageal echocardiography in the diagnosis of conditions mimicking aortic dissection. *Am Heart J* 1991, 122:495–504.

14. DeBakey ME, Henly WS, Cooley DA, *et al.*: Surgical management of dissecting aneurysm of the aorta. *J Thorac Cardiovasc Surg* 1965, 49:130–149.

15. Miller DC, Mitchell RC, Oyer PE, *et al*: Independent determinants of operative mortality for patients with aortic dissections. *Circulation* 1984, 70(suppl I):153.

16. Glower DD, Fann JI, Spier RH, *et al.*: Comparison of medical and surgical therapy for uncomplicated descending aortic dissection. *Circulation* 1990, 82(suppl 5):IV-39–IV-46.

17. Eagle KA, DeSanctis RW: Diseases of the aorta. In *Heart Disease: A Textbook of Cardiovascular Medicine*, edn 4. Edited by Braunwald E. Philadelphia: Saunders; 1992: 1528–1557.

18. Dake MD, Kato N, Mitchell RS, *et al.*: Endovascular stent-graft placement for the treatment of acute aortic dissection. *N Engl J Med* 1999, 340:1546–1552.

19. Grubb BP, Sirio C, Zelis R: Intravenous labetalol in acute aortic dissection. *JAMA* 1987, 258:78–79.

20. Haverick A, Miller DC, Scott WC, *et al.*: Acute and chronic aortic dissections: determinants of long-term outcome for operative survivors. *Circulation* 1985, 72(suppl II):II-22–II-34.

21. White RD, Ullyot DJ, Higgins CB: MR imaging of the aorta after surgery for aortic dissection. *Am J Roentgenol* 1988, 150:87–92.

22. Doroghazi RM, Slater EE, DeSanctis RW, *et al.*: Long-term survival of patients with treated aortic dissection. *J Am Coll Cardiol* 1984, 3:1026–1034.

3 — Arterial Occlusive Diseases of the Extremities

CHAPTER

Alan T. Hirsch

The arterial occlusive diseases of the lower extremities represent a spectrum of disorders encompassing myriad etiologies. The normal "end-organ" functions of the lower and upper extremities are (1) to permit independent ambulation, and (2) to manipulate objects; thus, diseases that alter normal limb function may potentially elicit major disabilities. Although the most common cause of lower extremity arterial occlusive disease in Western societies remains atherosclerosis, other disorders may perturb normal limb perfusion. The extremity arteries are susceptible to congenital, inflammatory, and degenerative diseases, including fibromuscular dysplasia, thromboangiitis obliterans (Buerger's disease), vascular entrapment syndromes, and both arterial thromboembolism and atheroembolism. The consideration of a broad differential diagnosis is essential for establishing an effective diagnostic and individualized treatment plan.

Atherosclerosis remains the most prevalent disorder affecting the arterial circulation in the lower extremity. Focal atherosclerotic stenoses develop with a predilection for anatomic sites in the distal abdominal aorta, and iliac, femoral, and infrapopliteal arteries. The risk of progressive atherosclerotic arterial disease of the legs correlates with the presence of the classic risk factors for progressive atherosclerosis in the coronary arteries. The clinical presentation of the patient with atherosclerotic peripheral arterial disease (PAD) depends on the rate of disease progression, the severity of the decrease in limb blood flow, the propensity for development of collateral blood flow, and the potential sudden occurrence of focal thrombosis. Thus, patients with anatomically comparable degrees of arterial occlusive disease may be asymptomatic or may present with symptoms that range from mild claudication to rest pain to frank gangrene.

The natural history of lower extremity arterial occlusive disease has been examined carefully. The progression of PAD may be slow, and over 75% to 85% of patients with intermittent claudication will manifest stable symptoms over a 5-year period. However, eventual symptomatic worsening develops in about 15% to 20% of these individuals, ischemic tissue necrosis and/or progression to rest pain (usually requiring percutaneous or surgical revascularization) may occur in an additional 3% to 5% of claudicating limbs annually, and amputation ultimately may be required in 1% of patients per year. Whereas the amputation rate may appear small, when these events are summed over 5 to 10 years of follow-up, a 5% to 10% amputation rate for this prevalent disease is notable.

The noninvasive vascular laboratory provides tools to establish the anatomic localization and quantification of the physiologic consequences of specific arterial stenoses; these techniques can be performed at a modest cost with minimal risk to the patient. Although angiographic procedures also provide important diagnostic data, these invasive procedures are performed primarily to define the anatomic details necessary to guide subsequent percutaneous or surgical revascularization procedures.

Ideal vascular therapeutic efforts are usually fostered through the clinical collaboration of specialists in vascular medicine, cardiology, interventional radiology, and vascular surgery. Effective medical therapies (risk factor normalization and use of antiplatelet therapy) should be prescribed to improve the natural history of PAD, to forestall the onset of limb-threatening events, and to increase the long-term success of surgical or percutaneous interventional therapies. Both exercise rehabilitation and pharmacotherapies should be applied to diminish the morbidity of these disorders. There is compelling evidence to support use of aggressive atherosclerotic risk factor modification strategies and antiplatelet therapies to improve long-term patient survival by decreasing the risk of coronary and cerebrovascular ischemic events.

EPIDEMIOLOGY OF PERIPHERAL ARTERIAL DISEASE

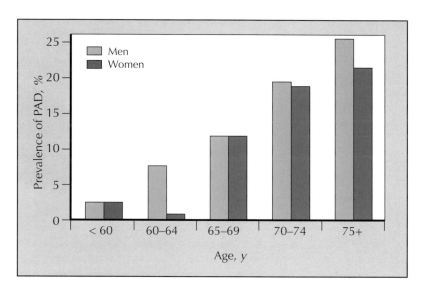

FIGURE 3-1. Age-dependent prevalence of peripheral arterial disease (PAD). The prevalence of PAD, as defined by an abnormal ankle-brachial index, increases with age, especially for individuals over 60 years of age. At 60 years of age, the prevalence of this atherosclerotic syndrome is approximately 2% to 3%, and increases to 20% to 25% of the population over 70 years of age. Although PAD is less common in younger individuals, it is known to be prevalent in those over 50 years of age who have common atherosclerotic risk factors (eg, smoking, diabetes). The prevalence of PAD rises in both men and women as they age, but it is more common in women after menopause. (Adapted from Criqui et al. [1].)

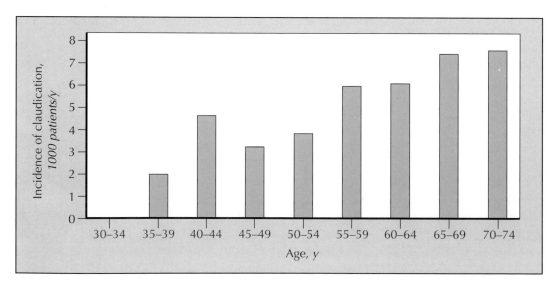

FIGURE 3-2. Claudication. Claudication, the subjective manifestation of symptomatic peripheral arterial disease (PAD), increases in incidence with advancing age. The incidence of claudication rises from 2% to 7% of adults between the third and seventh decades of life. Classic symptoms of claudication include a feeling of fatigue, aching, heaviness, or frank pain in the muscles of the calves, thighs, and buttocks that occurs reproducibly with exercise and resolves promptly with rest. Claudication can be differentiated from pain due to other causes by the reproducible stop-start nature of the symptoms in relation to exercise. Individuals with claudication usually experience the onset of symptoms at approximately the same distance, termed the initial claudication distance. Inasmuch as claudication represents the symptom induced by the mismatch of muscle blood flow supply and demand with exercise, claudication is experienced by only a fraction of those individuals with PAD. Their description of claudication symptoms may not be easily recognized due to the presence of other concomitant exercise limitations. Sedentary individuals with moderate to severe PAD may not experience claudication. (Adapted from [2].)

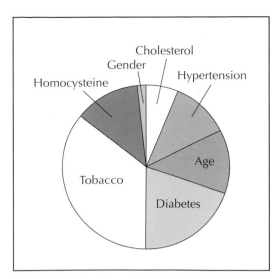

FIGURE 3-3. Risk factors for peripheral arterial disease (PAD). Risk factors for atherosclerosis (tobacco use [6.25], diabetes [3.5], age [2.2], hypertension [2.0], hypercholesterolemia [1.1], gender [1.0], and hyperhomocystinemia [2.2]) confer an increased relative risk for development of PAD, analogous to the associated risk for development of coronary artery disease (CAD). The numbers represent the relative risk of developing PAD conferred by each risk factor. Although risk factors for PAD and CAD are similar, the exact relative risk of each factor is not identical for PAD as compared to CAD. Use of any tobacco product is the most powerful predictor of PAD risk. Data from the Cardiovascular Health Study [3] demonstrate a greater than sixfold increase in PAD incidence in individuals who smoke. Diabetes is also a powerful contributor to the incidence of PAD (three- to fourfold increased risk). Elevated blood cholesterol also confers increased risk, albeit with less power than for CAD. Every 10% rise in total cholesterol confers a 10% increased risk of PAD. (*Adapted from* Newman *et al.* [3].)

ANNUAL INCIDENCE OF CLAUDICATION ACCORDING TO CIGARETTE CONSUMPTION

		INCIDENCE (RATE PER 10,000/y)	
AGE, y	CIGARETTES/d, n	MEN	WOMEN
45–54	None	10	0.2
	< 20	13	4
	> 20	25	11
55–64	None	28	18
	< 20	44	22
	> 20	108	33

FIGURE 3-4. Annual incidence of claudication according to cigarette consumption. Tobacco use is a particularly powerful predictor of increased rates of claudication, conferring a two- to fivefold increase in symptom incidence in the Framingham study population [4]. The increased risk is present even when individuals smoke less than one pack per day, and this risk rises steeply with both number of cigarettes smoked and the age of the individual.

Lower Extremity Arterial Anatomy, Limb Blood Flow, and Symptoms

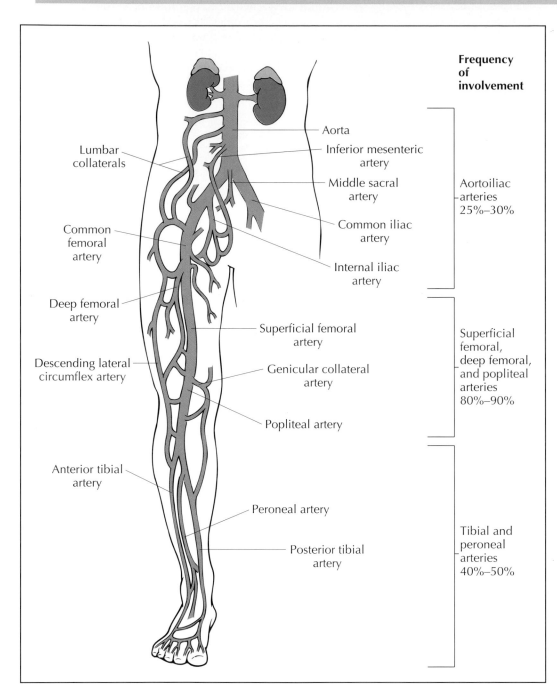

Frequency of involvement

Lumbar collaterals

Common femoral artery

Deep femoral artery

Descending lateral circumflex artery

Anterior tibial artery

Aorta

Inferior mesenteric artery

Middle sacral artery

Common iliac artery

Internal iliac artery

Superficial femoral artery

Genicular collateral artery

Popliteal artery

Peroneal artery

Posterior tibial artery

Aortoiliac arteries 25%–30%

Superficial femoral, deep femoral, and popliteal arteries 80%–90%

Tibial and peroneal arteries 40%–50%

Figure 3-5. Normal lower extremity arterial anatomy. Lower extremity atherosclerosis may cause focal or segmental arterial narrowing in the distal aorta and proximal iliofemoral arteries, the superficial femoral, deep femoral, and popliteal arteries, and the infrapopliteal tibial and peroneal arteries. A pattern of more distal disease is common in diabetic patients. The site of arterial stenosis often correlates with the site of clinical symptoms (*eg*, muscles affected by claudication or presence of rest pain or nonhealing wounds). For example, distal aortic and common iliac peripheral arterial disease is associated with gluteal or thigh claudication. Peripheral arterial disease of the superficial femoral artery, as it traverses Hunter's canal, may elicit calf claudication, and multisegmental superficial femoral, popliteal, and infrapopliteal stenoses may be associated with severe or critical limb ischemia.

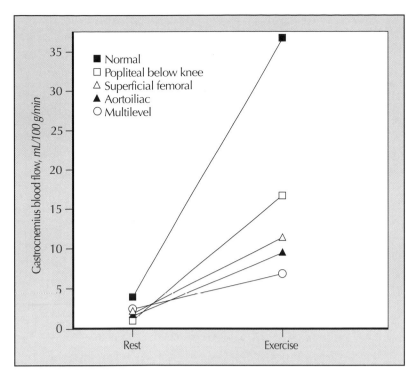

FIGURE 3-6. Limb blood flow at rest and during exercise. Although lower extremity arterial stenoses may limit blood flow at rest, nutritive blood flow may still be adequate to permit normal muscle metabolism, preserve skin integrity, and elicit minimal symptoms in patients in the nonstressed state. Exercise in normal subjects is associated with a five- to tenfold increase in blood flow to the exercising muscles. The ability of limb blood flow to increase in response to the demands of exercise depends on the anatomic site and number of stenoses that are present. In general, more proximal (aortoiliac) and multilevel stenoses result in the greatest blunting of blood flow changes with exercise [5]. (*Adapted from* Strandness and Zierler [5].)

NATURAL HISTORY AND PROGNOSIS

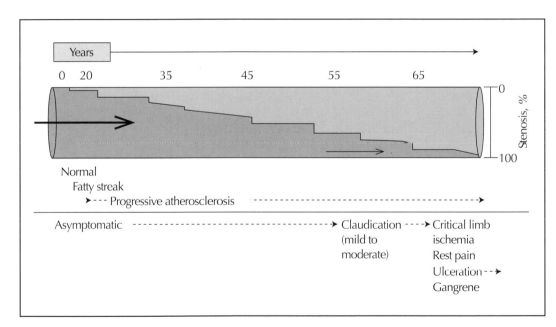

FIGURE 3-7. The natural history of peripheral arterial disease (PAD). Peripheral arterial disease is usually considered an indolent, slowly progressive disease. Decreased exercise capacity is often accepted as a consequence of aging and is not attributed to concomitant PAD and limb ischemia. Atherosclerosis of lower extremity arterial segments is thought to progress slowly over the lifetime of an individual from an early fatty streak, to complex arterial plaque, to high-grade stenosis, and this process remains largely clinically "silent." Recognition of overt PAD therefore is often delayed until moderate to severe claudication or manifestations of critical limb ischemia (*eg*, rest pain, ischemic ulceration, or gangrene) supervene late in the natural history of this disease. Early PAD detection should permit the initiation of risk factor reduction to decrease the rate of disease progression. The sudden onset of severe limb symptoms or conversion of stable claudication to rest pain suggests superimposed thrombosis, which invariably accompanies severe atherosclerotic disease [6].

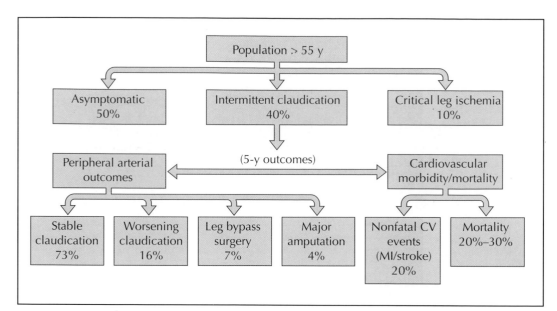

FIGURE 3-8. Natural history of peripheral arterial disease (PAD). For any population of adults with PAD, the clinical presentation represents a spectrum that includes individuals who are asymptomatic, who have claudication, or who have critical limb ischemia. Over the next 5 years of observation, these patients all face a high risk of fatal and nonfatal myocardial infarction (MI) and stroke, as well as a range of limb outcomes. Long-term clinical care should be guided by efforts to intervene beneficially to both reduce the systemic risk (heart attack and stroke) and to improve quality of life (decrease claudication symptoms and avoid amputation) [7,8]. CV–cardiovascular.

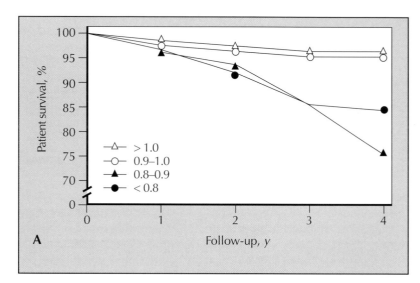

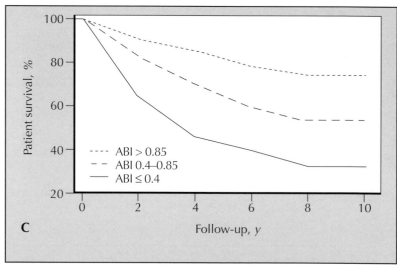

FIGURE 3-9. Ankle-brachial index (ABI) and mortality. The high mortality of patients with claudication who present for surgical arterial revascularization procedures has long been appreciated. The relationship between the presence of peripheral arterial disease and mortality in community-based (nonreferral) populations has been more obscure. Epidemiologic studies have confirmed the inverse relationship between the ABI and subsequent patient survival [9–11]. **A,** Vogt *et al.* [9] have demonstrated the predictive relationship between a low ABI and 4-year mortality in white women over 65 years of age (*n* = 1492). It is notable that the high mortality in the low ABI (ABI < 0.90) cohorts occurred irrespective of the predominant asymptomatic character of this population.

B, The ABI also predicted subsequent total and cardiovascular mortality in the hypertensive elderly men and women (*n* = 1537) followed in the Systolic Hypertension in the Elderly Program (SHEP). In this study, an abnormal ABI was associated with a three- to fourfold increased relative risk of death [10].

C, McKenna *et al.* [11] have documented 5-year mortality rates of approximately 30% and 50% in patients with ABIs of 0.85 and 0.40, respectively. This prognostic information provides a

predictor of survival similar to that obtained via use of the ejection fraction or left ventricular end-diastolic diameter for patients with heart failure. Despite the increasing use of more sophisticated vascular diagnostic tests (*eg*, arterial duplex), only the ABI presently yields such vital predictive cardiac event rate and survival data. CHD—coronary heart disease; RR—relative risk. (*Panel A adapted from* Vogt *et al.* [9]; *panel B adapted from* Newman *et al.* [10]; *panel C adapted from* McKenna *et al.* [11].)

Clinical Presentation

CLINICAL PRESENTATION OF CLAUDICATION

Exertional pain, cramping, tightness, fatigue

Occurs in muscle groups, not joints

Reproducible from day to day (consistent level of walking ability)

Resolves completely in 3–4 min

Occurs at same distance once activity resumes

FIGURE 3-10. Clinical presentation of claudication. The pain of claudication is similar in character to that experienced at the limit

of normal exertion. Muscle fatigue and frank pain may occur in the buttocks, thigh, calf, or foot, and the location of discomfort often correlates with a more proximal flow-limiting stenosis. In contrast to the leg discomfort caused by spinal stenosis ("pseudoclaudication"), vascular claudication rarely occurs with mere standing or bending, and is relieved reproducibly by relatively brief periods of rest (< 10 minutes). Not all patients with peripheral arterial disease should be expected to describe classic descriptions of claudication, just as not all patients with angina describe chest discomfort with a positive Levine sign. The development of rest pain is an ominous sign that basal limb blood flow is critically diminished. Leg perfusion may be improved if the limb is maintained in the dependent position; in contrast, leg elevation may provoke symptoms severe enough to interfere with sleep.

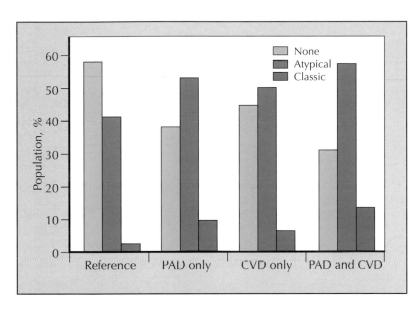

FIGURE 3-11. Frequency of leg symptoms in the PARTNERS (PAD [peripheral arterial disease] Awareness, Risk and Treatment: New Resource for Survival) study. Traditionally, it has been assumed that a high percentage of patients with PAD might be identified by the presence of typical claudication symptoms. The PARTNERS study recruited nearly 7000 patients from primary care office practices and evaluated them for the presence of classic claudication, atypical leg symptoms, or no symptoms as assessed by the standardized San Diego Claudication Questionnaire. Individuals were stratified post-hoc into those with no clinical evidence of atherosclerosis (reference population), those with PAD alone, those with other cardiovascular disease (CVD) alone, and those with both PAD and CVD. In this elderly community-derived population study, fewer than 10% of individuals with PAD as their only manifestation of atherosclerosis suffered classic claudication, while 53% had more atypical leg symptoms. These data imply that individuals with PAD suffer a range of leg symptoms and that the ankle-brachial index or other objective testing would be required to detect PAD in this high-risk population [12].

CLINICAL EXAMINATION OF THE PATIENT WITH PAD

Measure blood pressure in both arms

Auscultate abdomen for presence of bruits

Palpate for presence of abdominal aortic aneurysm

Palpate and record pulses (femoral, popliteal, posterior tibial, dorsalis pedis)

Evaluate for elevation pallor and dependent rubor

Inspect feet for ulcers, fissures, calluses, tinea, tendonous xanthomas; evaluate overall skin care

Measure ankle-brachial index

FIGURE 3-12. Clinical examination of the patient with peripheral arterial disease (PAD). A careful vascular physical examination is of great value for patients with suspected or diagnosed PAD.

Blood pressure should be measured in both arms. An abdominal examination should be performed in an attempt to palpate an aortic aneurysm, and the abdomen and flank evaluated for bruits. Femoral, popliteal, dorsalis pedis, and posterior tibial pulses should be palpated and recorded. The feet should always be carefully inspected for skin integrity or wounds.

The leg examination in most patients with PAD will demonstrate only decreased or absent lower extremity pulses. With more advanced PAD, deconditioning may induce visible induced muscle atrophy. With yet more severe PAD, there may be dependent rubor and a loss of skin integrity, with ischemic ulcers and/or frank gangrene. If supine leg perfusion pressure distal to an arterial stenoses is quite low (< 50 mm Hg), leg elevation may result in elevation pallor; resumption of the horizontal position will elicit reactive hyperemia (dependent rubor). A complete vascular physical examination should include (1) directed palpation for an abdominal aneurysm; (2) auscultation for bruits; (3) a complete pulse examination; (4) an assessment of skin integrity; and (5) an ankle-brachial index measurement.

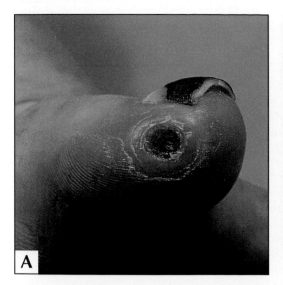

A

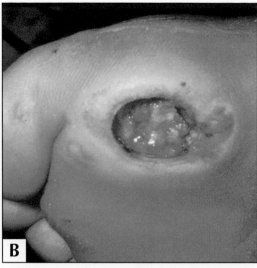

B

FIGURE 3-13. Ischemic toe (**A**) and metatarsal (**B**) ulceration. Ischemic skin ulceration is likeliest to occur on the heel, the lateral malleoli, and at the base of the toes since these sites are subjected to repeated trauma during ambulation. The propensity for development of ischemic wounds may be decreased markedly by the use of well-fitting, protective footwear at all times, proper trimming of nails, lubrication of dry skin, and avoidance of accidental injury.

DIAGNOSTIC EVALUATION

NONINVASIVE VASCULAR TESTS

NONINVASIVE VASCULAR TESTING FOR PAD			
TEST	DISEASE LOCALIZATION	QUANTITATION OF DISEASE SEVERITY	RELATIVE COST
ABI	–	++	+
Segmental pressure analysis	++	++	+
Pulse volume recordings	+	+	+
Transcutaneous oximetry	+	+++	++
Doppler waveform analysis	+++	++	++
Arterial duplex	+++	++	+++
Exercise Doppler	–	+++	+++

FIGURE 3-14. Noninvasive testing. The noninvasive vascular laboratory provides powerful tools to assess objectively the location and physiologic significance of lower extremity arterial disease, and thereby accelerate the delineation of a therapeutic plan. Compared with angiographic methods, these studies are relatively inexpensive, can be performed with negligible risk, and provide prognostic information. Noninvasive vascular examinations of the lower extremity arterial circulation are performed to achieve the following goals: (1) to objectively establish the presence of arterial occlusive disease; (2) to assess quantitatively the severity of disease; (3) to localize lesions to specific arterial segments of the limb; and (4) to determine the temporal progression of disease or its response to specific therapy. ABI—ankle-brachial index; PAD—peripheral arterial disease.

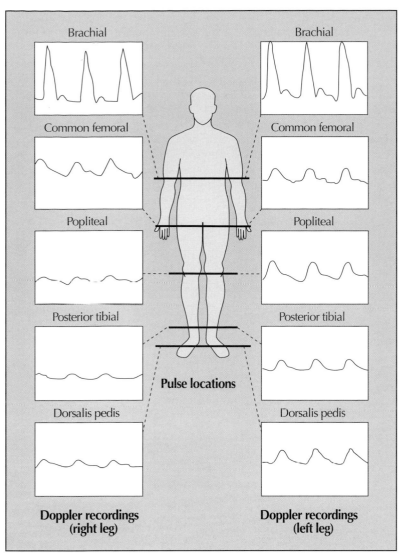

Brachial

Common femoral

Popliteal

Posterior tibial

Dorsalis pedis

**Doppler recordings
(right leg)**

Brachial

Common femoral

Popliteal

Posterior tibial

Dorsalis pedis

**Doppler recordings
(left leg)**

Pulse locations

FIGURE 3-15. Doppler waveform analysis. Continuous-wave Doppler waveform analysis can also provide important information to assess arterial patency or to localize arterial occlusive lesions. In many circumstances a change in peak blood velocity and/or pulse waveform provides reasonably accurate information about the location and extent of specific lower extremity lesions. The normal Doppler profile demonstrates a brisk upstroke, triphasic waveform, and moderate peak blood velocities. The blood flow profile will demonstrate a characteristic increase in peak velocity within and immediately distal to a significant stenosis; the Doppler profile decreases in amplitude and the waveform becomes biphasic or monophasic distal to the limiting lesion. Doppler waveform analyses are reliable even in highly calcified vessels that are not amenable to systolic pressure determinations. The continuous-wave Doppler profiles displayed here demonstrate normal bilateral brachial blood acceleration profiles. Doppler profiles are decreased in amplitude and monophasic in both common femoral and more distal arteries, suggesting aortic or bilateral arterial occlusive disease and possible right superficial femoral or popliteal arterial disease.

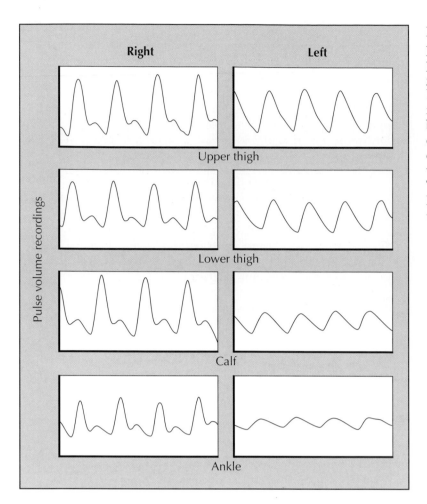

Right / **Left**

Pulse volume recordings

Upper thigh

Lower thigh

Calf

Ankle

FIGURE 3-16. Pulse volume recordings. Pulse volume recordings provide a method to evaluate the arterial pressure waveform profile qualitatively via the use of either a pneumoplethysmograph or a mercury-in-Silastic (polymeric silicone) strain gauge. Both of these devices can be applied in a segmental manner from the thigh to the ankle to assess the change in limb volume between diastole and systole. The subsequent recording of such data and analysis of the pulse volume amplitude provide an index of large vessel patency and correlate with blood flow. The pulse volume recordings are normal in the right leg of this patient. There are progressively abnormal pulse volume recordings at the left thigh, calf and ankle of this patient with sequential lesions of the left iliac and superficial femoral arteries.

SEGMENTAL PRESSURE MEASUREMENTS

ARM BLOOD PRESSURE, *mm Hg*		RIGHT 155/86		LEFT 154/85	
CUFF POSITION	DP	PT	DP	PT
Upper thigh	—	98	150	—
Lower thigh	—	88	100	—
Upper calf	—	83	95	—
Lower calf	70	80	65	50
ABI	0.45	0.52	0.42	0.32

FIGURE 3-17. Segmental pressure measurements. Arterial systolic pressures can be measured noninvasively using sphygmomanometric cuffs placed sequentially along the limb at various levels (*eg*, the upper thigh, the lower thigh, the upper calf, and the lower calf above the ankle). In contrast to simple ankle-brachial index (ABI) studies, the segmental pressure analysis often is able to determine accurately the location of individual arterial stenoses. In most laboratories, any gradient greater than 10 to 15 mm Hg between adjacent sites may represent a physiologically important focal stenosis. However, segmental pressure measurements may be elevated artifactually or may be uninterpretable in patients with calcified, noncompressible vessels, as is the case with simple ABI determinations. In this example, segmental pressure measurements demonstrate the following: a 57-mm Hg gradient between the brachial systolic pressure and the right upper thigh, denoting right iliofemoral arterial disease; a 50-mm Hg mid-left thigh gradient, suggesting superficial femoral artery occlusive disease; and a 30- to 45-mm Hg gradient between the left upper and lower calf, suggesting infrapopliteal disease. DP—dorsalis pedis; PT—posterior tibial.

	ARM BLOOD	RIGHT	LEFT	RIGHT	LEFT
PROTOCOL TIME	PRESSURE, mm Hg	PT	DP	ABI	ABI
Rest	155/86	145	123	0.94	0.79
Immediately postexercise	195/90	40	70	0.21	0.36
1 min postexercise	170/88	65	84	0.38	0.49
5 min postexercise	165/70	83	90	0.50	0.54
10 min postexercise	145/80	138	118	0.95	0.81

EXERCISE DOPPLER STUDY: AORTOILIAC DISEASE

FIGURE 3-18. Exercise Doppler stress testing. It is commonly thought that patients with peripheral arterial disease cannot be evaluated effectively by cardiovascular treadmill testing. Standard exercise testing protocols may be inordinately arduous for many patients with claudication, but less vigorous treadmill testing protocols may be extremely useful in objectively documenting the magnitude of claudication symptoms in patients with mild to moderate disease prior to initiating exercise, pharmacologic, or revascularization procedures. These studies afford the opportunity to record the time of onset of limiting leg symptoms, to note the total walking time, and to determine if associated coronary ischemic symptoms or electrocardiographic abnormalities are provoked during usual activities. The addition of a Doppler recording of the ankle systolic blood pressures before and after exercise yields objective data to grade the dynamic functional significance of limb arterial stenoses. Patients with true vasculogenic claudication are characterized by a reproducible fall in the postexercise ankle-brachial index (ABI) compared with its baseline value. In contrast, the patient with pseudoclaudication due to spinal stenosis will demonstrate a normal postexercise ABI, despite limiting symptoms that would otherwise suggest arterial insufficiency.

This figure illustrates the expected results for a patient with aortoiliac disease and buttock, thigh, and calf claudication whose resting ABIs are near normal. Exercise reproduced typical symptoms with a marked fall in the postexercise ABI and a delay in ABI recovery time. The patient exercised for 10.4 minutes using a modified Bruce protocol. He developed typical right > left thigh claudication at 4 minutes and bilateral calf claudication at 6 minutes. No angina or ischemic electrocardiographic changes were noted. DP—dorsalis pedis; PT—posterior tibial.

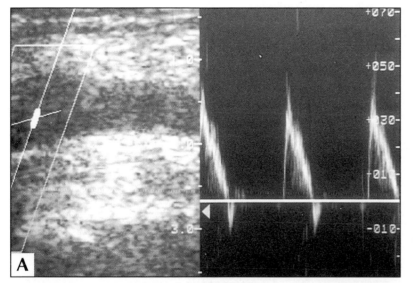

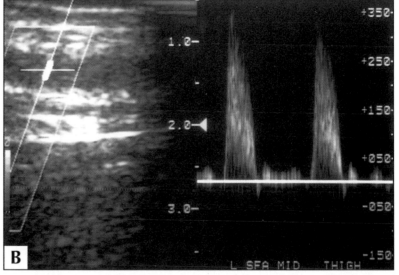

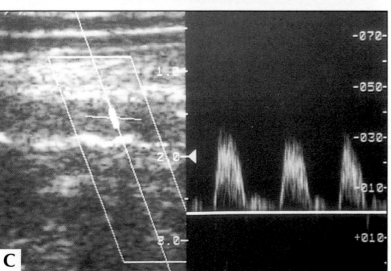

FIGURE 3-19. Duplex ultrasound scanning. Duplex ultrasound scanning uses dual imaging (*left panels*) and Doppler waveform (*right panels*) analysis to assess lower extremity arterial anatomy and perfusion. Duplex studies can assess plaque morphology and surgical graft patency, and can establish the presence of arteriovenous fistulae. Although duplex scanning can provide diagnostic information in a majority of patients, this technique requires a technically proficient examiner, may require extensive time for a complete examination, and is significantly more expensive than most physiologic testing. Duplex testing should be reserved for specific indications in which the precise anatomic information obtained by this technique is likely to be useful (*eg*, the assessment of proximal iliofemoral stenoses) and to evaluate the patency of saphenous vein and prosthetic arterial grafts, angioplasty sites, and intravascular stents.

A, In this example, interrogation of the normal left common femoral artery demonstrates the preserved triphasic Doppler waveform, a sharply defined spectral envelope, and peak velocity of 40 cm/s. **B,** In contrast, Doppler evaluation of the mid-left superficial femoral artery at the site of a high-grade stenosis shows a biphasic waveform, marked spectral broadening, and increased peak velocity of 300 cm/s. **C,** Examination below the stenosis in the distal superficial femoral artery demonstrates a low velocity (30 cm/s) and monophasic waveform.

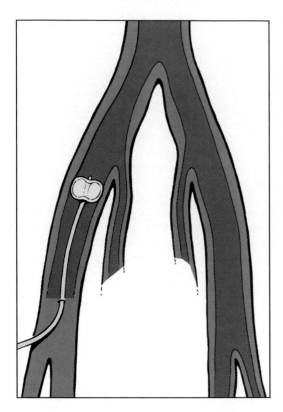

FIGURE 3-20. Lower extremity arteriography to define the detailed extent of arterial occlusive disease. The lower extremity arteries may be visualized via a puncture of either femoral artery in order to complete both pelvic angiographic and lower extremity "runoff" images. Alternatively, greater angiographic detail may be obtained via performance of the balloon occlusion technique (shown here), in which contrast media are injected selectively into a single leg distal to a balloon inflated in the common femoral artery.

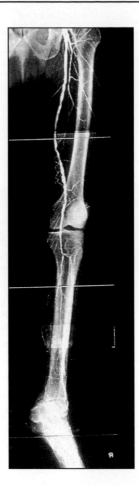

FIGURE 3-21. Lower extremity angiography in peripheral arterial disease. Angiogram of the left lower extremity was performed in a 62-year-old man who presented with limiting calf and foot claudication. Diffuse atherosclerotic disease of the superficial femoral artery, profunda femoral artery, and popliteal artery is evident. The mid-superficial femoral artery is occluded discretely in its midportion and the origins of the anterior tibial artery and posterior tibial-peroneal trunk are also diseased.

Atherosclerotic Lower Extremity Peripheral Arterial Disease

Medical Therapy

MANAGEMENT OF PAD

RISK FACTOR MODIFICATION

Smoking cessation

Goal: complete cessation

Lipid management

Goal: LDL < 100 mg/dL

Blood pressure control

Goal: < 130/85 mm Hg

Blood sugar control in patients with diabetes

Goal: HbA_{1c} < 7%

ANTIPLATELET THERAPIES

Aspirin, clopidogrel

Goal: reduction in risk of MI, stroke

SYMPTOM-DIRECTED THERAPIES

Supervised exercise rehabilitation

Cilostazol, pentoxifylline

Selective use of revascularization (PTA, bypass)

GENERAL SUPPORTIVE CARE

Foot care

Psychosocial support

FIGURE 3-22. Management of peripheral arterial disease (PAD). Optimal care for all patients with PAD should be comprehensive. Risk factor modification should be effective in blunting cardiovascular ischemic event rates, and perhaps the rate of progression of PAD. Long-term patency rates of arterial revascularization procedures are known to be improved by tobacco abstinence. Smoking cessation, effective lipid management (low-density lipoprotein [LDL] cholesterol < 100 mg/dL), normalization of blood pressure (< 130/85 mm Hg), and normalization of blood sugar (HbA_{1c} < 7.0%) should be achieved in all patients with PAD. Antiplatelet medications (clopidogrel or aspirin) should be prescribed uniformly unless otherwise contraindicated. For patients with limb symptoms, supervised exercise training (rehabilitation), use of pharmacotherapies, or selective use of revascularization may improve symptoms. Attention to foot care will diminish the incidence of ischemic wounds and amputation. Peripheral arterial disease may be debilitating, disrupting employment and family dynamics. Many patients may benefit from professional psychosocial support. MI—myocardial infarction; PTA—percutaneous transluminal angioplasty.

RISK OF ISCHEMIC EVENTS IN ATHEROSCLEROTIC SYNDROMES*

SITE OF INITIAL ISCHEMIC EVENT/CONDITION	INCREASE IN RISK VS GENERAL POPULATION	
	GREATER RISK OF MI	GREATER RISK OF STROKE
MI	5–7× (includes death)	3–4× (includes TIA)
Stroke	2–3× (includes angina, sudden death)	9×
PAD	4× (includes only fatal MI and other CHD death)	2–3× (includes TIA)

*Epidemiologic data show that patients with atherosclerosis are at increased risk of both MI and stroke [13–15].

FIGURE 3-23. Risk of ischemic events in atherosclerotic syndromes: the rationale for aggressive secondary prevention. Secondary prevention of cardiovascular events is recognized to be an essential component of care for patients with established coronary heart disease (CHD). Patients with documented atherosclerotic peripheral arterial disease (PAD) should also be aggressively treated to lower their risk of subsequent myocardial infarction (MI) and stroke, and thus to prolong event-free survival.

Patients with PAD suffer increased risk of ischemic CHD events and stroke, as is the case for patients with documented cerebrovascular disease or CHD itself. Thus, risk factor reduction interventions and use of antiplatelet medications should be initiated in any patient with PAD, whether the patient is asymptomatic (ankle-brachial index < 0.90), suffers claudication, or has undergone previous arterial reconstructive procedures [13–16]. TIA—transient ischemic attack.

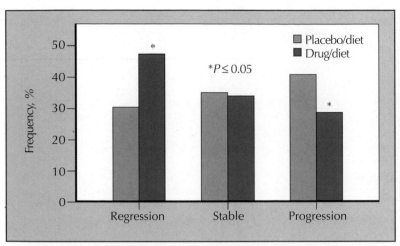

FIGURE 3-24. Feasibility of regression of femoral atherosclerosis. The Cholesterol Lowering Atherosclerosis Study (CLAS) of Barndt et al. [17] assessed the rates of both coronary and femoral atherosclerotic disease progression in a cohort of 162 middle-aged, nonsmoking men in a double-blind, placebo-controlled study of dietary versus aggressive lipid-lowering drug treatment. Patients were treated either by combined dietary modification and colestipol and niacin therapy, or by dietary management alone over a relatively brief 2-year study period. These data demonstrated that the rate of femoral arterial atherosclerotic disease progression, as assessed by paired quantitative angiography, was blunted, and femoral arterial disease regression was greater in those subjects who achieved optimal effective lipid lowering. (*Adapted from* Barndt *et al.* [17].)

LIPID-LOWERING THERAPY AND INTERMITTENT CLAUDICATION: RESULTS OF THE POSCH STUDY

EVENT	CONTROL	ILEAL BYPASS	P VALUE
Mortality	62	49	0.164
CHD/MI	300	195	**0.001**
Claudication	71	52	**0.038**
CVA	15	14	0.69

FIGURE 3-25. Lipid-lowering therapy and intermittent claudication. Data from POSCH (Program on the Surgical Control of the Hyperlipidemias) show that lipid lowering has clinical benefits. Most medical lipid-lowering clinical trials have been performed with follow-up extended for less than 3 years, and claudication symptom endpoints have not been assessed. The POSCH study achieved optimal, long-term normalization of serum lipids by ileal bypass surgery, and extended the benefits of treatment through 10 years of follow-up. Study subjects ($n = 838$) had one prior myocardial infarction (MI), blood pressure less than 180/105 mm Hg, and cholesterol levels of more than 220 mg/dL. As in the CLAS (Cholesterol Lowering Atherosclerosis Study) trial, the rate of both coronary and femoral arterial atherosclerosis disease progression was diminished; more impressively, this intervention improved coronary heart disease (CHD)/MI event rates and also reduced the rate of development of symptomatic claudication by 27% [18]. CVA—cerebrovascular accident. (*Adapted from* Buchwald *et al.* [18].)

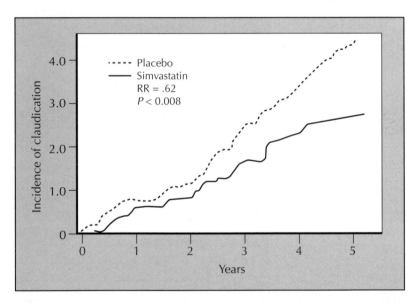

FIGURE 3-26. Effect of aggressive lipid normalization with simvastatin on the development of claudication. Whereas CLAS (Cholesterol Lowering Atherosclerosis Study) and other studies have shown that aggressive low-density lipoprotein (LDL) lowering is associated with both plaque stabilization (less progression) as well as frank regression of femoral atherosclerosis, additional data suggest that the new or worsening claudication symptoms can be diminished by lipid-lowering therapy. In patients with coronary artery disease who were treated aggressively to normalize LDL cholesterol, as was accomplished in 4S (Scandinavian Simvastatin Survival Study), the development of symptomatic claudication was decreased [19]. RR—relative risk.

SPECIFIC GOALS OF LIPID-LOWERING THERAPY IN PATIENTS WITH ATHEROSCLEROTIC VASCULAR DISEASE

LDL cholesterol < 100 mg/dL

Increase HDL cholesterol as much as possible by nonpharmacologic means, and consider benefits of HDL raising on choices of drug therapies

Decrease triglycerides to < 200 mg/dL, or perhaps to < 150 mg/dL for diabetic patients

FIGURE 3-27. Goals of lipid-lowering therapy for peripheral arterial disease (PAD). Effective lipid management should be considered a mandatory component of the medical therapy of patients with objective evidence of lower extremity arterial occlusive disease. This strategy has been sanctioned by the recent National Cholesterol Education Panel (NCEP) guidelines, which recommend that patients with objective evidence of PAD (symptomatic or objective evidence, such as a reduced ankle-brachial index) be treated by a therapeutic lifestyle modification and/or pharmacologic therapy to achieve an LDL (low-density lipoprotein) cholesterol below 100 mg/dL [20]. Secondary treatment goals include measures to raise HDL (high-density lipoprotein) cholesterol and to normalize fasting serum triglycerides. Such efforts should achieve a decreased rate of both cardiac and vascular ischemic events in this high-risk population.

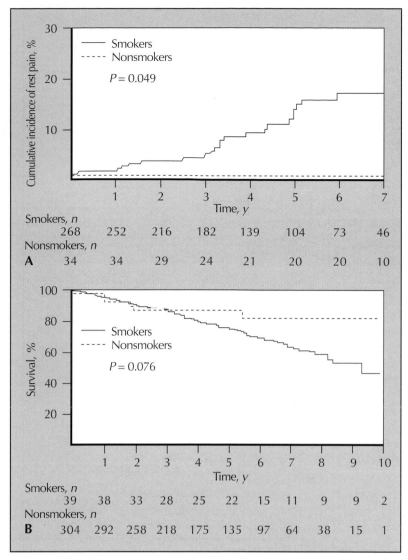

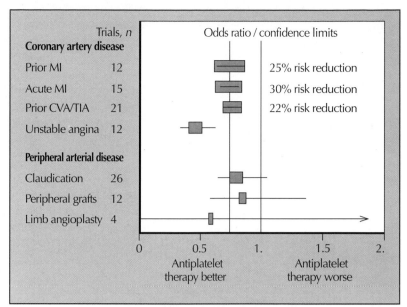

FIGURE 3-29. Role of antiplatelet therapies. The benefits of antiplatelet therapies (aspirin, clopidogrel, ticlopidine) have been demonstrated in the secondary prevention of recurrent myocardial infarction (MI), stroke, and cardiovascular death in patients who have survived prior myocardial ischemic events. These trials have evaluated large patient cohorts over an extensive number of years to show a 22% to 29% risk reduction for these coronary ischemic events. Whereas over 42 investigations have evaluated antiplatelet therapies in patients with claudication or after limb arterial reconstructive procedures, these trials have usually been limited in size and duration of follow-up, and thus the confidence limits of these trials have been wide, not reaching statistical significance. Presently available data suggest that antiplatelet therapy yields comparable coronary protective benefits in patients with peripheral arterial disease [24]. *Horizontal lines* represent 95% confidence intervals. CVA—cerebrovascular accident; TIA—transient ischemic attack. (*Adapted from* [25].)

FIGURE 3-28. Importance of tobacco abstinence. All patients with peripheral arterial disease should be strongly encouraged to discontinue tobacco use in order to decrease the rate of limb atherosclerosis progression and symptomatic worsening. **A,** As many as 18% of patients with claudication who continue to smoke cigarettes may develop rest pain over the subsequent 5 years of observation [21]. In contrast, those patients who quit smoking rarely progress to this painful endpoint. **B,** Successful tobacco cessation also has major effects on patient survival in this population [22,23]. The numbers below the graphs indicate the patients at risk at each time interval. The 5-year mortality rates for patients with claudication who continue to smoke may be as high as 40% to 50%. In contrast, tobacco abstinence in this population is associated with markedly decreased rates of myocardial infarction and stroke, resulting in an impressive improvement in survival. (*Panel A adapted from* De Felice *et al.* [24]; *panel B adapted from* Jonason and Bergstrom [21].)

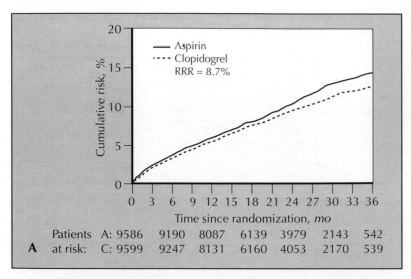

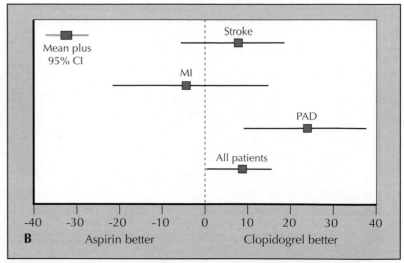

FIGURE 3-30. The CAPRIE (Clopidogrel versus Aspirin in Patients at Risk of Ischaemic Events) trial. The relative benefits of aspirin and clopidogrel on the combined endpoint of myocardial infarction (MI), stroke, and vascular death were studied in the prospective international CAPRIE study [26]. The study recruited patients with various manifestations of atherosclerosis, including patients who had suffered a recent MI or ischemic stroke, or had established peripheral arterial disease (PAD). Investigators hypothesized that individuals with prior stroke, MI, or PAD suffer comparably high rates of subsequent MI, stroke, and vascular death. The study included 6452 patients with PAD, making it one of the largest prospective trials ever performed to evaluate any medical therapy

for PAD. In CAPRIE, PAD was defined as either self-reported claudication with an ankle-brachial index less than 0.85, or a history of prior lower extremity arterial revascularization procedures (either angioplasty or vascular surgery) or amputation. **A**, Clopidogrel treatment was more effective than standard aspirin, eliciting an overall relative risk reduction (RRR) of 8.7% in preventing subsequent ischemic stroke, MI, or vascular death in the total study population. **B**, Patients with PAD benefited from clopidogrel therapy, with a 23.8% RRR compared to aspirin in this subgroup. Current clinical data therefore suggest that all patients with documented PAD should receive antiplatelet therapy unless otherwise contraindicated.

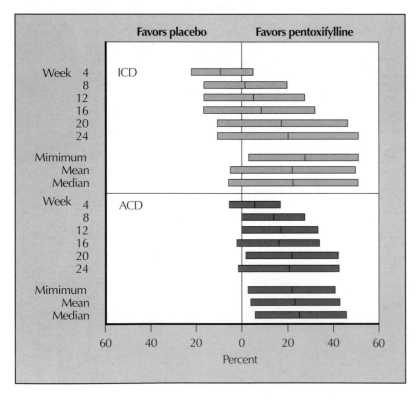

FIGURE 3-31. Role of pentoxifylline therapy. Pentoxifylline was the first medication approved for treatment of patients with peripheral arterial disease to improve symptoms of claudication. The mechanism of benefit is reported to be a reduction in blood viscosity and improved erythrocyte deformability. This figure demonstrates the expected 20% to 30% improvement from pentoxifylline therapy on intermittent claudication distance (ICD) and absolute claudication distance (ACD) in a series of clinical trials [27]. The ICD represents the treadmill distance walked until the first onset of claudication. The ACD represents the maximal, limiting treadmill distance until walking must be terminated. Thus, pentoxifylline elicits only a small improvement in walking distances, and other therapies are considered more effective. This agent is well tolerated, only infrequently eliciting adverse effects (*eg*, flushing, dizziness, gastrointestinal distress). (*Adapted from* Lindgarde *et al.* [27].)

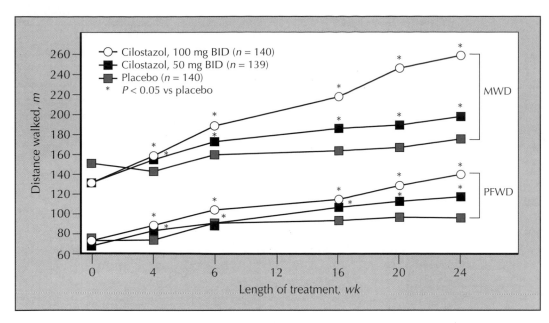

FIGURE 3-32. Role of cilostazol therapy for claudication. Cilostazol was approved for the treatment of claudication in 1999. This medication is a phosphodiesterase III inhibitor that increases intracellular cyclic AMP (cAMP) in platelets and vascular smooth

muscle cells, thereby decreasing platelet aggregation and inducing microvascular vasodilation [28]. Cilostazol use is also associated with small increases in serum high-density lipoprotein and decreases in serum triglyceride values. This figure demonstrates the dose-dependent increase in both pain-free walking distance (PFWD) and maximal walking distance (MWD) observed when treatment is continued for at least 12 weeks, with additional benefit accruing over 24 weeks. A single trial (not shown) has demonstrated superiority of cilostazol over pentoxifylline. Cilostazol is also well tolerated, but adverse effects include headache, palpitations, nausea, or loose stools. Due to a potential class effect of long-term oral administration of phosphodiesterase inhibitors, cilostazol is absolutely contraindicated in patients with heart failure [29–32].

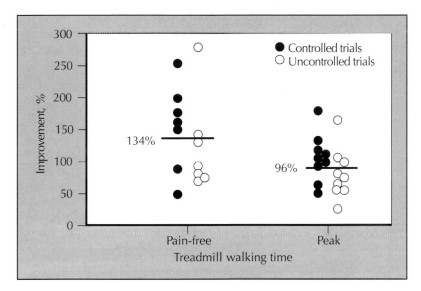

FIGURE 3-33. Supervised exercise rehabilitation for the patient with claudication. The efficacy of claudication exercise training has been well established by numerous investigators [33–35]. These studies of the efficacy of exercise training have demonstrated an improvement in both pain-free walking time (mean increase 134%, represented by the *horizontal line*) and maximal walking time (mean increase 96%). The mechanism(s) by which exercise training improves functional capacity likely is multifactorial, inclusive of improvement in blood viscosity, by promoting a change in walking techniques to more biomechanically efficient techniques, by altering the ischemic pain threshold or tolerance, or by improving abnormal skeletal muscle oxidative metabolism. There is no evidence to support the hypothesis that exercise training improves collateral blood flow.

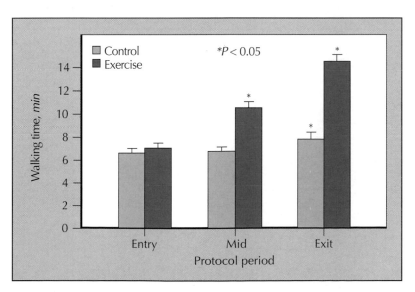

FIGURE 3-34. Exercise training in peripheral arterial disease (PAD); effect of a 12-week training program. These data from Hiatt [34] demonstrate the functional benefit of exercise training in PAD patients who entered a 12-week supervised walking program compared with a control group. Total treadmill walking time was evaluated at study entry, after 6 weeks of training or observation, and at study exit. The doubling of walking time is typical of the benefits of exercise rehabilitation for patients with claudication [34]. (*Adapted from* Hiatt [34].)

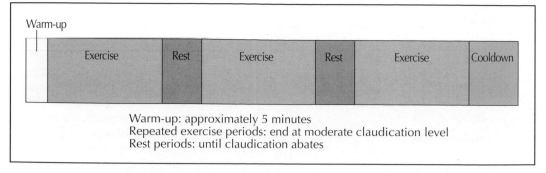

Warm-up

| Exercise | Rest | Exercise | Rest | Exercise | Cooldown |

Warm-up: approximately 5 minutes
Repeated exercise periods: end at moderate claudication level
Rest periods: until claudication abates

FIGURE 3-35. Claudication exercise training. Exercise reproducibly elicits an improvement in pain-free and maximal walking distance when repeated exercise sessions are performed on a regular schedule, which has been demonstrated to be effective only in supervised settings. Therapeutic exercise for claudication is outlined by Current Procedural Terminology (CPT) code 93668, which outlines use of 45- to 60-minute exercise sessions and a motorized treadmill or track to permit each patient to achieve their symptom-limited claudication [36]. Sessions are usually supervised by an exercise physiologist, nurse, or physical therapist, who documents the patient's claudication threshold and other cardiovascular limitations. Periods of alternating exercise and rest are then performed in sessions scheduled at least three times weekly for a minimum of 12 weeks.

PERCUTANEOUS THERAPY

CLINICAL APPROACH TO REVASCULARIZATION

What are the therapeutic goals?
Claudication, rest pain, wound healing, or threatened limb

Localize the physiologically important anatomic disease
Aortoiliac vs iliofemoral vs infrapopliteal

Determine the optimal revascularization techniques
for that site (initial success and long-term patency rates)
Thrombolysis vs PTA vs in situ or PTFE bypass (or combination)

What is the impact of revascularization on cardiovascular
homeostasis?

What is the comorbidity of the revascularization technique?

FIGURE 3-36. Clinical approach to revascularization. Revascularization may be indicated to improve leg ischemic symptoms if severe claudication is refractory to medical therapy or if critical limb ischemia (rest pain, nonhealing ischemic wounds, or rest pain) supervene. The advent of catheter-based therapies has profoundly improved the treatment of lower extremity arterial occlusive disease, permitting a nonsurgical method for restoration of limb perfusion. The rapid evolution of percutaneous and surgical techniques may permit either a percutaneous or surgical revascularization approach alone or in combination. Therefore, the choice of revascularization techniques and the likelihood of achieving clinical success are dependent on the unique features of the individual patient. The clinician should define a precise therapeutic goal, attempt to correct the most physiologically severe arterial lesions, and be cognizant of local success rates for the desired revascularization procedure. The relative short- and long-term cardiovascular risk of the revascularization procedure should be considered prior to initiating a limb revascularization strategy.

Long-term clinical success should be defined by the degree of symptom improvement, not merely by the angiographic patency rate for a selected improvement. PTA—percutaneous transluminal angioplasty; PTFE—polytetrafluoroethylene.

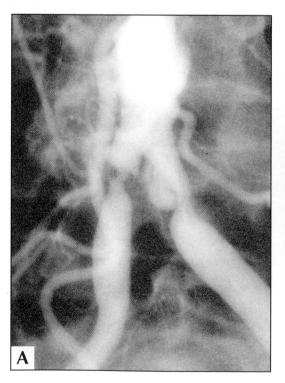

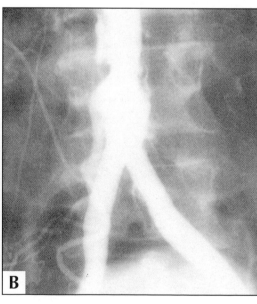

FIGURE 3-37. Iliac angioplasty. **A,** The distal aorta and proximal segments of both common iliac arteries are diseased in this 65-year-old man with severe thigh claudication. **B,** Balloon angioplasty was successful in decreasing the severity of the stenoses in both iliac arteries, with complete alleviation of the patient's exercise limitation.

INDICATIONS FOR ENDOVASCULAR ILIAC STENTS

Ineffective angioplasty
  Residual stenosis > 30%
  Residual gradient > 10–20 mm Hg
Refractory restenosis
Total iliac artery occlusions
Ulcerated plaque

FIGURE 3-38. Indications for endovascular stents. Despite the relative success of iliac angioplasty to achieve revascularization of the more proximal limb circulation, this success remains tempered by residual long-term restenosis rates. Considerable effort has led to the development of metallic endovascular prostheses (stents) that may be placed percutaneously at stenotic arterial sites to further improve long-term patency rates. The indications for placement of the iliac stents include an ineffective primary angioplasty (defined by a significant residual stenosis or pressure gradient), refractory restenosis due to elastic recoil or severe intimal hyperplasia, revascularization of long occluded iliac artery segments, and regions of marked iliac ulceration.

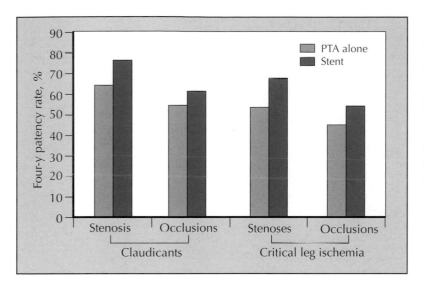

FIGURE 3-39. Percutaneous transluminal angioplasty (PTA) patency rates with and without stents for aorto-iliac disease. Bosch and Hunink [37] performed a meta-analysis of six PTA studies inclusive of 1300 patients and eight stent studies inclusive of 816 patients to summarize procedural success. Four-year primary patency rates were 65% for stenoses and 54% for occlusions after PTA to treat claudication. Primary patency rates were 53% for stenoses and 44% for occlusions to treat critical limb ischemia. Patency rates for both stenoses and occlusions in both claudication and critical limb ischemia were increased whenstent placement was used.

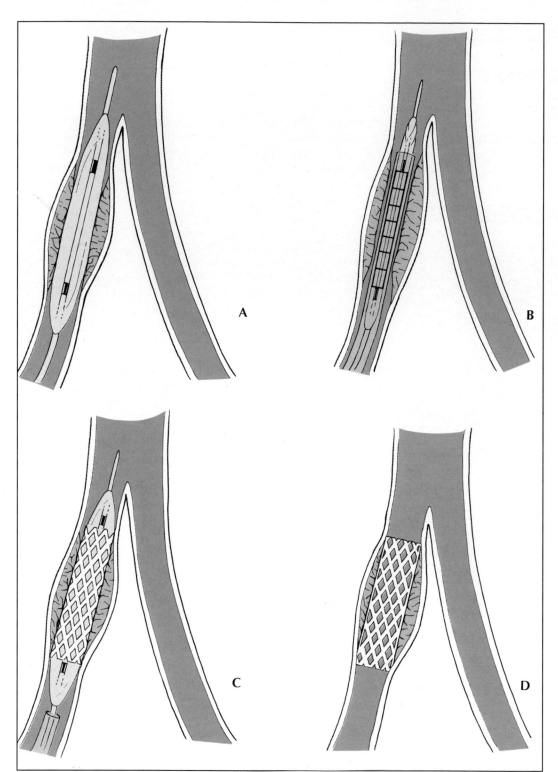

FIGURE 3-40. Placement of iliac stents for the treatment of iliac disease. **A,** Standard balloon angioplasty is used initially to decrease the diameter of the iliac stenosis. **B,** The stent is then loaded onto a balloon catheter and guided to the diseased arterial segment. **C,** Balloon inflation permits the stent to enlarge to its maximal diameter. **D,** After removal of the catheter, the stent retains its position and intima will eventually grow to encompass the metallic mesh.

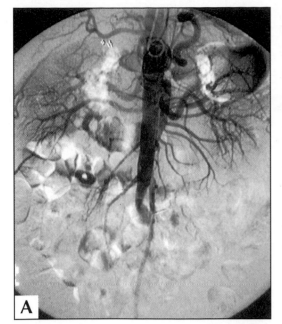

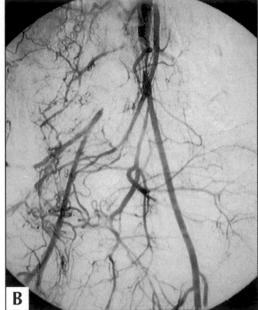

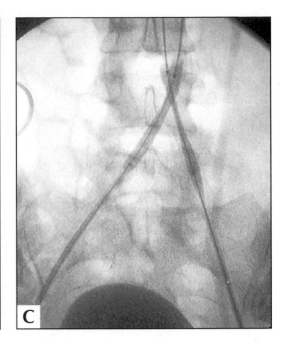

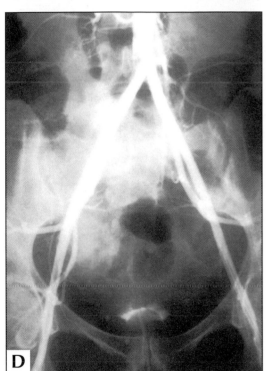

FIGURE 3-41. Bilateral iliac revascularization using multiple Palmaz stents (Cordis Corp., Miami, FL). The combined use of angioplasty and endovascular stent placement has been used successfully to achieve bi-iliac revascularization. These pelvic angiograms show a 32-year-old woman who presented with severe, bilateral claudication of the thighs, calves, and feet, with great toe ischemic ulceration. **A,** On initial contrast injection, the distal aorta is noted to taper, and little filling of the common iliac arteries is observed. **B,** A later film demonstrates a long occluded segment of the right common iliac system and high-grade stenosis at the origin of the left common iliac artery. **C,** Guidewires were placed across these two diseased segments from distal puncture sites, and the "kissing balloon" technique was used to treat both arterial segments simultaneously; serial Palmaz stents were placed using the same technique. **D,** The patency of both iliac segments is demonstrated in the final angiogram at the conclusion of this procedure.

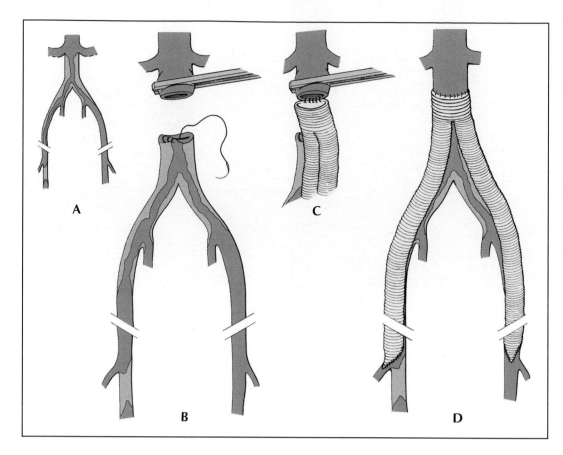

FIGURE 3-42. Aorto-bifemoral bypass. The surgical placement of a prosthetic aorto-bi-iliac bypass graft from the infrarenal aorta to the femoral arteries is the most frequently employed surgical approach for aortoiliac disease. **A,** Schematic preoperative angiogram. **B,** Resection of the diseased aorta with oversewing of the distal aortic stump. **C,** End-to-end anastomosis of the aorta to the proximal bypass graft. **D,** The entire aorto-bifemoral graft in place [38]. (*Adapted from* Brewster [38].)

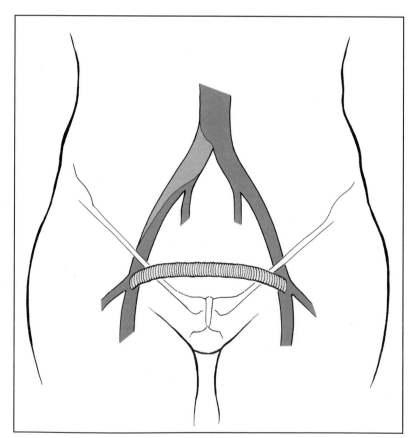

FIGURE 3-43. Femoral-femoral bypass. A femoral-femoral bypass graft may be placed to treat unilateral iliac occlusive disease if the contralateral iliac arteries are free of significant stenoses [38]. (*Adapted from* Brewster [38].)

PATENCY RATES FOR SURGICAL LIMB BYPASS PROCEDURES

SITE	1-Y PATENCY, %	5-Y PATENCY, %
Aorto-bifemoral bypass	90–95	80–90
Above-knee SVG	80–90	60–80
Below-knee SVG	70–90	50–80

FIGURE 3-44. Patency rates for aorto-bifemoral and saphenous vein bypass grafts (SVGs). Many factors contribute to the durability of all surgical revascularization procedures. These factors include anatomic characteristics, such as the adequacy of both the inflow of blood into the graft and the outflow (runoff) distal to the bypass graft, as well as patient-related factors, such as the presence of diabetes or continued tobacco use.

THROMBOANGIITIS OBLITERANS AND FIBROMUSCULAR DYSPLASIA

CLINICAL HALLMARKS OF THROMBOANGIITIS OBLITERANS

Prevalence: 13/100,000

Demographic profile: Young age (< 40 y); M:F ratio: 7:3; tobacco users predominate

Pathology: Affects small and medium-sized arteries and veins; segmental, inflammatory obliterative panarteritis; associated thrombosis with variable organization; rare giant cells

FIGURE 3-45. Clinical hallmarks of thromboangiitis obliterans (TAO). Thromboangiitis obliterans (Buerger's disease) is a well-defined clinicopathologic entity that may cause an obliterative arteritis affecting the upper or lower extremity of young adults. It affects primarily young adults (< 40 years of age), with a male predominance. Thromboangiitis obliterans elicits a segmental, inflammatory vasculitis affecting small to medium-sized arteries and veins. Associated thrombosis, the presence of occasional giant cells, and fibrosis are common histopathologic hallmarks.

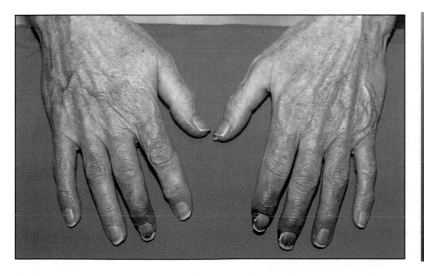

FIGURE 3-46. Digital ischemia in upper extremity arterial occlusive disease. Gangrene of the fingertips is an unfortunate and common clinical presentation of thromboangiitis obliterans.

DIAGNOSIS OF THROMBOANGIITIS OBLITERANS

Clinical
    Young patient with distal arterial occlusive disease
    Associated superficial thrombophlebitis
    Digital ischemic syndromes
Angiographic
    Distal small and medium-sized arteries affected
    Abrupt segmental occlusive lesions
    Absence of atherosclerotic irregularities
Confirmed by histopathology

FIGURE 3-47. Establishing the diagnosis of thromboangiitis obliterans (TAO). The diagnosis of TAO is often considered empirically when young, tobacco-using patients present with severe distal upper or lower extremity ischemia. However, establishment of a definitive diagnosis requires the presence of associated clinical, angiographic, or histopathologic features.

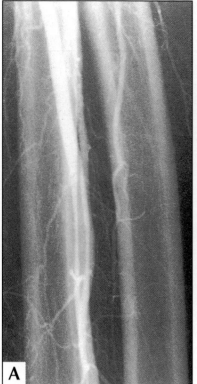
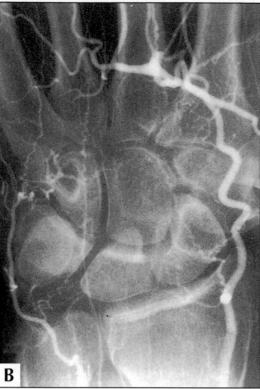
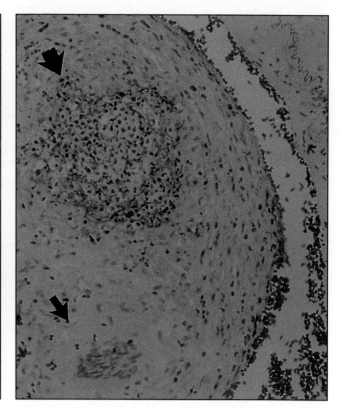

FIGURE 3-48. Angiographic presentation of thromboangiitis obliterans (TAO). Angiographic studies provide essential information that may aid in confirming the diagnosis of TAO, in delineating the extent of occlusive disease to guide revascularization, and to localize promising sites for arterial biopsy. **A,** In this patient the proximal brachial arteries appear normal, but the vessels demonstrate focal tubular stenoses in their midportion. Generous collateral vessels are also present. **B,** The hand angiogram demonstrates truncation of the radial artery at the wrist, disruption of the palmar arch, and occlusion of multiple digital arteries. Prominent corkscrew collaterals are also noted.

FIGURE 3-49. Histopathology of thromboangiitis obliterans (TAO). The distinctive histopathologic features of TAO were described by Buerger in his original report of this disease [39]. The initial lesion is characterized by a lymphocytic infiltration of the media and adventitia, with occasional giant cells (*arrows*) and rare eosinophils. The arterial lumen may be occluded initially by a cellular thrombus, which may recanalize in older lesions. Although a reactive fibrosis may result in late lesions, the elastic laminae are often spared.

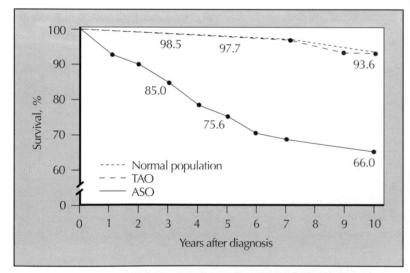

FIGURE 3-50. Contrasting patterns of patient survival for thromboangiitis obliterans (TAO) versus arteriosclerosis obliterans (ASO). The presence of severe arterial disease in young adults may be due to either TAO or premature atherosclerosis (ASO). This differentiation of etiology has important prognostic implications. McPherson *et al.* [40] have noted that the survival of patients with TAO is comparable to that of an age-matched normal population, whereas those patients with severe premature atherosclerosis were likely to experience foreshortened survival due to ischemic cardiac and cerebral events. (*Adapted from* McPherson *et al.* [40].)

TREATMENT OF THROMBOANGIITIS OBLITERANS

Total abstinence from all tobacco use
Surgical revascularization
Anticoagulation and antiplatelet therapies
Calcium channel antagonists or PGE_1 infusion
Amputation

FIGURE 3-51. Treatment of thromboangiitis obliterans (TAO). Although the mechanism(s) by which tobacco contributes to the etiology of TAO remain obscure, complete abstinence from use of all forms of tobacco is essential. Patients who successfully stop smoking require amputation at a markedly diminished rate. Continued tobacco use bodes unremitting limb ischemia and amputation. Inasmuch as TAO tends to cause distal arterial occlusions, surgical revascularization may often be difficult. Intravenous heparin has been advocated in early disease stages to diminish the thrombotic contribution to limb ischemia, and antiplatelet therapies are indicated for long-term treatment. The role of calcium channel antagonists has not been defined by controlled clinical trials, although their use has been advocated. Infusion of prostaglandin E_1 (PGE_1) has been reported to improve digital wound healing rates in TAO in one clinical trial.

FIBROMUSCULAR DYSPLASIA

CLINICAL HALLMARKS OF FIBROMUSCULAR DYSPLASIA

ETIOLOGY

Congenital hyperplastic disease that affects medium-sized and small arteries

Sites of involvement: renal > carotid > subclavian, iliac, coronary, mesenteric arteries

Three subtypes based on predominant involvement of the intima, media (hyperplasia or fibroplasia), or periadventitia

CLINICAL PRESENTATION

More prevalent in young adults (ages 20–40 y)

Females > males (8:1 in nonpediatric patients)

Presenting symptoms vary by region affected

ANGIOGRAPHIC ASSESSMENT

Classic appearance as a "string of beads"; may cause focal occlusions or poststenotic dilatation

FIGURE 3-52. Clinical hallmarks of fibromuscular dysplasia. Fibromuscular dysplasia is a congenital hyperplastic disease that affects primarily medium and small-sized arteries, and may cause serial eccentric stenoses and dilatation of the diseased artery [41]. Ninety percent of adult patients with fibromuscular dysplasia are female. The most common sites of involvement are the renal and carotid arteries, but coronary, subclavian, mesenteric, and iliac arterial involvement may occur. At least three distinct histopathologic variants have been described based on the predominant involvement of the intima, media, or periadventitial arterial layers. The clinical presentation is dependent on the anatomic site of the affected arterial segment. fibromuscular dysplasia in each regional arterial bed produces symptoms identical to those caused by arterial occlusive disease of other etiologies.

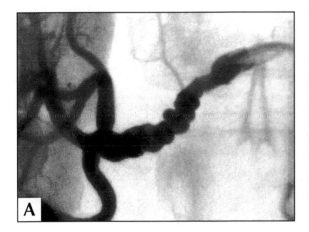

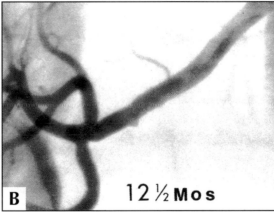

FIGURE 3-53. Angiographic presentation of fibromuscular dysplasia. Fibromuscular dysplasia may appear as a classic "string of beads," in which areas of stenosis alternate with areas of aneurysmal dilatation. **A,** This angiogram demonstrates fibromuscular dysplasia affecting the distal right renal artery in a 34-year-old woman with renovascular hypertension. **B,** This lesion was successfully treated by balloon angioplasty of the affected arterial segment.

POPLITEAL ENTRAPMENT SYNDROME

POPLITEAL ARTERY ENTRAPMENT SYNDROME: DIAGNOSIS

CLINICAL PRESENTATION

Young male or female without atherosclerosis

Exercise-induced calf claudication

Differential diagnosis includes popliteal adventitial cyst

PHYSICAL EXAMINATION

Ankle extension: normal ankle pulses

Ankle flexion: decreased ankle pulses

ANGIOGRAPHY

Popliteal artery occlusion, medial deviation, or poststenotic dilatation

Obtain views with ankle dorsiflexion and plantar flexion

FIGURE 3-54. Principal features of the popliteal entrapment syndrome. The popliteal entrapment syndrome is caused by a congenital abnormality in the relationship between the popliteal artery and the medial head of the gastrocnemius (or associated) muscle. The true incidence of this anatomic variation is unknown. The diagnosis of popliteal entrapment is most commonly considered in active males who present with exercise-induced calf claudication, although the syndrome may also be present in athletic women. This variant of normal popliteal artery anatomy may be present without symptoms or may elicit either acute or chronic lower extremity ischemic symptoms (including distal limb thromboemboli). The possibility of popliteal adventitial cyst disease should be considered in the differential diagnosis. Evidence for bilateral entrapment should be sought. The presence of normal ankle pulses (or Doppler blood flow pattern) with the ankle in a neutral position and the subsequent decrease in these pulses with ankle flexion supports this diagnosis. Angiographic studies may demonstrate segmental occlusion of the mid-popliteal artery, medial deviation of the vessel, poststenotic dilatation, or popliteal aneurysm formation.

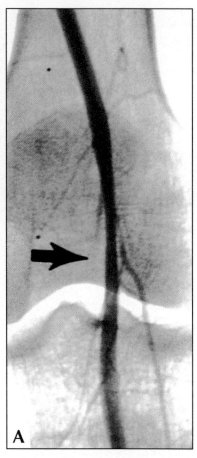 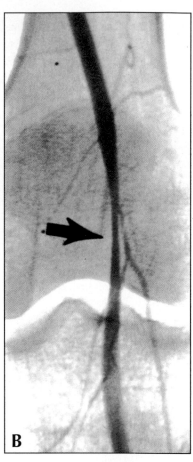

A **B**

FIGURE 3-55. Angiographic presentation of popliteal entrapment syndrome. **A,** This digital angiogram of the left popliteal artery was performed during slight plantar flexion of the foot. In this position, there is only slight narrowing of a short segment of the mid-popliteal artery (*arrow*). **B,** With complete plantar flexion of the foot, the lumen of the popliteal artery has become progressively narrower (*arrow*). In some affected individuals, such ankle flexion maneuvers may provoke total popliteal arterial occlusion. (*Courtesy of* A.W. Stanson, MD, The Mayo Clinic, Rochester, MN.)

POPLITEAL ARTERY ENTRAPMENT SYNDROME: OPERATIVE TREATMENT

Release of the muscular origin of the medial head of the gastrocnemius or popliteus muscle

Vein graft bypass if the popliteal artery is chronically occluded

FIGURE 3-56. Treatment of popliteal entrapment syndrome. Operative treatment should be considered in both symptomatic individuals as well as in asymptomatic individuals who may be at risk for subsequent limb-threatening ischemic complications. Operative release of the entrapped artery, thrombolysis of occluded segments, and/or vein graft bypass procedures are indicated in these patients.

FIGURE 3-57. Clinical presentation of acute arterial occlusion. The classic clinical presentation of acute arterial occlusion is characterized by the five "Ps": limb pain, paresthesias, pallor, pulselessness, and paralysis. Viable limbs are characterized by the lack of rest pain, adequate skin capillary blood flow, the presence of audible pedal arterial Doppler flow signals, and ankle systolic pressures greater than 30 mm Hg (SVS/ISCVS [Society for Vascular Surgery/International Society for Cardiovascular Surgery] class I). Threatened limbs that may be salvageable with prompt treatment are more likely to present with ischemic rest pain, mild sensory or motor neurologic deficits, and absent arterial Doppler flow signals (but intact venous flow) (class II). Major, irreversible ischemia is likely in limbs in which there is profound sensory and/or motor dysfunction, absent skin capillary blood flow, and neither arterial nor venous Doppler flow signals (class III) [42].

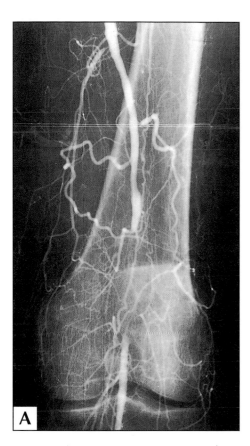
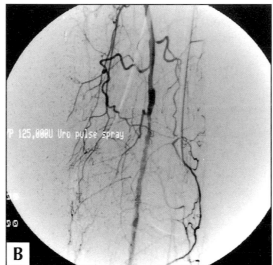
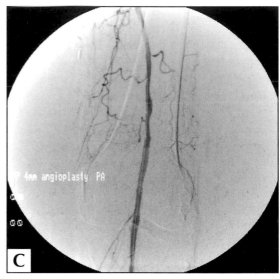

FIGURE 3-58. Radiographic presentation of acute arterial occlusion. A 62-year-old woman presented with a 3-day history of rapidly progressive left calf claudication. The left ankle-brachial index was diminished to 0.48 from her prior baseline value of 0.87. **A,** Angiography demonstrated an occlusion of the distal superficial femoral and proximal popliteal arteries, with spare bridging collaterals. **B,** An infusion catheter was placed to permit local administration of urokinase for 6 hours, yielding a patent vessel. A focal distal superficial femoral artery stenosis was present at the origin of the occluded segment with minor residual local thrombus remaining. **C,** The stenotic segment was then treated by angioplasty to achieve complete patency and normal antegrade flow through the previously occluded segment.

ETIOLOGIES OF ACUTE ARTERIAL OCCLUSION

Emboli

In situ thrombosis: high-grade native-vessel stenoses, graft stenoses

Vascular inflammatory diseases

Trauma: external compression, dissection, compartment syndrome

Severe venous diseases: phlegmasia cerulea dolens

Other: hypercoagulable states, intravenous drug abuse

FIGURE 3-59. Etiologies of acute arterial occlusion. Acute arterial occlusion is most commonly a consequence of the atherosclerotic disease process. An embolus is usually a consequence of atherosclerotic disease at a central arterial site (*eg*, a thrombus originating from the heart, the aorta, or a proximal ulcerated arterial plaque). In contrast, in situ thrombosis may result from the low flow and disrupted endothelium present in high-grade atheroma. Alternative etiologies may contribute to the occurrence of acute arterial occlusion, and include arterial inflammatory diseases, vascular trauma, and primary hypercoagulable states.

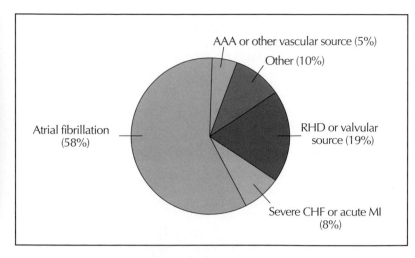

FIGURE 3-60. Cardiovascular etiologies of acute arterial thromboembolism. Essentially all thromboemboli are the result of underlying medical diseases. Atrial fibrillation remains the most common cardiac etiology contributing to the pathogenesis of distal acute arterial occlusions. Valvular heart disease, congestive heart failure (CHF), or acute myocardial infarction (MI), and abdominal aortic aneurysms (AAA) account for etiology of the majority of the remainder of cases. RHD—rheumatic heart disease.

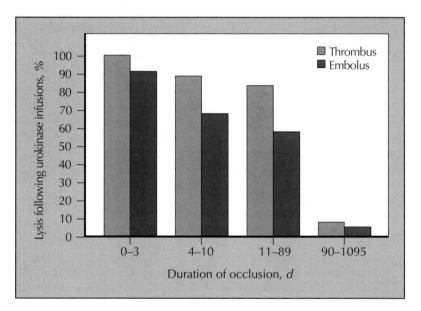

FIGURE 3-61. Intra-arterial thrombolysis: efficacy relative to duration and etiology of occlusion. The duration of arterial occlusion predicts the response to thrombolytic treatment. One study evaluated the relative rates of clot lysis based on the duration of symptoms before treatment and the thrombotic versus embolic etiology of the arterial occlusion. Although the youngest clots were more likely to be lysed by thrombolytic therapy, successful clot lysis was often possible even in limbs suspected to be occluded between 1 week and 3 months. Thrombotic occlusions were more likely to undergo complete clot lysis than embolic lesions. (*Adapted from* McNamara and Fischer [43].)

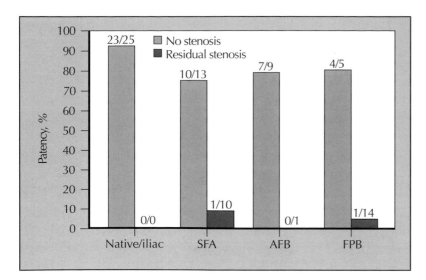

FIGURE 3-62. Intra-arterial thrombolysis: 6-month patency rates. Although the efficacy of early clot lysis depends on the cause and duration of arterial occlusion, the long-term patency rate is dependent on correction of underlying factors that might impede antegrade blood flow. In the absence of a residual stenosis in the native iliac vessels, the 6-month patency rate was excellent. Six-month patency rates were somewhat less in superficial femoral arteries (SFA), aortofemoral bypass grafts (AFB), and femoropopliteal bypass grafts (FPB). In contrast, patency rates were poor at all native and graft sites in this study if a residual stenosis was left untreated [44]. (*Adapted from* McNamara and Bomberger [44].)

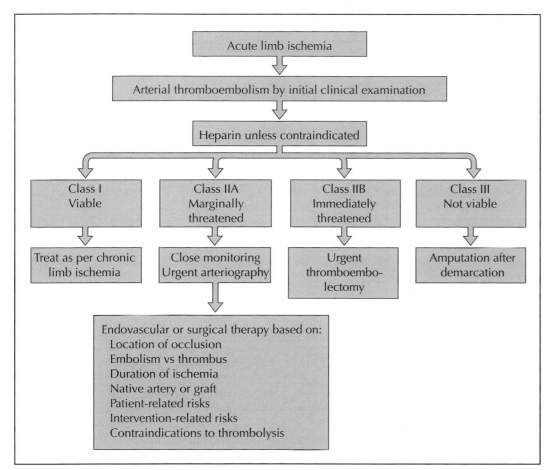

FIGURE 3-63. Thrombolysis versus surgery for acute limb ischemia. The relative efficacy of thrombolytic versus surgical revascularization of acute arterial occlusion was assessed prospectively in two trials. The STILE (Surgery versus Thrombolysis for Ischemia of the Lower Extremity) trial evaluated 393 patients who presented with limb ischemia of less than 6 months' duration, randomizing subjects to optimal surgical revascularization versus intra-arterial, catheter-directed thrombolysis with either tissue plasminogen activator or urokinase [45]. Outcome assessment included death, ongoing/recurrent ischemia, major amputation, or major morbidity (*eg*, bleeding). In this study, surgical revascularization was more effective than thrombolysis in patients with less than 6 months of ischemia, with similar safety profiles for the two interventions. For patients with acute limb ischemia of less than 14 days' duration, a higher rate of amputation-free survival and shorter hospital stays were observed for the thrombolysis groups. The TOPAS (Thrombolysis or Peripheral Arterial Surgery) trial randomized 548 patients with leg ischemia of less than 14 days' duration to vascular surgery or catheter-directed intra-arterial thrombolysis (urokinase). The primary endpoint of this study was amputation-free survival, with secondary endpoints of 1-year amputation-free survival and survival free of the following events: open surgical procedures at 6 months, clot lysis, increase in ankle-brachial index, and hemorrhagic events [46]. TOPAS demonstrated high rates of recanalization (67.9% complete clot dissolution), and both treatments led to similar 6-month amputation-free survival (71.8% and 74.8% for thrombolysis and surgery, respectively). Patients treated by urokinase underwent fewer open operative procedures, but suffered a greater incidence of major hemorrhage. The results of these two studies and others have led to this algorithm for care [47], in which clinical examination and classification of the degree of limb ischemia (per Society for Vascular Surgery classes) is followed by a choice of arteriography and endovascular or surgical therapy (choice based on an individual patient risk-benefit assessment), urgent thromboembolectomy, or amputation.

CLINICAL HALLMARKS OF ATHEROEMBOLISM

ETIOLOGY

Macroembolism of atherosclerotic debris (erythrocytes, platelet aggregates, fibrin) to distal arteries

Microembolism of cholesterol crystals to arteriolar beds

Event may be spontaneous or triggered by specific events (*eg*, catheterization, surgery, anticoagulation/thrombolysis)

CLINICAL PRESENTATION

More common in individuals with advanced atherosclerosis

Limb ischemia, single-organ dysfunction, or multi-organ system failure

Presenting symptoms vary by region affected

FIGURE 3-64. Etiology and clinical presentation of atheroembolism. The syndrome of atheromatous embolization remains frequently misdiagnosed and unrecognized. It is caused by the embolization of atherosclerotic debris and cholesterol crystals from proximal arterial plaques to distal organ systems. Although these atheroembolic episodes may occur spontaneously, it is increasingly recognized that specific iatrogenic events (arterial instrumentation, major surgery, initiation of anticoagulant or thrombolytic therapies) may precipi-

tate an atheroembolic shower. The syndrome is more common in elderly men with advanced atherosclerosis. The clinical syndrome may include nonspecific symptoms and signs suggesting a systemic illness (*eg*, fever, malaise, anorexia, weight loss, myalgias, headache), or atheroembolism may provoke acute, catastrophic organ system failure. The varied clinical presentations of atheroembolism have earned the syndrome the moniker "the great masquerader."

DIAGNOSIS OF ATHEROEMBOLISM

PHYSICAL EXAMINATION

Blue toe syndrome, livedo reticularis, ulceration, gangrene

LABORATORY EVALUATION

Elevated ESR, leukocytosis, anemia

Elevated BUN, creatinine, active urine sediment

Elevated hepatic transaminases or amylase

Eosinophilia and hypocomplementemia

FUNDOSCOPIC EXAMINATION AND TISSUE BIOPSY

Retinal arterial cholesterol emboli (Hollenhorst plaque)

Skin or muscle (gastrocnemius or quadriceps) biopsy

Pathognomonic needle-shaped cholesterol clefts

FIGURE 3-65. Diagnosis of atheroembolism. Because there are few signs or symptoms that are specific for atheroembolism, it is frequently overlooked. Recognition begins with a high index of clinical suspicion. Atheroembolism should be suspected when patients with advanced atherosclerotic disease present with new limb ischemia (especially "blue toe syndrome," livedo reticularis, or ischemic ulcers), renal failure, amaurosis fugax, transient ischemic attacks, or angina that is not explained by local large artery occlusive disease. Although the laboratory findings may also be nonspecific in these patients, elevations in erythrocyte sedimentation rate (ESR), leukocytosis, anemia, and azotemia are common. Confirmation of atheroembolism may be established by direct fundoscopic examination or muscle biopsy, which may demonstrate pathognomonic cholesterol crystals in the retinal artery branches or in the small vessels of affected tissues. BUN—blood urea nitrogen.

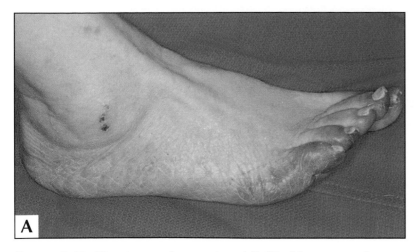

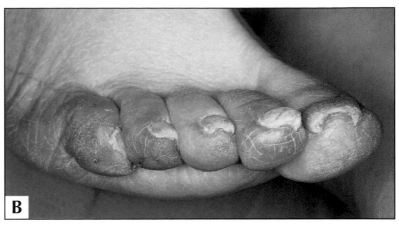

FIGURE 3-66. Blue toe syndrome. **A** and **B**, The blue toe syndrome is caused by occlusion of the small digital arteries that supply the toes. Such end-arterial occlusion may elicit mild cyanosis or frank digital ischemic ulceration or necrosis.

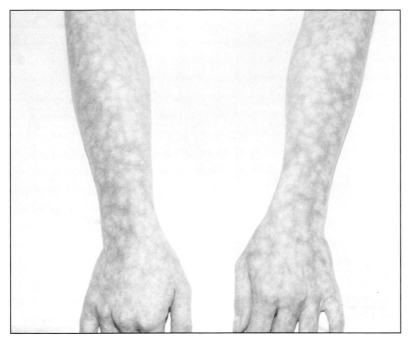

FIGURE 3-67. Livedo reticularis. Although livedo reticularis may be provoked by an atheroembolic shower to the dermal vessels, this striking cutaneous finding is not specific for this condition. As in this example of livedo reticularis affecting this patient's forearms, the skin demonstrates a netlike pattern of confluent, cyanotic skin surrounding areas of normal skin color.

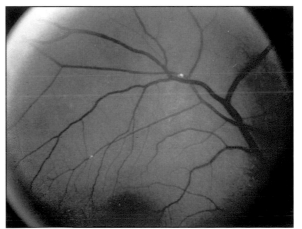

FIGURE 3-68. Retinal atheroemboli: Hollenhorst plaque. This is the appearance of a refractile cholesterol atheroembolus in a branch retinal arteriole.

TREATMENT OF ATHEROEMBOLISM

SYMPTOMATIC CARE OF AFFECTED END-ORGANS

Local foot care, debridement, limited amputation

Avoidance of nephrotoxic drugs

TREATMENT OF THE ATHEROEMBOLIC SOURCE

Resection of thoracic or abdominal aortic aneurysms

Resection or stenting of ulcerated iliac plaque

Avoid thrombolytic or anticoagulant therapies

Aspirin (?)

SECONDARY PREVENTION OF CARDIAC DEATH

Patients who survive an episode of systemic atheroembolism have a high risk of subsequent cardiovascular death; attention and treatment of ischemic cardiac symptoms is merited

FIGURE 3-69. Treatment of atheroembolism. The time course of onset and resolution of the signs and symptoms of atheroembolism are quite variable. Conservative care is mandated and is directed primarily at treatment of affected end-organs. Ischemic, ulcerated, or gangrenous toes may require debridement or limited amputation. If an obvious atheroembolic source can be discerned (aortic aneurysms or aorto-iliac ulcerated plaque), definitive treatment may be attempted via surgical resection or local arterial stenting. However, the relative risk of acute precipitation of additional ischemic events versus the potential benefit of long-term risk reduction must be considered carefully. These patients suffer a high rate of cardiovascular death in the years after an initial atheroembolic event, and treatments should also be directed at prolonging overall survival.

REFERENCES

1. Criqui MH, Fronek A, Barrett-Connor E, *et al*.: The prevalence of peripheral arterial disease in a defined population. *Circulation* 1985, 1:510–515.

2. TransAtlantic Inter-Society Consensus (TASC). Management of peripheral arterial disease. *J Vasc Surg* 2000, 31(1):S9.

3. Newman AB, Siscovick DS, Manolio TA, *et al*.: Ankle-arm index as a marker of atherosclerosis in the Cardiovascular Health Study. *Circulation* 1993, 88:837–845.

4. Kannel WB, Wolf PA, Garrison RJ, eds: The Framingham Study: an epidemiologic investigation of cardiovascular disease, Section 34. National Technical Information Service, 1987, NIH publication No. 87-2703.

5. Strandness DE, Zierler RE: Exercise ankle pressure measurements in arterial disease. In *Noninvasive Diagnostic Techniques in Vascular Disease*, edn 3. Edited by Bernstein EF. St. Louis: Mosby; 1985:575–583.

6. Hirsch AT, Rooke TW: Peripheral vascular diseases. In *Cardiovascular Medicine*, edn 2. Edited by Cohn JN, Willerson JT. New York: Churchill-Livingstone; 2000:1398–1416.

7. Weitz JI, Byrne J, Clagett P, *et al*.: Diagnosis and treatment of chronic arterial insufficiency of the lower extremities: a critical review. *Circulation* 1996, 94:3026–3049.

8. McDaniel MD, Cronenwett JL: Basic data related to the natural history of intermittent claudication. *Ann Vasc Surg* 1989, 3:273–277.

9. Vogt MT, Cauley JA, Newman AB, *et al*.: Decreased ankle/arm blood pressure index and mortality in elderly women. *JAMA* 1993, 270:465–469.

10. Newman AB, Sutton-Tyrrell K, Vogt MT, Kuller LH: Morbidity and mortality in hypertensive adults with a low ankle/arm blood pressure index. *JAMA* 1993, 270:487–489.

11. McKenna M, Wolfson S, Kuller L: The ratio of ankle and arm blood pressure as an independent risk factor of mortality. *Atherosclerosis* 1991, 87:119–128.

12. Hirsch AT, Criqui MH, Treat-Jacobson D, *et al*.: Peripheral arterial disease, detection, awareness, and treatment in primary care. *JAMA* 2001, 286:1317–1324.

13. National Cholesterol Education Program. Second Report of the Expert Panel on Detection, Evaluation, and Treatment of High Blood Cholesterol in Adults (Adult Treatment Panel II). *Circulation* 1994, 89(3):1333–1445.

14. Kannel WB: Risk factors for atherosclerotic cardiovascular outcomes in different arterial territories. *J Cardiovasc Risk* 1994, 1(4):333–339.

15. Wilterdink JL, Easton JD: Vascular event rates in patients with atherosclerotic cerebrovascular disease. *Arch Neurol* 1992, 49(8):857–863.

16. Criqui MH, Langer RD, Fronek A, *et al*.: Mortality over a period of 10 years in patients with peripheral arterial disease. *N Engl J Med* 1992, 326(6):381–386.

17. Barndt R, Blankenhorn DH, Crawford DW, Brooks SH: Regression and progression of early femoral atherosclerosis in treated hyper-lipoproteinemic patients. *Ann Intern Med* 1977, 86:139–146.

18. Buchwald H, Varco RL, Matts JP, *et al*.: Effect of partial ileal bypass on mortality and morbidity from coronary heart disease in patients with hypercholesterolemia: report of the Program on the Surgical Control of the Hyperlipidemias. *N Engl J Med* 1990, 323:946.

19. Pedersen TR, Kjekshus J, Pyorala K, *et al*.: Effect of simvastatin on ischemic signs and symptoms in the Scandinavian simvastatin survival study (4S). *Am J Cardiol* 1998, 81:333–335.

20. Executive Summary of The Third Report of the National Cholesterol Education Program (NCEP) Expert Panel on Detection, Evaluation, and Treatment of High Blood Cholesterol in Adults (Adult Treatment Panel III). *JAMA* 2001, 285:2486–2497.

21. Jonason T, Bergstrom R: Cessation of smoking in patients with intermittent claudication: effects on the risk of peripheral vascular complications, myocardial infarction and mortality. *Acta Med Scand* 1987, 221:253–260.

22. Faulkner KW, House AK, Castleden WM: The effect of cessation of smoking on the accumulative survival rates of patients with symptomatic peripheral vascular disease. *Med J Aust* 1983, 1:217–219.

23. Lassila R, Lepantalo M: Cigarette smoking and the outcome after lower limb arterial surgery. *Acta Chir Scand* 1988, 154:635–640.

24. De Felice M, Gallo P, Masotti G: Current therapy of peripheral obstructive arterial disease: the nonsurgical approach. *Angiology* 1990, 41:1–11.

25. Collaborative meta-analysis of randomised trials of antiplatelet therapy for prevention of death, myocardial infarction, and stroke in high-risk patients. *Br Med J* 2002, 324:71–86.

26. A randomized, blinded, trial of clopidogrel versus aspirin in patients at risk of ischaemic events (CAPRIE). *Lancet* 1996, 348:1329–1339.

27. Lindgarde F, Jelnes R, Bjorkman H, *et al.*: Conservative drug treatment in patients with moderately severe chronic occlusive peripheral arterial disease: Scandinavian Study Group. *Circulation* 1989, 80:1549–1556.

28. Kimura Y, Tani Y, Knabe T, Watanabe K: Effect of cilostazol on platelet aggregation and experimental thrombosis. *Arzneimittelforschung* 1985, 35:1144–1149

29. Dawson DL, Cutler BS, Meissner MH, *et al.*: Cilostazol has beneficial effects in treatment of intermittent claudication: results from a multicenter, randomized, prospective, double-blind trial. *Circulation* 1998, 98:678–686.

30. Money SR, Herd JA, Isaacsohn JL, *et al.*: Effect of cilostazol on walking distances in patients with intermittent claudication caused by peripheral vascular disease. *J Vasc Surg* 1998, 27:267–274.

31. Beebe HG, Dawson DL, Cutler BS, *et al.*: A new pharmacological treatment for intermittent claudication: results of a randomized, multicenter trial. *Arch Intern Med* 1999, 159:2041–2050.

32. Dawson DL, Cutler BS, Hiatt WR, *et al.*: A comparison of cilostazol and pentoxifylline for treating intermittent claudication. *Am J Med* 2000, 109(17):523–530.

33. Larsen O, Lassen N: Effect of daily muscular exercise in patients with intermittent claudication. *Lancet* 1966, II:1093–1096.

34. Hiatt WR: Benefit of exercise conditioning for patients with intermittent claudication. *Circulation* 1990, 81:602–609.

35. Gardner AW, Poehlman ET: Exercise rehabilitation programs for the treatment of claudication pain. *JAMA* 1995, 274:975–980

36. Current Procedural Terminology (CPT) 2001. Chicago: American Medical Association; 2001.

37. Bosch JL, Hunink MG: Meta-analysis of the results of percutaneous transluminal angioplasty and stent placement for aortoiliac occlusive disease. *Radiology* 1997, 204(1):87–96.

38. Brewster DC: Clinical and anatomical considerations for surgery in aortoiliac disease and results of surgical treatment. *Circulation* 1991, 83(suppl I):I-42–I-52.

39. Buerger L: Thromboangiitis obliterans: a study of the vascular lesions leading to pre-senile, spontaneous gangrene. *Am J Med Sci* 1908, 136:56.

40. McPherson JR, Juergens JL, Gifford RW: Thromboangiitis obliterans and arteriosclerosis obliterans: clinical and prognostic differences. *Ann Int Med* 1963, 59:288–296.

41. Luscher TF, Lie JT, Stanson AW, *et al.*: Arterial fibromuscular dysplasia. *Mayo Clin Proc* 1987, 62:931–952.

42. Rutherford RB, Flanigan DP, Gupta SK, *et al.*: Suggested standards for reports dealing with lower extremity ischemia. *J Vasc Surg* 1986, 4:80–94.

43. McNamara TO, Fischer JR: Thrombolysis of peripheral arterial and graft occlusions: improved results using high-dose urokinase. *Am J Radiol* 1985, 144:169–175.

44. McNamara TO, Bomberger RA: Factors affecting initial and 6-month patency rates after intra-arterial thrombolysis with high dose urokinase. *Am J Surg* 1986, 152:709–712.

45. Results of a prospective trial evaluating surgery versus thrombolysis for ischemia of the lower extremity. The STILE trial. *Ann Surg* 1994, 220(3):251–268.

46. Ouriel K, Vieth FJ, Sasahra AA: A comparison of recombinant urokinase with vascular surgery as initial treatment for acute arterial occlusion of the legs. Thrombolysis or Peripheral Arterial Surgery (TOPAS) Investigators. *N Engl J Med* 1998, 338:1105–1111.

47. TransAtlantic Inter-Society Consensus (TASC): Management of peripheral arterial disease. *J Vasc Surg* 2000, 31(1):S162.

CHAPTER 4

RENAL ARTERY DISEASE

Jeffrey W. Olin

Renal artery stenosis (RAS) is most commonly due to either fibromuscular dysplasia or atherosclerosis. Fibromuscular dysplasia is found most commonly in young women with hypertension, while atherosclerosis usually is found in individuals over age 55 years presenting with hypertension, renal failure (ischemic nephropathy), or congestive heart failure. Renal artery stenosis may be discovered incidentally (atrophic or small kidney) during imaging studies for other reasons or at autopsy. Incidental RAS is quite common, while renovascular hypertension occurs only in 1% to 5% of all patients with hypertension.

The presence of anatomic RAS does not necessarily establish that the hypertension or renal failure is caused by RAS. Many patients have had essential (primary) hypertension for years and then develop atherosclerotic RAS later in life.

Screening tests for RAS have improved considerably over the past decade. While captopril renography was utilized almost exclusively in the past, duplex ultrasound of the renal arteries or magnetic resonance angiography have replaced other modalities as the screening tests of choice in many centers. Rarely does an arteriogram have to be performed for diagnostic purposes only.

Management of RAS consists of three possible strategies: medical management, surgical management, or percutaneous therapy with balloon angioplasty and stent implantation. The treatment of choice to control hypertension in patients with fibromuscular disease is percutaneous angioplasty. Renal artery stenting has replaced surgical revascularization for most patients with atherosclerotic disease who require an intervention. Indications for revascularization include at least a 70% stenosis of one or both renal arteries and inability to adequately control blood pressure despite a good antihypertensive regimen, or chronic renal insufficiency not related to another clear-cut cause (disease should be bilateral or stenosis to a solitary functioning kidney). Other indications for revascularization include dialysis-dependent renal failure in a patient without a definite cause of end-stage renal disease, and recurrent congestive heart failure or flash pulmonary edema not attributed to a cardiac cause. The treatment of elevated serum creatinine with unilateral disease is controversial, and there are no good clinical trials to help guide the clinician.

In patients with long-standing hypertension, a cure with surgical or percutaneous intervention is unlikely. However, 50% to 80% of patients do experience improvement in blood pressure control. While there is compelling evidence to suggest that stent implantation can improve or at least stabilize renal function in many patients, there remain 15% to 20% of patients in whom renal function deteriorates after percutaneous intervention. Reasons for this deterioration include contrast injury, atheromatous embolization, or renal failure caused by an etiology other than RAS, *ie*, nephro-sclerosis. It is may be difficult to predict which patients will exhibit a decline in renal function after percutaneous intervention.

Risk factor modification is important for all patients with RAS. Patients should be advised to stop smoking, lose weight, and exercise. Control of diabetes and appropriate management of hyperlipidemia are equally important. Since the majority of lesions are attributable to atherosclerosis or fibromuscular dysplasia, comments regarding therapy will focus on these two diseases.

ETIOLOGY OF RENOVASCULAR DISEASE

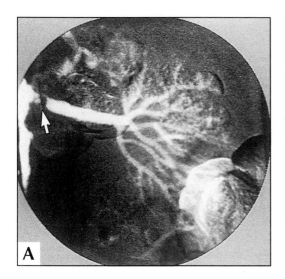 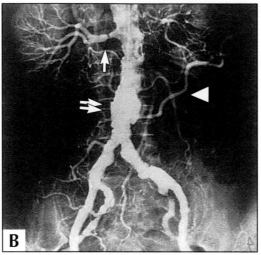

FIGURE 4-1. Examples of severe renal artery stenosis (RAS) in a solitary functioning kidney. Approximately 90% of all renovascular lesions are secondary to atherosclerosis (see Fig. 9-1). While atherosclerotic RAS may be isolated to the renal artery alone, it is more commonly a manifestation of generalized atherosclerosis involving the aorta, coronary, cerebral, and peripheral vessels. Atherosclerotic RAS most often occurs at the ostium or at the proximal 2 centimeters of the renal artery. **A**, Angiogram of a patient who underwent a right nephrectomy 15 years earlier. At age 62, she presented with malignant hypertension and acute renal failure. There is a subtotal stenosis (*arrow*) to a solitary kidney. The patient underwent percutaneous transluminal angioplasty and was able to come off dialysis until a fatal complication occurred. **B**, Arteriogram of the aorta, renal, and iliac arteries. Note severe aortic and renal artery atherosclerosis. The left renal artery is occluded, and the right renal artery has a severe stenosis in the proximal portion (*arrow*). The distal abdominal aorta has severe ulcerated plaques (*double arrows*). The wandering artery of Drummond (*arrowhead*) indicates that there is severe disease or occlusion to either the superior mesenteric artery or inferior mesenteric artery. (*Panel A from* Olin and Wholey [1]; with permission; *panel B from* Olin and Begelman [2]; with permission.)

CLASSIFICATION OF FIBROMUSCULAR DYSPLASIA

CLASSIFICATION	FREQUENCY, %	PATHOLOGY	ANGIOGRAPHIC APPEARANCE
Medial dysplasia			
Medial fibroplasia	75–80	Alternating areas of thinned media and thickened fibromuscular ridges containing collagen; internal elastic membrane may be lost in some areas	"String of beads" appearance where the diameter of the "beading" is larger than the diameter of the artery
Perimedial fibroplasia	10–15	Extensive collagen deposition in the outer half of the media	"Beading" in which the "beads" are smaller than the diameter of the artery
Medial hyperplasia	1–2	True smooth muscle cell hyperplasia without fibrosis	Concentric smooth stenosis (similar to intimal disease)
Intimal fibroplasia	< 10	Circumferential or eccentric deposition of collagen in the intima; no lipid or inflammatory component; internal elastic lamina fragmented or duplicated	Concentric focal band; long, smooth narrowing
Adventitial (periarterial) fibroplasia		Dense collagen replaces the fibrous tissue of the adventitia and may extend into surrounding tissue	

FIGURE 4-2. Classification of fibromuscular dysplasia (FMD). Fibromuscular dysplasia is a nonatherosclerotic, noninflammatory disease that most commonly affects the renal arteries and is the second most common cause of renal artery stenosis (RAS). The most common clinical presentation is that of hypertension in a young woman. Fibromuscular dysplasia has been demonstrated in virtually every vascular bed. Renal artery involvement occurs in 60% to 75% of patients with FMD, followed by involvement of the cervicocranial arteries in 25% to 30%, visceral arteries in 9%, and arteries of the extremities in approximately 5% of patients. Fibromuscular dysplasia may present as a systemic disease (affecting a combination of the carotids, mesenteric, subclavian, and/or extremity vessels) in up to 28% of patients. The diagnosis rarely is made pathologically, but usually is determined by its typical angiographic appearance. Fibromuscular dysplasia characteristically involves the distal two thirds of the renal artery and may involve the branches.

The lesions of FMD are thought to be congenital dysplasias with maldevelopment of the fibrous, muscular, and elastic tissues of the renal artery. They are subcategorized according to the layer of the arterial wall involved. This classification is important since each type of fibrous dysplasia has distinct histologic and angiographic features, and each type occurs in a different clinical setting. Most patients with FMD respond well to balloon angioplasty alone and do not require stent implantation [3–5]. (*Adapted from* Begelman and Olin [4].)

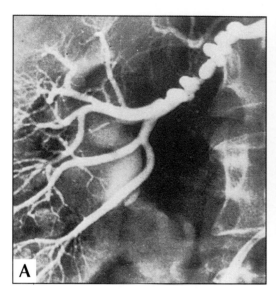

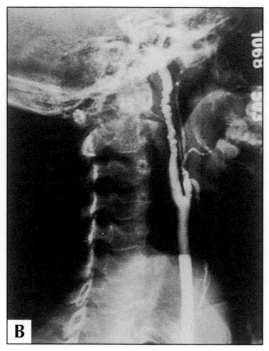

Microscopically, the internal elastic membrane is thinned variably and disappears. Within the alternating thickened areas, much of the muscle is replaced by collagen, hence the term medial fibroplasia. In other areas, thinning of the media occurs to the point of complete loss, and microaneurysms can be seen as saccules lined by only the external elastica. In extreme cases, giant aneurysms may be found in association with medial fibroplasia. Progression to total occlusion is rare in this subtype. This type of FMD also occurs commonly in the extracranial carotid **(B)** or vertebral arteries. Note that FMD occurs several centimeters from the carotid bifurcation, whereas atherosclerosis occurs most often at the carotid bifurcation. There is an increased risk of cerebral aneurysm in patients with medial fibroplasia, especially when it involves the carotid or vertebral arteries. All patients with cervicocranial FMD should have a cerebral arteriogram performed at the time of the arteriogram of the carotid and vertebral arteries. If a standard angiogram is not indicated, a magnetic resonance angiogram should be performed to eliminate the possibility of a central nervous system aneurysm. (*Panel A from* Olin and Novick [6]; with permission.)

FIGURE 4-3. Medial fibromuscular dysplasia (FMD). Medial FMD has been further divided into medial hyperplasia, perimedial dysplasia, and medial fibroplasia. Medial fibroplasia is the histologic finding in nearly 80% of all cases of FMD. It tends to occur in 25- to 50-year-old women and often involves both renal arteries. It has a "string of beads" appearance angiographically, with the "bead" diameter larger than the proximal, unaffected artery **(A)**.

The areas of stenosis are often overshadowed by contrast medium in the microaneurysms, making the degree of actual stenosis difficult to assess. This beading is due to thickening of the media, interspersed by areas of aneurysmal dilatation.

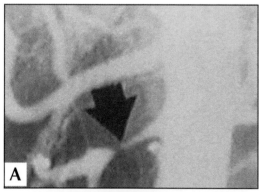

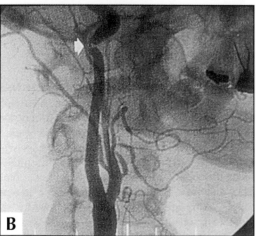

FIGURE 4-4. Intimal fibroplasia. Intimal fibroplasia occurs in children and young adults, and accounts for approximately 10% of the total number of fibrous lesions. This lesion is characterized by a circumferential accumulation of collagen inside the internal elastica lamina. Disruption and duplication of the elastica internal occur more often in younger patients, with dissecting hematomas as a complication in some patients. Intimal fibroplasia with complicating medial dissection is characterized pathologically by large dissecting channels in the outer one-half of the media. Arteriography in intimal fibroplasia reveals either a smooth long area of narrowing or a concentric band-like focal stenosis, usually involving the midportion of the vessel or its branches.
A, Long, smooth narrowing of the right renal artery in a patient with intimal fibroplasia. **B**, Note the concentric band in the distal internal carotid artery in the young woman with intimal fibroplasia. In intimal disease, progressive renal artery obstruction and ischemic atrophy of the involved kidney may occur. Although intimal fibroplasia most commonly affects the renal arteries, it may also occur as a generalized disorder with concomitant involvement of the carotid, upper and lower extremities, and mesenteric vessels, and may mimic a necrotizing vasculitis [7,8]. (*Panel B from* Begelman and Olin [4]; with permission.)

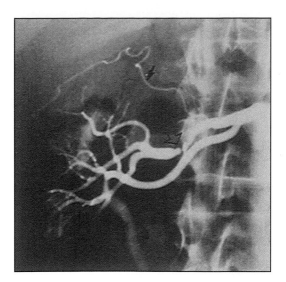

FIGURE 4-5. Perimedial fibroplasia. Perimedial fibroplasia occurs predominantly in 15- to 30-year-old women. Of all fibrous lesions, 10% to 15% are perimedial fibroplasias. These tightly stenotic lesions only occur in the renal artery and consist pathologically of a collar of dense collagen enveloping the renal artery for variable lengths and thickness. The collagen is deposited in the outer border of the media and usually replaces a considerable portion of it; in some areas, collagen may completely replace the media. The arteriogram of perimedial fibroplasia may give the appearance of arterial beading, but careful observation shows that the "bead" does not exceed the caliber of the normal segment of the vessel. This fact, along with the frequent occurrence of external collateral circulation, differentiates this lesion angiographically from that of medial fibroplasia. (*From* Olin and Novick [6]; with permission.)

FIGURE 4-6. Less common causes of renal artery disease.

LESS COMMON CAUSES OF RENAL ARTERY DISEASE

Renal artery aneurysm

Renal artery dissection

Atheromatous embolization

Thromboembolization

Large artery vasculitis (Takayasu's arteritis or giant cell arteritis)

Arteriovenous malformation, fistula or trauma (*ie*, radiation, lithotripsy, direct injury, or surgery)

Neurofibromatosis

Retroperitoneal fibrosis

PREVALENCE OF RENAL ARTERY DISEASE

PREVALENCE OF ATHEROSCLEROTIC RAS IN 395 CONSECUTIVE ARTERIOGRAMS

≥ 50% STENOSIS	AAA (n = 108) (%)	AOD (n = 21) (%)	PAD (n = 189) (%)	RAS (n = 76) (%)
All patients	41 (38)	7 (33)	74 (39)	53 (70)*
Diabetic	6 (50)	1 (33)	34 (50)†	10 (71)
Nondiabetic	35 (36)	6 (33)	40 (33)	43 (69)*

*P < 0.01 compared with other three groups.
†P < 0.02 compared with nondiabetic patients with PAD.

FIGURE 4-7. Prevalence of atherosclerotic renal artery stenosis (RAS). Atherosclerotic RAS is common in patients with atherosclerosis elsewhere in the body. The renal arteries were evaluated in 395 patients undergoing arteriography for various reasons. Arteriography was performed in 108 patients while they were investigated for the presence of an abdominal aortic aneurysm (AAA); 21 patients underwent arteriography while being investigated for aortoiliac occlusive disease (AOD); and 189 patients underwent arteriography while they were investigated for peripheral arterial disease (PAD). None of the aforementioned groups had clinical indications for the presence of renal artery disease. One or more clues for the presence of renal artery disease were found in 76 patients. Of those patients who had clues to suggest renal artery disease (RAS group), 53 of 76 (70%) in fact did have RAS. However, in the three groups of patients without clinical clues to suggest the presence of RAS, RAS was present in 33% to 39% of those patients. Renal artery stenosis was found in 50% of the patients with diabetes mellitus in the PAD group [9].

Other studies have confirmed this very high prevalence of RAS in patients with evidence of atherosclerosis elsewhere in the body [10]. However, it should be noted that the mere presence of RAS does not mean that the RAS is causing the hypertension. Dustan et al. [11] showed that only 50% of the patients with significant RAS had hypertension.

Renal artery stenosis is also associated with coronary artery disease. Several studies have demonstrated that 14% to 30% of all patients undergoing cardiac catheterization had greater than 50% RAS. In the series by Harding et al. [12], of the 30% of patients with RAS, only 15% had greater than 50% stenosis. Of these 15%, 11% had unilateral disease and 4% had bilateral disease [11].

PREVALENCE OF BILATERAL RENAL ARTERY STENOSIS

STUDY	STENOTIC ARTERIES, n	BILATERAL, n (%)	METHOD
Holley et al. [13]	159	105 (66)	Autopsy
Wollenweber et al. [14]	109	67 (61)	Arteriogram
Dean et al. [15]	41	14 (34)	Arteriogram
Olin et al. [9]	175	67 (38)	Arteriogram
Tollefson and Ernst [16]	48	14 (29)	Arteriogram
Harding et al. [12]	192	52 (27)	Arteriogram
Total	724	319 (44)	

FIGURE 4-8. Prevalence of bilateral renal artery stenosis (RAS). Six studies reported on the prevalence of bilateral RAS. Of 319 patients, 44% had bilateral disease. Patients with bilateral disease or disease to a solitary functioning kidney are at risk for ischemic nephropathy, end-stage renal disease, recurrent bouts of congestive heart failure, or flash pulmonary edema as the predominant presentation of RAS. (*Adapted from* Rimmer and Gennari [17].)

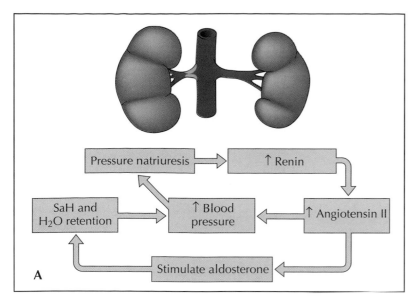
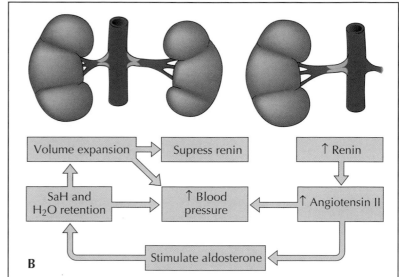

FIGURE 4-9. Pathogenesis of hypertension in renovascular disease. In 1934 Goldblatt *et al.* [18] first demonstrated that constriction of the renal artery in a dog produced a sustained increase in blood pressure. **A**, Example of the 2 kidney, 1 clip (2K, 1C) model of renovascular hypertension. It is analogous to unilateral renal artery stenosis (RAS). In the 2K, 1C model, decreased renal blood flow stimulates the production of renin. Renin cleaves the proenzyme angiotensinogen to form angiotensin I, which, in the presence of angiotensin-converting enzyme (ACE), is converted to angiotensin II (AII). Angiotensin II has several important functions: (1) it elevates blood pressure directly by causing systemic vasoconstriction; (2) it stimulates aldosterone secretion, causing sodium reabsorption, and potassium and hydrogen ion secretion in the cortical collecting duct; and (3) it changes the intrarenal hemodynamics, by decreasing glomerular capillary surface area and redistributing intrarenal blood flow. The salt and water retained due to excess aldosterone production is rapidly excreted by the contralateral (normal kidney) by pressure natruresis. This produces a cycle of renin-dependent hypertension. Administration of an ACE inhibitor blocks the vicious cycle and returns the blood pressure to normal early in the course of renovascular hypertension. There is decreased blood flow to the kidney with the clipped (stenotic) artery, increased renin secretion from the ischemic kidney, and suppressed renin secretion from the contralateral

kidney in the 2K, 1C model. This is the pathophysiologic mechanism by which captopril decreases renal blood flow and glomerular filtration rate on the ipsilateral side of an RAS when a captopril-stimulated renal flow scan is performed.

B, Example of the 1 kidney, 1 clip (1K, 1C) model of renovascular hypertension. It is analogous to either bilateral RAS or RAS to a solitary functioning kidney. In the 1K, 1C model of renovascular hypertension, there is a similar decrease in blood flow to the affected kidney(s), acutely causing the secretion of renin and synthesis of AII and aldosterone. Angiotensin II directly elevates blood pressure, and aldosterone causes salt and water retention. However, in this model, there is not a normal kidney that can sense the elevated blood pressure; therefore, no pressure natriuresis occurs. The increased aldosterone causes sodium and water retention and volume expansion. The expanded plasma volume suppresses plasma renin activity, thus converting the animal from renin-mediated hypertension to volume-mediated hypertension. During this stage, administration of an ACE inhibitor or AII antagonist does not decrease blood pressure or change renal blood flow. Dietary restriction of sodium or administration of diuretics will convert the animal to a renin-mediated form of hypertension, and the animal will then become sensitive to an ACE inhibitor or an AII antagonist. (*Adapted from* Olin and Novick [6].)

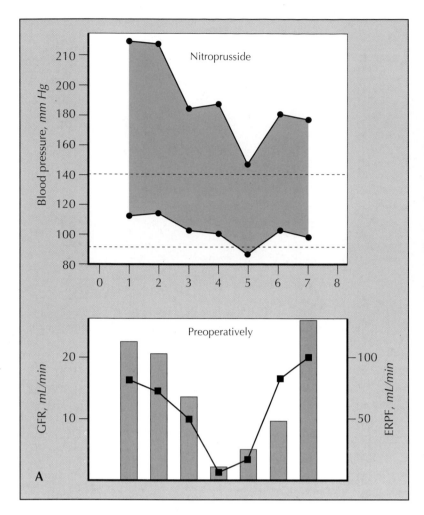

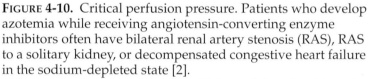

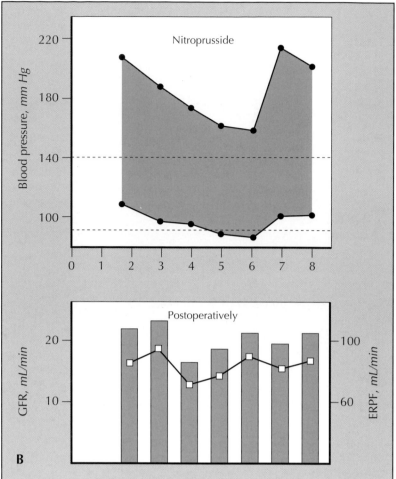

FIGURE 4-10. Critical perfusion pressure. Patients who develop azotemia while receiving angiotensin-converting enzyme inhibitors often have bilateral renal artery stenosis (RAS), RAS to a solitary kidney, or decompensated congestive heart failure in the sodium-depleted state [2].

There are two mechanisms by which renal functional impairment may occur with the use of antihypertensive agents. The first may occur with any antihypertensive agent when a critical perfusion pressure is reached below which the kidney no longer receives adequate perfusion. This has been shown by the infusion of sodium nitroprusside in patients with high-grade

bilateral RAS. **A,** Glomerular filtration rate (GFR) and effective renal plasma flow (ERPF) decrease markedly as the blood pressure is lowered with sodium nitroprusside in a patient with bilateral RAS. The exact pressure necessary to perfuse a kidney with RAS varies with the degree of stenosis and is different among different patients. **B,** Renal function impairment is reversible following unilateral renal artery revascularization. Note that there is no longer a decline in GFR or ERPF when nitroprusside brings the blood pressure down to the previous critical level. (*Adapted from* Textor *et al.* [19].)

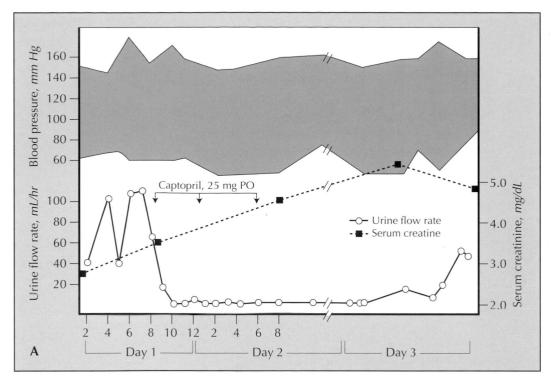

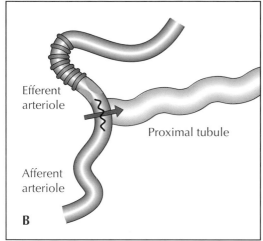

C. ROLE OF SODIUM BALANCE IN RENAL INSUFFICIENCY CAUSED BY ACE INHIBITORS

	SODIUM DEPLETION, DAY 1	SODIUM DEPLETION PLUS CAPTOPRIL, DAY 2	SODIUM REPLETION, DAY 4	SODIUM REPLETION PLUS CAPTOPRIL, DAY 5
Weight, *kg*	73.6	73.9	75.2	76.8
Serum creatinine, *mg/dL*	1.5	3.6	1.6	1.6
Inulin clearance, *mL/min*	73	37	62	53
PAH clearance, *mL/min*	339	238	420	386

FIGURE 4-11. Angiotensin-converting enzyme (ACE) inhibitor-induced acute renal failure. The second mechanism of acute renal failure is confined to patients receiving ACE inhibitors or angiotensin-receptor blocking agents and may occur despite no significant change in blood pressure. **A,** Schematic showing a patient with renal artery stenosis (RAS) to a solitary functioning kidney. Despite no change in the systemic blood pressure, there was abrupt cessation of urine output (*solid line*) and loss of filtration (*dotted line*) after the initial dose of ACE inhibitor. Patients with high-grade bilateral RAS or RAS to a solitary kidney may be highly dependent on angiotensin II for glomerular filtration. This is particularly common in patients who receive a combination of ACE inhibitor and diuretic, or in patients who are placed on a sodium-restricted diet. Under these circumstances, the constrictive effect of angiotensin II on the efferent arteriole allows for the maintenance of normal transglomerular capillary hydraulic pressure, thus allowing glomerular filtration to remain normal in the presence of markedly diminished blood flow (**B**). Glomerular filtration is highly dependent on angiotensin II in this instance. When an ACE inhibitor is administered, the efferent arteriolar tone is no longer maintained and glomerular filtration is therefore decreased. A similar situation occurs in patients with decompensated congestive heart failure who are sodium depleted. **C,** Hricik *et al.* [20] demonstrated the important role that sodium balance plays in the azotemia associated with bilateral RAS or RAS to a solitary functioning kidney. When an ACE inhibitor was given alone, there was no change in renal function. However, if the patient was sodium depleted and then an ACE inhibitor was administered, the patient demonstrated a marked increase in the serum creatinine, and a decrease in the glomerular filtration rate and effective renal plasma flow. This was rapidly reversed with restoration of plasma volume by the administration of intravenous fluids. PAH—para-aminohippurate. (*Panel A adapted from* Textor *et al.* [19]; *panel B adapted from* Olin and Novick [6]; *panel C adapted from* Hricik *et al.* [20].)

CLINICAL MANIFESTATIONS AND DIAGNOSIS OF RENAL ARTERY DISEASE

CLINICAL CLUES TO THE DIAGNOSIS OF RENOVASCULAR DISEASE

Onset of hypertension after age 55 years or before age 30 years

Exacerbation of previously well-controlled hypertension

Malignant hypertension

Resistant hypertension

Epigastric bruit (systolic and diastolic)

Unexplained azotemia

Azotemia while receiving ACE inhibitors or AII receptor blocking agents

Atrophic kidney or discrepancy in size between the kidneys

Atherosclerosis elsewhere

Flash pulmonary edema or recurrent congestive heart failure

FIGURE 4-12. Clinical clues to the diagnosis of renovascular disease. In healthy patients, the systolic blood pressure increases in an almost linear fashion as patients age. However, the diastolic blood pressure rises until the approximate age of 55 years, and then it begins to decline. Therefore, the onset of diastolic hypertension after age 55 years should be a very strong clue for the presence of atherosclerotic renal artery disease. Since most patients with primary (essential) hypertension have an onset of hypertension between ages 30 and 55 years, patients below age 30 years with high blood pressure (fibromuscular dysplasia) or above age 55 years (atherosclerosis) should be investigated for the presence of renal artery stenosis or another secondary cause of hypertension, especially if blood pressure cannot be adequately controlled with medical therapy. ACE—angiotensin-converting enzyme; AII—angiotensin II.

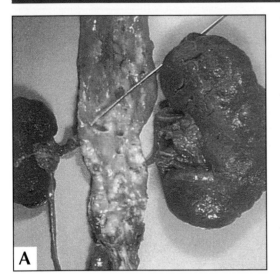

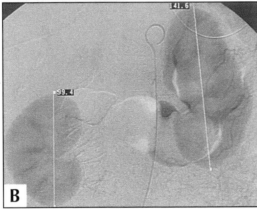

FIGURE 4-13. Atrophic kidney. **A,** If a kidney is atrophic or there is a difference in kidney size, the smaller kidney usually has a severe stenosis or occlusion of the renal artery supplying that kidney. However, more importantly, the contralateral (normal size kidney) renal artery is stenotic approximately 60% of the time. Therefore, discovery of a small kidney demands a thorough investigation for the presence of renal artery stenosis (RAS). Kidney sizes can be measured by an imaging procedure performed for some other reason. **B,** Nephrogram of both kidneys. The right kidney measured 9.9 cm while the left measured 14.2 cm. This should lead the clinician to suspect strongly the presence of RAS. However, the absence of a small kidney does not exclude RAS [21–23].

DIAGNOSTIC STUDIES TO EVALUATE FOR THE PRESENCE OF RENAL ARTERY STENOSIS

USEFUL	NOT USEFUL
Renal scintigraphy with captopril	Renal scintigraphy alone
Renal artery duplex	Intravenous urogram
CT angiography	Plasma renin activity
MR angiography	Captopril test
Intravascular ultrasound	Renal vein renin sampling
CO_2 angiography	
Angiography	

FIGURE 4-14. Diagnostic studies to evaluate for the presence of renal artery stenosis (RAS). The sensitivity and specificity of the tests on the right are too low to be of any value. Intravascular ultrasound, CO_2 angiography, and digital angiography are rarely used as the initial screening test for the diagnosis of RAS. Which test is used as an initial screening test depends in part on the "local" expertise available. Routine use of CT angiography is not recommended because it requires the intravenous admisistration of a bolus of contrast, a risk for a patient with azotemia. However, with rapid advances in CT technology using multiplanar CT scanners, this may change in the next few years. MR—magnetic resonance.

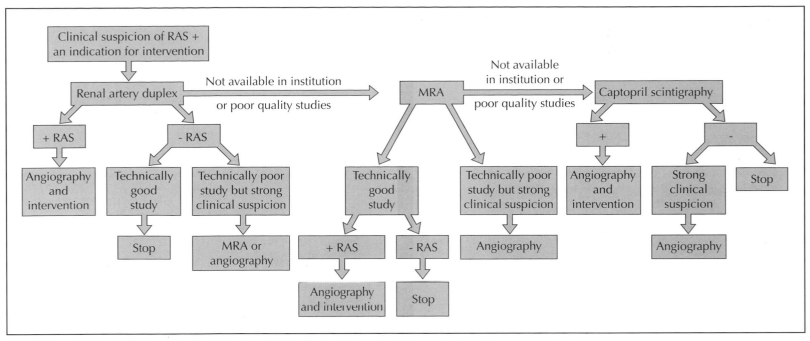

Figure 4-15. An approach to the imaging evaluation of patients with renal artery disease. (*Adapted from* Carman and Olin [24].)

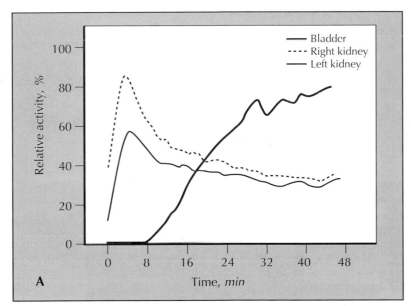

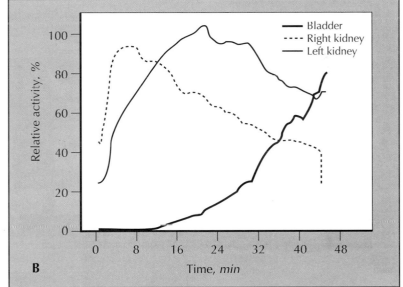

Figure 4-16. Captopril renal flow scan. When an angiotensin-converting enzyme (ACE) inhibitor such as captopril is added to isotope renography, the sensitivity and specificity of the test improves considerably, especially for patients with unilateral renal artery stenosis (RAS). In most instances of unilateral RAS, the glomerular filtration rate (GFR) of the stenotic kidney falls by approximately 30% after captopril administration. In contrast, the contralateral normal kidney exhibits an increase in GFR, urine flow, and salt excretion despite a reduction in systemic blood pressure. These expected physiologic changes within the stenotic and contralateral kidneys are the basis of the asymmetry of renal function following ACE inhibition detected by renal scintigraphy.

Oral hydration (water, 10 mL/kg) is encouraged on the morning of the test. A peripheral venous catheter for sampling and/or injection is inserted, and baseline blood pressure is measured and repeated at 15 to 20 minute intervals. Captopril (25–50 mg, crushed) is administered and a conventional radionuclide study of the kidneys is begun 60 minutes after captopril administration.

Both the scintigraphic images and computer-generated time-activity curves provide information about renal size, perfusion, and excretory capacity. Diagnostic criteria to suggest RAS include the following: delayed time to maximal activity (T_{max} more than 11 minutes after captopril); significant asymmetry of peak activity of each kidney; marked cortical retention of the radionuclide after captopril; and marked reduction in calculated GFR of the ipsilateral kidney after ACE [25–33]. (*Adapted from* Nally [25].)

SENSITIVITY, SPECIFICITY, AND PREDICTIVE VALUE OF CAPTOPRIL RENOGRAPHY

INVESTIGATORS	PATIENTS STUDIED, n	PATIENTS WITH RAS, n	RADIONUCLIDE USED	SENSITIVITY, %	SPECIFICITY, %	PREDICTIVE VALUE
Geyskes et al. [31]	34	15	^{131}I OIH	80	100	Yes (12/15)
Sfakianakis et al. [34]	31	16	^{131}I OIH	67	100	—
			Tc-DTPA	48		
Erbsloh-Moller et al. [35]	40	28	^{131}I OIH	96	95	Yes (10/11)
Svetkey et al. [36]	6	11	Tc-DTPA	74	44	—
			^{131}I OIH	71	41	
Setaro et al. [37]	90	44	Tc-DTPA	91	94	Yes (15/18)
Mann et al. [32]	55	35	Tc-DTPA	94	95	No (8/19)
			^{131}I OIH	83	85	
Fommei et al. [30]	472	259	Tc-DTPA	83	91	Yes (40/43)
			Tc-DTPA	83	100	
Dondi [38]	102	54	Tc-MAG$_3$	90	92	Yes
Elliott et al. [39]	100	59	Tc-pertechnetate	92	80	Yes (51/53)
van Jaarsveld et al. [33]	505	263	DTPA + MAG$_3$	68	90	—
Mittal et al. [40]	86	45	DTPA	82	98	100% (PPV)
						85% (NPV)
Miralles et al. [41]	60	44	?	87	87	74% (PPV)
						94% (NPV)
Johansson et al. [42]	98	18	DTPA	68	92	—

NPV—negative predictive value; PPV—positive predictive value.

FIGURE 4-17. Sensitivity, specificity, and predictive value of captopril renography. This figure represents a synopsis of captopril renography studies in hypertensive patients suspected of having renovascular disease. Overall, the accuracy of captopril renography in identifying patients with renovascular disease appears quite acceptable, with a sensitivity of approximately 85% to 90% (range 45 to 94) and specificity of approximately 93% to 98% (range 81 to 100). Those patients with unilateral disease and normal renal function would be best suited for a captopril renogram.

The presence of significant azotemia or bilateral renal artery stenosis may adversely affect the accuracy of captopril reno- graphy. Many investigators have excluded patients with serum creatinine exceeding 2.5 to 3.0 mg/dL. In patients with a serum creatinine $\geq$ 1.5 mg/dL and $\leq$ 3.0 mg/dL, Fommei et al. [30] reported a reduction in the positive predictive value from 88% to 57%, while there was a minimum reduction insensitivity/ specificity in patients with serum creatinine of 1.5 mg/dL.

While the captopril renogram was once the noninvasive diagnostic test of choice for patients with renal artery stenosis, it is now relegated to a secondary screening modality because the quality of the images of duplex ultrasound, magnetic resonance angiography, and CT angiography are excellent. (*Adapted from* Nally and Barton [27].)

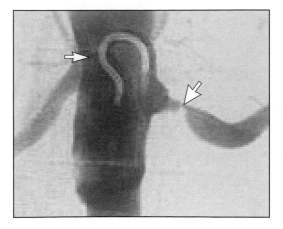

FIGURE 4-18. Renal aortic ratio. Duplex ultrasound, combining B-mode ultrasound with Doppler examination, has proven useful in the diagnosis of renal artery stenosis. Better ultrasound and transducer technology has led to better visualization of the renal arteries, allowing more precise Doppler interrogation of the entire renal artery. Duplex ultrasound is an excellent screening test for the presence of renal artery stenosis for several reasons: it provides information about the anatomic location of stenosis; it gives an accurate estimate of kidney size; it is not altered by antihypertensive medications so the antihypertensive regimen does not have to be discontinued before testing; it is noninvasive and not nephrotoxic so that it can be performed even in patients with significant azotemia; and it is less expensive than other tests such as CT angiography, magnetic resonance angiography, or digital subtraction angiography. Sensitivity and specificity has been estimated at 75% to 95% and 87% to 100%, respectively.

The examination should be performed using both an anterior and an oblique approach. An aortic velocity at the level of the renal arteries should be obtained in the longitudinal view. The maximum renal artery velocity is used to calculate the renal to aortic ratio, which is used to diagnose significant renal artery stenosis. *Small arrow,* aorta peak systolic velocity = 75 cm/s; *large arrow*, renal artery peak systolic velocity = 400 cm/s; renal artery ratio = 400/75 = 5.3.

CRITERIA FOR DIAGNOSIS OF RENAL ARTERY DISEASE

DUPLEX CRITERIA	STENOSIS, %
RAR < 3.5 and PSV < 200 cm/s	0–59
RAR ≥ 3.5 and PSV > 200 cm/s	60–99
RAR > 3.5 and EDV ≥ 150 cm/s	80–99
Absence of flow and low amplitude parenchymal signal	Occluded

FIGURE 4-19. Criteria used for the diagnosis of renal artery disease. The renal arteries are visualized with the B-mode image, then are interrogated with the Doppler using a 60° angle of insonance at the origin, proximal, mid, and distal renal arteries. The entire artery from the origin to the renal hilum should be surveyed. It is important to sweep the Doppler throughout the artery, as opposed to spot checking velocities, in an effort to identify any velocity shift that may occur.

If the ratio of the peak systolic velocity (PSV) in the renal artery to the PSV in the aorta (RAR) is 3.5 or greater, the degree of stenosis is classified between 60% and 99%. If the end diastolic velocity is 150 cm/s or greater, this suggests a high-grade lesion (greater than 80%). If the RAR is less than 3.5 and the PSV is less than 200 cm/s, the artery would be classified as 0% to 59% stenosis; if there is an absence of flow and a low-amplitude parenchymal signal, the artery is occluded.

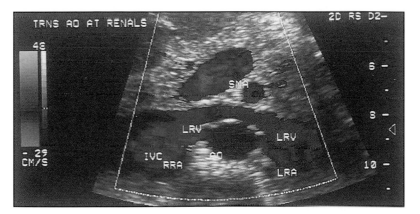

FIGURE 4-20. Ultrasound examination with transverse view of anatomic landmarks. From the anterior approach, the celiac axis, superior mesenteric artery, and left renal vein are identified. These serve as key landmarks for identifying the renal arteries. Note how the left renal vein crosses anterior to the aorta. Occasionally, a retroaortic renal vein will be present. AO—aorta; IVC—inferior vena cava; LRA—left renal artery; LRV—left renal vein; RRA—right renal artery; SMA—superior mesenteric artery. (*From* Olin [43]; with permission.)

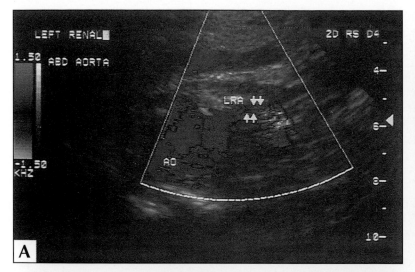

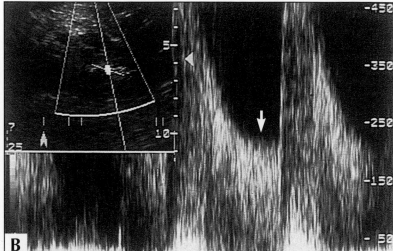

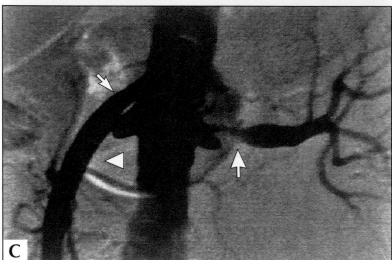

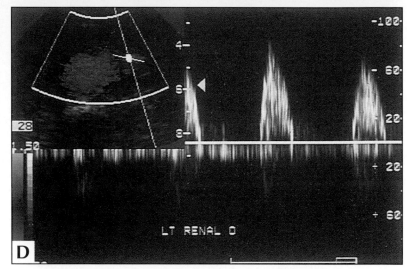

FIGURE 4-21. Renal artery duplex scanning. Not only is renal artery duplex an excellent technique for diagnosing patients with renal artery disease, it is a very valuable tool for following patients after renal artery stent implantation or surgical revascularization to identify restenosis should it occur. This 72-year-old woman presented with poorly controlled hypertension (170/96 mm Hg despite taking three antihypertensive medications) and a serum creatinine of 3.2 mg/dL.

A, Renal artery duplex scan demonstrating excellent visualization of the left renal artery from the origin in the anterior approach. Note the mosaic color pattern just distal to the arrows indicating turbulence of flow. This area should be carefully insonated with the Doppler.

B, The Doppler was placed in the proximal left renal artery at the correct angle of 60°. The peak systolic velocity was more than 450 cm/s and the end diastolic velocity (*arrow*) is 220 cm/s, indicating

a stenosis of over 80% of the left renal artery. The right renal artery could not be found and the right kidney was atrophic.

C, Aortogram showing a total occlusion of the right renal artery (*arrowhead*) and a severe eccentric stenosis of the left renal artery (*large arrow*) with post-stenotic dilatation. The superior mesenteric artery is also visualized (*small arrow*).

D, Duplex of the left renal artery after a renal artery stent was placed. Note normal velocities (peak systolic velocity 70 cm/s) compared with the markedly elevated velocities before the placement of the renal artery stent. The patient had normal blood pressure (130/82 mm Hg) while on two medications, and her serum creatinine decreased to 1.6 mg/dL after placement of the renal artery stent. She was followed with renal artery duplex on a yearly basis for 9 years; the stent remained widely patent and she continued to do well clinically. (*From* Olin and Begelman [2]; with permission.)

COMPARISON OF DUPLEX ULTRASOUND WITH ARTERIOGRAPHY

STENOSIS DIAGNOSED BY ULTRASOUND, %	STENOSIS DIAGNOSED BY ARTERIOGRAPHY, %				
	0–59	60–79	80–99	100	Total
0–59	62	0	*1*	*1*	64
60–99	*1*	31	67	0	99
100	0	*1*	*1*	22	24
Total	63	32	69	23	187

FIGURE 4-22. Comparison of duplex ultrasound with arteriography. This prospective blinded study compared duplex ultrasound of the renal arteries with angiography. Among 187 arteries, the duplex compared with angiography in 183 arteries. The numbers in italics represent the five arteries that were incorrectly diagnosed by duplex. The sensitivity was 0.98, specificity .98, positive predictive value .99, and negative predictive value .97. The sensitivity of identifying accessory renal arteries was approximately 67% in the one study that looked at this. If there is a high index of suspicion for renal artery stenosis and the duplex examination fails to reveal a significant stenosis, an accessory vessel may be suspected as the culprit.

The biggest criticism of renal artery duplex ultrasound imaging has been that the results from some of the larger centers are difficult to duplicate. This technique does have a steep learning curve but with good imaging equipment, persistence, effective training, and proper patient preparation (overnight fast), it is not unreasonable to expect results similar to those published. Even the obese patient can be adequately scanned under most circumstances using the oblique approach (22,44–46).

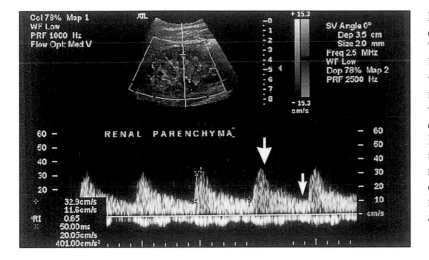

FIGURE 4-23. Assessment of intrarenal hemodynamics. During the duplex examination, parenchymal waveforms should be obtained. This usually is accomplished from the flank or oblique approach. Using a 0° angle, the Doppler is placed in the cortical blood vessels of the upper and lower poles, and the mid portion of the renal cortex and velocities are measured. The peak systolic velocity (*large arrow*) and end diastolic velocity (*small arrow*) are obtained and the resistive index (RI) is calculated by the formula PSV (peak systolic velocity) - EDV (end-diastolic velocity)/PSV. In this case, the RI equals 0.65. Values less than 0.80 are considered normal. A high RI implies that there is significant small vessel disease within the kidney. This increased resistance within the renal circulation may have a bearing on which patients improve after renal revascularization and which patients do not.

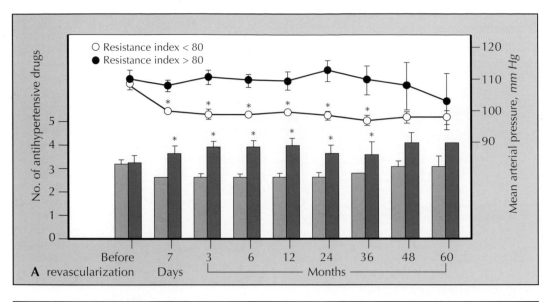

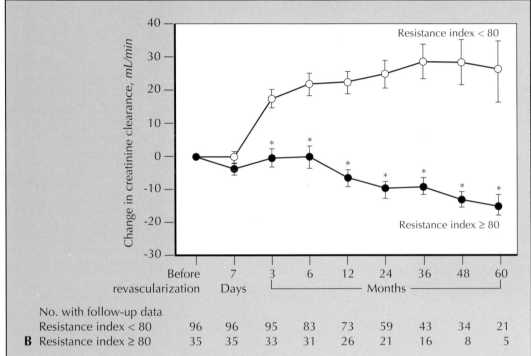

FIGURE 4-24. Resistance index and outcome of therapy. This study used duplex ultrasonography to predict the outcome of therapy in patients with renal artery stenosis (RAS). Renal artery angioplasty or surgery for blood pressure control or preservation of renal function was performed in 138 patients with greater than 50% stenosis of the renal artery. A renal resistance index of at least 80 accurately identified patients in whom angioplasty

or surgery was not associated with improved blood pressure, renal function, or kidney survival. No improvement in blood pressure was noted in 97% of patients with an increased renal resistance index, and 80% had no improvement in renal function. The authors suggest that the increased resistive index identifies structural abnormalities in the small vessels of the kidney. Such small vessel disease has been seen with long-standing hypertension associated with nephrosclerosis or glomerulosclerosis. If this study is confirmed, it could provide a method for predicting which patients would improve after percutaneous or surgical revascularization.

A, Mean (+ SE) change in mean arterial pressure and the number of antihypertensive drugs taken after the correction of RAS, according to resistance-index values before revascularization. In the group of patients with a resistance index of less than 80 before revascularization, mean (± SD) blood pressure was 150 ± 22/89 ± 12 mm Hg initially and 135 ± 14/80 ± 10 mm Hg at last follow-up visit (*P* < 0.001); the respective values in the group of patients with a resistance index of at least 80 before revascularization were 164 ± 21/83 ± 16 mm Hg and 163 ± 19/86 ± 10 mm Hg (*P* = 0.73). The antihypertensive drugs included angiotensin-converting enzyme inhibitors, angiotensin II-receptor blockers, β-blockers, calcium antagonists, α-blockers, direct vasodilators, diuretics, and nitrates. Asterisks indicate a significant difference (*P* < 0.05) between the two groups with use of an unpaired t-test with Bonferron's adjustment.

B, Mean (± SE) changes in the creatinine clearance after the correction of RAS, according to the resistance-index value before revascularization. Asterisks indicate a significant difference (*P* < 0.05) between the two groups with use of an unpaired t-test with Bonferron's adjustment. (*Adapted from* Radermacher *et al.* [47].)

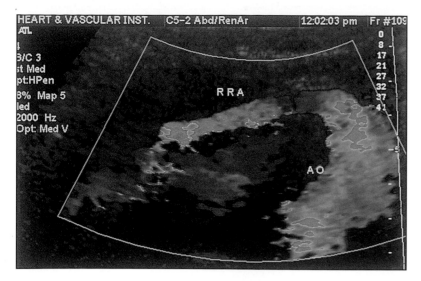

HEART & VASCULAR INST.   C5-2 Abd/RenAr   12:02:03 pm   Fr #109
ATL
3/C 3
st Med
pt:HPen
3% Map 5
led
2000 Hz
Opt: Med V

RRA

AO

0
8
17
21
27
32
37
41

FIGURE 4-25. Visualization via oblique approach. Note the renal artery from the kidney to the aorta using an oblique approach. The oblique approach is particularly useful in visualizing the renal artery distally from where it enters the kidney and following it to the aorta. By measuring Doppler velocities in two different views, one can be certain that a focal renal artery stenosis is not being overlooked. In addition, the oblique approach is particularly useful in patients with fibromuscular dysplasia, since this entity commonly occurs in the distal two thirds of the renal artery and its branches.

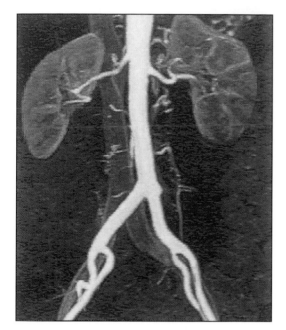

FIGURE 4-26. Magnetic resonance angiography (MRA). Magnetic resonance angiography is a useful screening test for renal artery stenosis. Time-of-flight, phase contrast, and maximal intensity projection are the most commonly used techniques for imaging the renal arteries. The images obtained can then be reconstructed and processed to provide both 2-dimensional and 3-dimensional images. In addition, intravenous contrast with gadolinium may overcome some of the flow-dependent loss of signal and provide better images of both the main renal arteries as well as accessory renal arteries. The 3-dimensional gadolinium-enhanced MRA shown was acquired with an 18-second breath hold. The sensitivity and specificity for detecting stenosis greater than 60% ranges from 73% to 100% and 76% to 100%, respectively. Thorton *et al.* [48] recently reported a sensitivity, specificity, and accuracy of 100%, 98%, and 99% using a gadolinium-enhanced breath hold method.

Like duplex ultrasound, MRA is dependent on the equipment and software used and the technical expertise of the specialist performing the MR examination. Quality does vary considerably from center to center based on institutional expertise in MR techniques. In addition, technical considerations such as respiratory artifact, peristaltic bowel motion artifact, and claustrophobia may contribute to a nondiagnostic study. Patients with metal clips or staples, pacemakers, or other metallic devices may not be candidates for examination.

Each examination should begin with acquisition of routine T_1- and T_2-weighted images to evaluate the kidneys, adrenal glands, and associated soft tissues. Time-of-flight and phase contrast are noncontrast techniques commonly used for vascular imaging. Software is available for both 2-dimensional and 3-dimensional imaging. The initial source images are completed in approximately 20 minutes. The reformatting process usually requires an additional 30 to 45 minutes. Maximum intensity projection and multiplanar reconstructions are the most commonly used postprocessing algorithms [48–50].

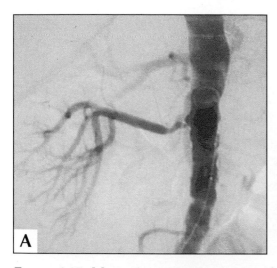

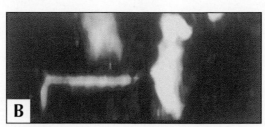

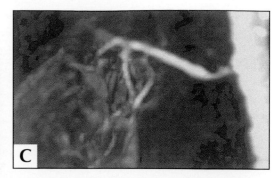

FIGURE 4-27. Magnetic resonance angiography (MRA). **A**, This digital subtraction arteriogram demonstrates a significant stenosis at the origin and proximal portion of the renal artery. The gradient measured 80 mm Hg across the lesion. **B**, A 3-dimensional phase contrast study in the same patient. One sees a pseudo-occlusion in the proximal right renal artery due to spin dephasing. **C**, An example of a gadolinium-enhanced 3-dimensional MRA in the same patient showing excellent correlation with the angiogram.

The spin dephasing does not occur when gadolinium is used as a contrast agent.

While the sensitivity and specificity of gadolinium-enhanced MRA is excellent in patients with atherosclerosis, it does not have the same sensitivity and specificity in patients with fibromuscular dysplasia. In fact, MRA can sometimes give the appearance of beading when no beading actually exists [22].

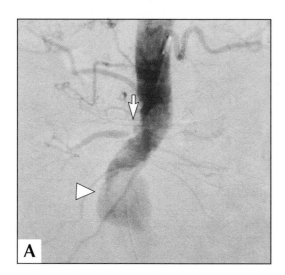

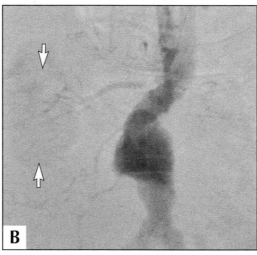

FIGURE 4-28. CO_2 angiography. Once a decision has been made to consider renal artery intervention, CO_2 or gadolinium can be used as a contrast agent in patients with chronic renal insufficiency because these agents are not nephrotoxic. **A**, The left renal artery is occluded. The right renal artery has a high-grade stenosis (*arrow*) and there is an infrarenal abdominal aortic aneurysm present (*arrowhead*). **B**, Later phase showing visualization of the common iliac arteries and a faint nephrogram of the right kidney (*arrows*).

When compared with contrast angiography, CO_2 angiography demonstrates a sensi-

tivity of 83% and a specificity of 99%. CO_2 is rapidly eliminated via the lungs, allowing repeated injections without increased risk of toxicity. The disadvantages of using CO_2 can be related to the buoyancy, compressibility, and solubility of the gas. Due to its buoyancy, CO_2 does not optimally visualize posteriorly placed structures. Large boluses may be necessary to completely displace the blood from the vessel and obtain quality images. This may be difficult because the compressibility of the gas can make injection difficult, and CO_2 dissolves rapidly in the blood; thus, the image degrades in a few seconds. While the use of CO_2 does prevent nephrotoxicity from contrast, the patient can still develop atheromatous embolization (from catheter manipulation in the aorta or renal artery) to the kidney. The major drawback in using CO_2 as a contrast agent is that the resolution and clarity are not as good as with iodinated contrast [51,52].

NATURAL HISTORY OF ATHEROSCLEROTIC RENAL ARTERY DISEASE

SERIES	FOLLOW-UP, mo	PATIENTS, n	PROGRESSION, n (%)	OCCLUSION, n (%)
Wollenweber et al. [14]	12–88	30	21 (70)	—
Meany et al. [53]	6–120	39	14 (36)	3 (8)
Dean et al. [15]	6–102	35	10 (29)	4 (11)
Schreiber et al. [54]	12–60	85	37 (44)	14 (16)
Tollefson and Ernst [16]	15–180	48	34 (71)	7 (15)
Total		237	116 (49)	28 (14)

FIGURE 4-29. Natural history of atherosclerotic renovascular disease. Knowledge of the natural history of atherosclerotic renovascular disease is extremely important in the subsequent management of these patients. It is not only important to study anatomic endpoints (*ie*, progression of stenosis), but also clinical endpoints (*ie*, frequency of chronic renal failure and end-stage renal disease). These clinical endpoints have been lacking in many reports.

Schreiber *et al.* [54] evaluated retrospectively 85 patients who had atherosclerotic renovascular disease. Thirty-seven patients (44%) were found to have anatomic progression of renal artery stenosis (RAS) on repeat angiography, and 14 patients (16%) progressed to complete occlusion. The mean angiographic follow-up was 52 months (range, 12 to more than 60 months). The rate of progression to total occlusion occurred more frequently (39%) when there was more than 75% stenosis on the initial renal arteriogram.

Tollefson *et al.* [16] studied 48 patients with 194 sequential aortograms over a mean period of 4.5 years. The RAS progressed in 34 of 48 patients, or 71%. Seven instances of RAS in seven patients (15%) progressed to complete occlusion. Crowley *et al.* [55] assessed progression in 1189 patients who had undergone renal angiography at the time of cardiac catheterization and later had a repeat cardiac catheterization. The disease progressed in 11.1% of patients.

Dean *et al.* [15] studied the rate of progression in a prospective fashion. Serial renal function studies were performed on 41 patients with atherosclerotic renal artery stenosis. The serum creatinine increased 25% to 120% in 19 (46%) patients. In 12 (29%) patients, the glomerular filtration rate decreased 25% to 50%. Fourteen (37%) patients lost more than 10% of renal length, and in four (12%) patients, severe stenosis progressed to occlusion. Seventeen (41%) patients had deterioration of renal function or loss of renal size that led to surgery. Of the 17 patients with deterioration, 15 had acceptable blood pressure control during nonoperative observation. (*Adapted from* Rimmer and Gennari [17].)

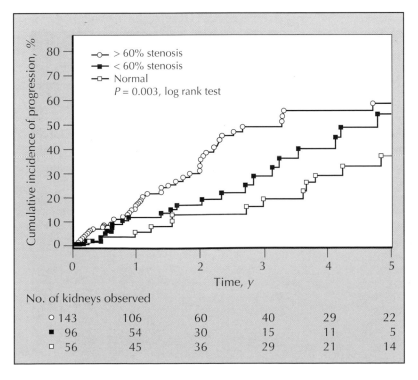

FIGURE 4-30. Progression of stenosis in patients with atherosclerotic renal artery disease. A total of 295 kidneys in 170 patients with atherosclerotic renal artery stenosis were followed prospectively by duplex ultrasound every 6 months. The mean follow-up period was 33 months. Overall, the cumulative incidence of progression was 35% at 3 years and 51% at 5 years. The cumulative 3-year incidence of progression was 18% in those classified as having normal renal arteries at baseline, 28% in those with less than 60% renal artery stenosis at baseline, and 49% in those with greater than 60% stenosis at baseline. There were only nine renal artery occlusions during the study, all of which occurred in renal arteries with greater than 60% stenosis at baseline. (*Adapted from* Caps *et al.* [56].)

RISK OF ATROPHY IN KIDNEYS WITH ATHEROSCLEROTIC RENAL ARTERY STENOSIS

DEGREE OF STENOSIS, %	2-Y CUMULATIVE INCIDENCE OF ATROPHY, %
Normal	5.5
< 60	11.7
≥ 60	20.8

FIGURE 4-31. Risk of atrophy in kidneys with atherosclerotic renal artery stenosis (RAS). Caps *et al.* [57] prospectively followed 204 kidneys in 122 patients with known RAS for a mean of 33 months. The 2-year cumulative incidence of renal atrophy was 5.5%, 11.7%, and 20.8% in kidneys with a baseline renal artery disease classification of normal, less than 60% stenosis, and greater than 60% stenosis, respectively ($P = 0.009$, log-rank test) [57].

In a study of 683 patients with end-stage renal disease, Mallioux *et al.* [58] showed that 83 (12%) patients had atherosclerotic RAS as the cause of end-stage renal disease [58].

SURVIVAL ESTIMATES FOR SELECTED RENAL DIAGNOSIS

DIAGNOSIS (*n*)	MEDIAN SURVIVAL, *mo*	LENGTH OF SURVIVAL			
		2 Y, %	5 Y, %	10 Y, %	15 Y, %
Polycystic kidney disease (56)	133	91	77	59	32
Malignant hypertension (23)	55	77	25	0	0
Renal vascular disease (83)	25	56	18	5	0

FIGURE 4-32. Survival estimates for selected renal diagnosis. This study demonstrated the extremely poor survival of patients who progress to end-stage renal disease from atherosclerotic renal artery stenosis (RAS). The median survival was only 25 months, compared with 133 months for patients with polycystic kidney disease and 55 months for malignant hypertension. The 2-year survival was 56%, 5-year survival 18%, 10-year survival 5%, and 15-year survival was 0 for patients with renal vascular disease. This is significantly worse than patients with polycystic kidney disease or malignant hypertension [59].

Connolly *et al.* [60] showed that the 2-year actuarial renal survival (percent of patients remaining off dialysis) was 97.3% for patients with unilateral RAS, 82.4% in patients with bilateral RAS, and 44.7% in patients with stenosis or occlusion to a solitary functioning kidney. Patients on dialysis have a shortened life expectancy. The average life expectancy for a patient over age 65 years with end-stage renal disease is only 2.7 years. (*Adapted from* Mailloux *et al.* [58].)

RENAL ARTERY STENOSIS: 2-YEAR ACTUARIAL SURVIVAL

DISEASE SEVERITY	SURVIVAL, %
Unilateral disease	96
Bilateral disease	74
Solitary disease	47

FIGURE 4-33. Survival in patients with renal artery stenosis (RAS). The mere presence of RAS, even before developing end-stage renal disease, portends an extremely poor prognosis. Patient survival decreases as the severity of RAS increases, with 2-year survival rates of 96% in patients with unilateral RAS, 74% in patients with bilateral RAS, and 47% in patients with stenosis or occlusion to a solitary functioning kidney [61].

Dorros *et al.* [62] demonstrated that as the serum creatinine increases, the survival decreases in patients with atherosclerotic RAS. The 3-year probability of survival was 92 + 4% for patients with a serum creatinine below 1.4 mg/dL, 74 + 8% for patients with a serum creatinine of 1.5 to 1.9 mg/dL, and 51 + 8% for patients with a serum creatinine above 2.0 mg/dL [62].

MEDICAL TREATMENT OF RENAL ARTERY DISEASE

Control blood pressure
  Follow recommendations of JNC VI
  ACE inhibitor ± diuretic for initial therapy
    for unilateral disease?
Preserve renal function
  Follow serum creatinine
  Follow renal size (ultrasound)
  Follow progression of renal artery stenosis with
    serial duplex ultrasound
Modify all cardiovascular risk factors

FIGURE 4-34. Medical treatment of renal artery disease. All patients should be treated medically, even those undergoing a revascularization procedure. The blood pressure should be well controlled following the guidelines of the Joint National Committee on the Evaluation, Prevention and Treatment of High Blood Pressure (JNC VI) [63]. Renal function should be carefully followed. Blood, urea, nitrogen, serum creatinine, and electrolytes should be measured every 3 months. A duplex ultrasound should be performed every 6 to 12 months to assess kidney size and progression of disease. A risk factor modification program should be instituted. This includes discontinuation of smoking, institution of an exercise program, achievement of ideal body weight, control of diabetes, and control of lipids with goal low-density lipid cholesterol below 100 mg/dL. The patient should be on an antiplatelet agent and perhaps an angiotensin-converting enzyme (ACE) inhibitor as well to prevent myocardial infarction, stroke, or cardiovascular death [63–65].

INDICATIONS FOR REVASCULARIZATION FOR ATHEROSCLEROTIC RENAL ARTERY STENOSIS

Inability to control blood pressure
Preservation of renal function
Control of congestive heart failure

FIGURE 4-35. Indications for revascularization for atherosclerotic renal artery stenosis (RAS). There has been a paradigm shift in management of atherosclerotic RAS. Before 1990, if a patient met the criteria for intervention, surgical renal artery revascularization was almost always performed. However, since the introduction of stents, surgical revascularization rarely is performed solely for the treatment of renal artery disease. Despite advances in the technical aspects of angioplasty and stent implantation, there has been a paucity of controlled clinical trials assessing the role of renal artery angioplasty and stenting to control hypertension or preserve renal function. Despite the lack of randomized controlled trials, the consensus of experts supports the use of angioplasty and stenting for most patients with atherosclerotic RAS who meet the criteria for intervention. Patients with fibromuscular dysplasia who meet criteria for intervention can be treated with angioplasty alone. Stent implantation in this subset of patients in usually not required or justified.

Blood pressure is considered uncontrolled when it cannot be normalized (< 140/90 mm Hg) with a good antihypertensive regimen consisting of at least three drugs of different mechanisms of action in near maximum doses. Other indications for revascularization include patients with side effects from multiple medications, or those patients who cannot afford their medications. Young patients with fibromuscular disease can be treated with percutaneous transluminal angioplasty when first diagnosed because this may be curative, thus precluding lifelong antihypertensive medication.

Patients requiring dialysis who have greater than 75% bilateral RAS or greater than 75% RAS to a solitary functioning kidney and no other readily explainable cause of end-stage renal disease should undergo renal artery stent implantation. It is best to intervene early, but there have been numerous cases in which renal function has been salvaged even when the serum creatinine was markedly increased.

The diagnosis of RAS should be considered in any patient with recurrent pulmonary edema or congestive heart failure without a readily explainable cause. This is especially important in patients with normal left ventricular function [66,67].

SURGICAL REVASCULARIZATION FOR THE TREATMENT OF RENOVASCULAR HYPERTENSION

SERIES	PATIENTS, n	CURED, n (%)	IMPROVED, n (%)	FAILED, n (%)
Van Bockel *et al.* [68]	105	19 (18)	64 (61)	22 (21)
Novick *et al.* [69]	180	55 (31)	110 (61)	15 (8)
Libertino *et al.* [70]	86	38 (44)	44 (51)	4 (5)
Hansen *et al.* [71]	152	22 (15)	116 (75)	14 (10)
Total	523	134 (26)	334 (64)	55 (10)

FIGURE 4-36. Surgical revascularization for the treatment of reno-vascular hypertension. Surgical revascularization has been used much less frequently than in the past. This is due in large part to the excellent technical results that can be achieved with angioplasty and stent implantation. Most patients can now undergo renal artery stent implantation as an outpatient procedure at a fraction of the cost of surgical revascularization and with less morbidity and mortality.

These series show the status of hypertension after renal artery revascularization. Current indications for surgical revascularization include the following: patients with branch disease from fibromus-cular dysplasia that cannot be adequately treated with balloon angioplasty; patients with recurrent stenosis after stenting (extremely rare); and patients who require simultaneous aortic surgery (abdominal aortic aneurysm repair or symptomatic aortoiliac disease). Even in this circumstance, it may be advisable to stent the renal artery first and then proceed with aortic reconstruc-tion. The mortality rate of aortic replacement with renal artery revascularization is higher than either procedure alone.

A variety of surgical revascularization techniques are available for treating patients with significant renal artery disease. Aortorenal bypass with autogenous saphenous vein was an excellent method in patients with a nondiseased abdominal aorta. However, severe aortic disease almost always accompanies atherosclerotic renal artery stenosis (RAS). Polytetrafluoroethylene aortorenal bypass grafts have been successfully employed, usually when an autogenous graft is not available. Renal endarterectomy also continues to be used to treat atherosclerotic renal artery disease. Patients with complex branch renal artery lesions can be managed with extracorporeal micro-vascular reconstruction and autotransplantation.

In older patients, severe atherosclerosis of the abdominal aorta may render an aortorenal bypass or endarterectomy technically difficult and potentially hazardous to perform. In such cases, alternate surgical approaches often allow renal revascularization to be safely and effec-tively accomplished while avoiding operation on a badly diseased aorta. The most effective alternate bypass techniques have been a splenorenal bypass for left renal revascularization and a hepatorenal bypass for right renal revascularization. The absence of occlusive disease involving the origin of the celiac artery is an important pre-requisite for these operations. Significant celiac artery stenosis may occur in up to 50% of patients with atherosclerotic RAS. This infor-mation underscores the importance of obtaining preoperative lateral aortography to evaluate the celiac artery origin in patients who are being considered for hepatorenal or splenorenal bypass. Use of the supraceliac or lower thoracic aorta for renal revascularization has also been performed successfully in patients with significant aortic disease. The supraceliac aorta is often relatively disease-free in such patients and can be used to achieve renovascular reconstruction with an interposition saphenous vein graft.

Reports from several large centers have demonstrated that surgical renal revascularization can be performed with operative mortality rates of 2.1%, 3.1%, 3.4%, and 6.1% in patients with atherosclerotic RAS. The mortality rate increases with bilateral simultaneous renal revascularizations, or when renal revascularization is performed with aortic replacement [6,68–73]. (*Adapted from* Olin and Novick [6].)

SURGICAL REVASCULARIZATION FOR ATHEROSCLEROTIC ISCHEMIC NEPHROPATHY

SERIES	PATIENTS, n	IMPROVED, n (%)	STABLE, n (%)	DETERIORATED, n (%)
Novick *et al.* [69]	161	93 (58)	50 (31)	18 (11)
Hallet *et al.* [74]	91	20 (22)	48 (53)	23 (25)
Hansen *et al.* [71]	70	34 (49)	25 (36)	11 (15)
Bredenberg *et al.* [75]	40	22 (55)	10 (25)	8 (20)
Libertino *et al.* [70]	91	45 (49)	31 (35)	15 (16)
Total	453	214 (47)	164 (36)	75 (17)

FIGURE 4-37. Surgical revascularization for atherosclerotic ischemic nephropathy. Patients who are at a markedly increased risk for atherosclerotic ischemic nephropathy are those with greater than 75% bilateral renal artery stenosis (RAS) or severe stenosis to a single func-tioning kidney. In this patient subgroup, the risk of total occlusion of the renal artery is significant, and if it occurs, the clinical outcome is a critical decrease in functioning renal mass with resulting renal failure.

The benefit of undertaking revascularization for preservation of renal function in patients with unilateral RAS and a normal contralateral renal artery is not established. If the contralateral kidney is anatomically and functionally normal, revascularization for this purpose is clearly not warranted. If the opposite kidney is func-tioning but involved with some type of parenchymal disorder, revas-cularization of the ischemic kidney may benefit some patients, but specific indications for this approach are not well defined.

Patients who develop acute renal failure shortly after the initiation of antihypertensive therapy often require intervention to preserve renal function [15,19,76]. (*Adapted from* Olin and Novick [6].)

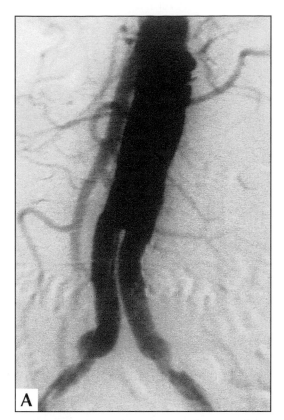

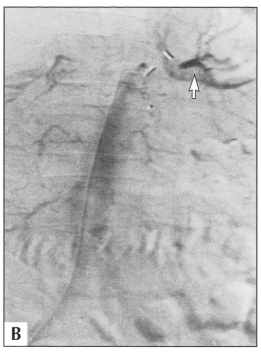

Figure 4-38. Restoration of renal function in totally occluded renal arteries. **A,** Angiogram of a patient who underwent an aortoiliac bypass graft with a bypass to the left renal artery. The bypass is occluded and a kidney is not visualized. The right renal artery was chronically occluded. **B,** On a later view, when contrast has washed out of the aorta, distal reconstitution of the left renal artery can be seen (*arrow*), indicating that the left kidney may be salvageable. This late visualization of the renal artery is a good prognostic sign. **C,** Angiogram showing a severe stenosis of the left renal artery. Note the presence of a nephrogram on the left (*arrows*), which is a good prognostic sign. (*Panels A and B from* Olin *et al.* [77]; with permission.)

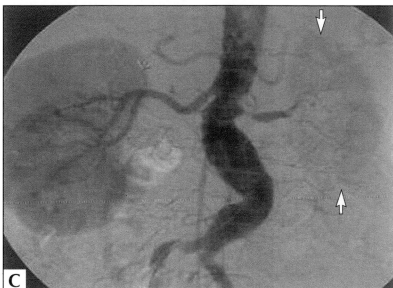

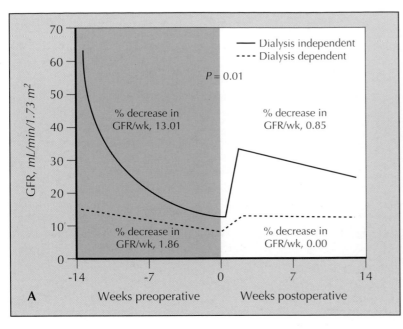
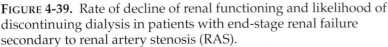
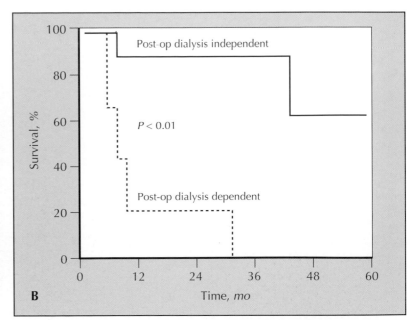

A Weeks preoperative — Weeks postoperative

B Time, *mo*

FIGURE 4-39. Rate of decline of renal functioning and likelihood of discontinuing dialysis in patients with end-stage renal failure secondary to renal artery stenosis (RAS).

Several anecdotal reports show that restoration of renal function in patients with totally occluded renal arteries with either endovascular therapy or surgical revascularization is feasible. Kaylor *et al.* [78] reported on nine patients who were on dialysis from 1 week to 13 months secondary to atherosclerotic RAS. Reversal of end-stage renal failure occurred in all nine patients who underwent surgical revascularization. The serum creatinine at 1 month ranged from 1.1 to 4.2 mg/dL, with a mean of 2.5 mg/dL. **A**, Hansen *et al.* [79] have also shown that it is possible to restore renal function with surgical revascularization in some patients who have been on chronic hemodialysis therapy. In their

study from 1987 to 1993, 340 patients underwent surgical renal revascularization. Twenty patients were receiving hemodialysis before renal artery repair. Hemodialysis was discontinued in 16 of the 20 patients (80%). Two of the 16 patients resumed dialysis 4 and 6 months after surgery. A favorable response in this series occurred in those patients who had a relatively rapid decline in their glomerular filtration rate (GFR) in the 14 weeks preceding renal revascularization [79].

B, The long-term survival was better in patients who were dialysis independent compared to those who required ongoing dialysis therapy. There were only two late deaths among the 14 patients not receiving dialysis (*solid line*) compared with five late deaths among the six patients who continued to receive dialysis after surgical revascularization (*dotted line*) (*P* < 0.01).

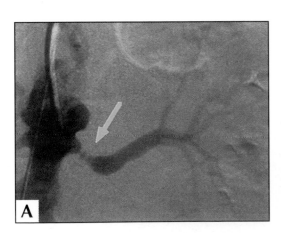
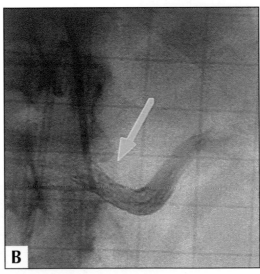

FIGURE 4-40. Renal artery stenting for atherosclerotic renal artery stenosis. Due to the very high restenosis rate with angioplasty alone, stents offer a significant advantage over percutaneous transluminal angioplasty (PTA) in patients with atherosclerotic disease, especially those with ostial stenosis. The degree of stenosis post-stenting approaches

zero, and most dissection flaps caused by PTA alone are successfully sealed with stents. There are a few important technical caveats when stenting the renal arteries: the shortest stent to adequately cover the lesion should be used; the stent must extend 1 to 2 mm into the aorta in patients with ostial disease; and the stent must be fully expanded.

A, Angiogram showing marked atherosclerosis in the abdominal aorta. Note the severe stenosis (*arrow*) in the ostial and proximal portion of the left renal artery with post-stenotic dilatation. The guiding catheter comes from above in this case due to the angle of the take off of the left renal artery. **B**, Excellent angiographic result after renal artery stenting (*arrow*). Note that the stent extends 1 to 2 mm into the aorta, which is perfect position in patients with ostial renal artery stenosis. (*Courtesy of* J. Michael Bacharach, MD, MPH.)

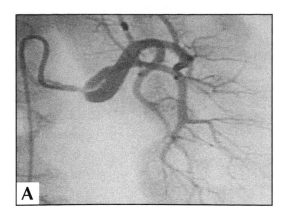 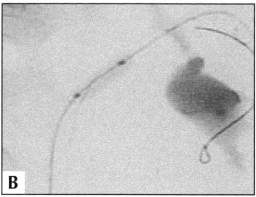 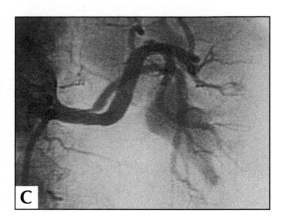

FIGURE 4-41. Complex renal artery stenting. Renal artery stenting of complex lesions is becoming commonplace thanks to better catheters, balloons, low-profile stents, and operators that are more experienced. **A**, Angiogram showing a severe stenosis in the proximal renal artery that extends distally to the bifurcation of the renal artery. **B**, The two main branches are protected with wires while the main renal artery undergoes percutaneous transluminalangioplasty and stent implantation. **C**, Post-stenting angiogram showing an excellent result. The smaller superior branch is still patent although the origin is covered by the stent (stent jail). (*Courtesy of* J. Michael Bacharach, MD, MPH.)

CLINICAL AND ANGIOGRAPHIC FOLLOW-UP IN RENAL ARTERY STENT PLACEMENT

INVESTIGATORS	PATIENTS, n	STENT	TECHNICAL SUCCESS, %	FOLLOW-UP, mo	HYPERTENSION CURE, %	IMPROVED, %	RENAL FUNCTION IMPROVED, %	STABLE, %	RESTENOSIS, %
Wilms et al. [80]	11	Wallstent[*]	83	7	30	40	0	0	29
Kuhn et al. [81]	10	Strecker[†]	80	11	29	43	50	NM	25
Rees et al. [82]	28	Palmaz[‡]	96	7	11	54	36	36	39
Hennequin et al. [83]	21	Wallstent[*]	100	32	14	86	17	50	20
van de Ven et al. [84]	24	Palmaz[‡]	100	6	68	5	36	64	13
Henry et al. [85]	59	Palmaz[‡]	100	14	19	57	20	NM	9
Iannone et al. [86]	63	Palmaz[‡]	99	10	4	35	36	45	14
Blum et al. [87]	68	Palmaz[‡]	100	27	16	62	NM	NM	11
Boisclair et al. [88]	33	Palmaz[‡]	100	13	6	61	41	35	—
Harden et al. [89]	32	Palmaz[‡]	100	6	NM	NM	34	34	13
White et al. [90]	100	Palmaz[‡]	99	6	NM	NM	20	NM	19
Rundback et al. [91]	45	Palmaz[‡]	94	17	NM	NM	NM	NM	25
Shannon et al. [92]	21	Palmaz[‡]	100	9	NM	NM	43	29	0
Doros et al. [93]	163	Palmaz[‡]	100	48	3	51	NM	NM	—
Total	678		98*	16*	20*	49*	30	38	17

[*] Boston Scientific, Natick, MA.
[†] Medi-Tech International, Miami, FL.
[‡] Cordis, Miami, FL.
[§]Mean based on random-effects model.
NM—not measured

FIGURE 4-42. Clinical and angiographic follow-up in patients who underwent renal artery stent placement. A meta-analysis of 14 studies compared the technical and clinical efficacy of renal artery percutaneous transluminal angioplasty (PTA) and stent implantation. The patients who received stents had a higher technical success rate and a lower restenosis rate when compared with patients only receiving PTA (98% vs 77% and 17% vs 26%; $P < 0.001$).

Among the 14 studies involving 698 patients, the technical success rate was 98% and the mean follow-up was 16 months. Hypertension was improved or cured in 69% of patients, and renal function improved or stabilized in 68% of patients. The mean restenosis rate was 17%, with a range from zero (study involving 21 patients followed for 9 months) to 39% (study involving 28 patients followed for 7 months). The restenosis rate in most contemporary series involving larger numbers of patients was between 9% and 20%.

The complication rate varies considerably among centers; high-volume centers generally can perform renal artery stenting with minimal morbidity and mortality. Although all studies reported use of an antithrombotic agent during the procedure, and most patients were discharged on an antiplatelet agent, the regimens varied.

Two recent studies evaluated the effect that renal artery stent implantation had on preserving renal function. Both studies used the reciprocal of the serum creatinine to determine the rate of decline or improvement in renal function. Harden et al. [89] placed renal artery stents in 32 patients (33 arteries) and reported that renal function improved or stabilized in 22 (69%) patients. In 25 patients with complete follow-up, Watson et al. [94] demonstrated that they all exhibited a negative slope to the reciprocal of the serum creatinine. After stent placement, the slopes were positive in 18 patients and less negative in seven patients. (*Data from* Leertouwer et al. [95].)

A. COMPLICATIONS ASSOCIATED WITH RENAL ARTERY STENT IMPLANTATION*

COMPLICATION	PERCENT
Renal failure	4.3
Segmental renal infarction	1.1
Perinephric hematoma	1.1
Renal artery thrombosis or occlusion	0.8
Stent misplacement	0.6
Brachial arterial occlusion	0.1
Mismatch of stent and vessel	0.1
Cholesterol embolism to lower extremities	0.1
Dissection of iliac artery	0.1
Brachial artery bleeding	0.1
Total major complications	8.9
Hematoma and access site complications	5.0
Total minor complications	5.0

*n = 678 patients, 799 treated arteries;
mortality rate was 1.0% (95% confidence interval 0–2).

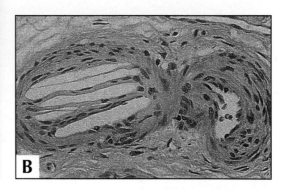

B

FIGURE 4-43. Complications associated with renal artery stent implantation. **A**, Common complications that occurred most frequently were contrast-induced acute renal failure and hematoma at the access site. Potentially devastating complications include atheromatous embolization to the kidneys (**B**), bowel and lower extremities, acute renal artery or stent thrombosis, and renal artery dissection. An experienced operator can limit many of these serious complications. Pseudoaneurysm at the access site can be treated with ultrasound-guided thrombin injection. (*Panel A adapted from* Leertouwer *et al.* [95].)

EFFECTS OF RENAL ARTERY STENTING ON RENAL FUNCTION IN PATIENTS WITH CONGESTIVE HEART FAILURE

BASELINE SERUM CREATININE, *mg/dL*	PATIENTS, *n*	IMPROVED, *n*	UNCHANGED, *n*	WORSE, *n*
1.1–1.9	9	2	5	2
2.0–2.9	12	7	3	2
3.0–3.9	8	5	2	1
> 4.0	10	6	0	4
Total	39	20 (51.4%)	10 (25.6%)	9 (23%)*

*Three patients required dialysis.

FIGURE 4-44. Effects of renal artery stenting on renal function in patients with congestive heart failure (CHF). This table demonstrates the serum creatinine values in a group of patients who improved (20 of 39 patients, 51%), remained unchanged (10 of 30 patients, 26%), or worsened (nine of 39 patients, 23%). The mean + SD serum creatinine prior to renal artery stenting was 3.2 + 1.6 mg/dL compared with 2.7 + 1.9 mg/dL post-procedure (P = 0.06). It should be noted that seven of 12 patients (58%) with a serum creatinine of 2.0 to 2.9, five of eight patients (63%) with a serum creatinine of 3.0 to 3.9, and six of 10 patients (60%) with a serum creatinine greater than 4.0 demonstrated improvement in renal function after renal artery stenting. Of the three patients who progressed to end-stage renal disease, the serum creatinine prior to the procedure was quite high (4.3, 5.5, and 7.9 mg/dL); this was a last effort to improve cardiac and renal function [96].

There have been several case reports and small series describing patients with bilateral renal artery stenosis (RAS) or RAS to a solitary functioning kidney who present with recurrent CHF or flash pulmonary edema [96–102]. Many of these patients have benefited from percutaneous transluminal angioplasty, stent implantation, or surgical revascularization.

All patients undergoing renal artery angioplasty and stenting in the Cleveland Clinic Foundation's peripheral intervention laboratory were prospectively entered into a peripheral vascular registry. Between 1991 and 1997, 207 patients underwent stenting of the renal arteries for atherosclerotic RAS. Thirty-nine of these patients had recurrent episodes of CHF and/or flash pulmonary edema. This represented 19% of all patients undergoing renal artery stenting in the peripheral interventional laboratory. Eighteen patients had bilateral RAS and 12 (66.6%) underwent bilateral stenting. Twenty-one patients had RAS to a solitary functioning kidney; all of these patients underwent unilateral stenting. Renal artery angioplasty and stenting was technically successful in all patients. Twenty of 39 patients (51%) had normal or mild left ventricular dysfunction on echocardiogram prior to intervention. Twelve patients (31%) had moderate and seven patients (18%) had severe systolic left ventricular dysfunction prior to stent implantation. The mean ± SD blood pressure before artery stenting was 174/85 ± 32/23 mm Hg compared with 148/72 ± 24/14 mm Hg after renal artery stenting (P < 0.001). There was a decrease in the number of blood pressure medications (3.0 ± 1 to 2.5 ± 1) necessary after renal artery stenting (P = 0.006). Twenty-eight patients (72%) demonstrated an improvement in blood pressure control.

EFFECTS OF RENAL ARTERY STENTING ON CONTROL OF CONGESTIVE HEART FAILURE

HOSPITALIZATIONS FOR CHF	BEFORE STENTING, n (%)	AFTER STENTING, n (%)
0	—	30 (76.9)
1	13 (33.3)	6 (15.4)
2	13 (33.9)	1 (2.6)
3	6 (15.4)	—
4	3 (7.7)	—
5	2 (5.1)	—
6	2 (5.1)	—

FIGURE 4-45. Effects of renal artery stenting on control of congestive heart failure (CHF). This study demonstrated that renal artery stenting decreased the severity of CHF, the frequency of flash pulmonary edema, and the need for hospitalization in most patients. The mechanism of CHF in these patients is not fully understood. Despite recurrent episodes of flash pulmonary edema and CHF, 51% of patients had normal left ventricular function or mild left ventricular dysfunction. Thirteen of 39 patients (33%) had a systolic blood pressure below 160 mm Hg at the time of congestive heart failure presentation. The mean + SD number of hospital admissions in the preceding year due to CHF prior to renal artery stent placement was 2.3 + 1.4 (range, 1 to 6). The mean number of hospitalizations post-procedure was 0.3 + 0.7 (range, 0 to 3) throughout the entire follow-up period (mean 21.3 months, P < 0.001). Thirty of 39 patients (77%) had no hospitalizations for CHF after renal artery stent implantation during a mean period of follow-up of 21.3 months. New York Heart Association Functional Class decreased from 2.9 + 0.9 before renal artery stent placement to 1.5 + 0.9 post-renal artery stent placement (P < 0.001). The American Heart Association Functional Class improved in 23 of 30 patients (77%) and remained stable in seven patients.

Four patients (four arteries) had greater than 60% stenosis on duplex ultrasound during follow-up. This was confirmed with selective arteriography and shown to be in-stent hyperplasia. All patients underwent repeat angioplasty and stenting with excellent results and no evidence of recurrent restenosis at latest follow-up. The mean period of follow-up for the entire cohort was 21.3 months (range, 1 to 61 months). Nine patients died during the course of follow-up from cardiovascular events. Eight of the nine patients died within 1 year. Seven of these nine patients (78%) had moderate to severe left ventricular dysfunction on echocardiography at baseline. Using Kaplan-Meier estimates, the mean + SE demonstrated that 95 + 4% were alive at 1 month, 87 + 5% at 6 months, 77 + 7% at 12 months, 77 + 7% at 24 months, and 72 + 8% at 36 months [96].

REFERENCES

1. Olin JW, Wholey M: Rupture of the renal artery nine days after percutaneous transluminal angioplasty. *JAMA* 1987, 257:518–519.

2. Olin JW, Begelman SM: Renal artery disease. In *Textbook of Cardiovascular Medicine*, edn 4. Edited by Topol E. Philadelphia: Lippincott Raven; 2002:2139–2159.

3. Gray BH, Young JR, Olin JW: Miscellaneous arterial diseases. In *Peripheral Vascular Diseases*, edn 4. Edited by Young JR, Olin JW, Bartholomew JR. St. Louis: CV Mosby; 1996:425–440.

4. Begelman S, Olin JW: Fibromuscular dysplasia. *Curr Opin Rheumatol* 2000, 12:41–47.

5. Harrison EG, McCormack LJ: Pathologic classification of renal arterial disease in renovascular hypertension. *Mayo Clin Proc* 1971, 46:161–167.

6. Olin JW, Novick AC: Renovascular disease. In *Peripheral Vascular Diseases*, edn 2. Edited by Young JR, Olin JW, Bartholomew JR. St. Louis: CV Mosby; 1996:321–342.

7. Stanley JC, Gewertz BL, Bove EL, *et al.*: Arterial fibroplasia, histopathologic character and current etiologic concepts. *Arch Surg* 1975, 110:561–566.

8. Stokes JB, Bonsib SM, McBride JW: Diffuse intimal fibromuscular dysplasia with multiorgan failure. *Arch Intern Med* 1996, 156:2611–2614.

9. Olin JW, Melia M, Young JR, *et al.*: Prevalence of atherosclerotic renal artery stenosis in patients with atherosclerosis elsewhere. *Am J Med* 1990, 88:46N–51N.

10. Scoble JE: The epidemiology and clinical manifestations of atherosclerotic renal disease. In *Renal Vascular Disease*. Edited by Novick A, Scoble J, Hamilton G. London: WB Saunders; 1996:143–149.

11. Dustan HP, Humphries AW, De Wolfe VG, *et al.*: Normal arterial pressure in patients with renal arterial stenosis. *JAMA* 1964, 187:1028-1029.

12. Harding MB, Smith LR, Himmelstein SI, *et al.*: Renal artery stenosis: prevalence and associated risk factors in patients undergoing routine cardiac catheterization. *J Am Soc Nephrol* 1992, 2:1608–1616.

13. Holley KE, Hunt JC, Brown AL, *et al.*: Renal artery stenosis: a clinical-pathologic study in normotensive and hypertensive patients. *Am J Med* 1964, 37:14–22.

14. Wollenweber J, Sheps SG, Davis GD: Clinical course of atherosclerotic renovascular disease. *Am J Cardiol* 1968, 21(1):60–71.

15. Dean RH, Kieffer RW, Smith BM, *et al.*: Renovascular hypertension. *Arch Surg* 1981, 116:1408–1415.

16. Tollefson DFJ, Ernst CB: Natural history of atherosclerotic renal artery stenosis associated with aortic disease. *J Vasc Surg* 1991, 14:327–331.

17. Rimmer JM, Gennari FJ: Atherosclerotic renovascular disease and progressive renal failure. *Ann Intern Med* 1993,118:712–719.

18. Goldblatt H, Lynch J, Hanzal RF, Summerville WW: Studies in experimental hypertension. I. The production of persistent elevation of systolic blood pressure by means of renal ischemia. *J Exp Med* 1934, 59:347–379.

19. Textor SC, Tarazi RC, Novick AC, *et al.*: Regulation of renal hemo-dynamics and glomerular filtration rate in patients with reno-vascular hypertension during converting enzyme inhibition with captopril. *Am J Med* 1984, 76:29–37.

20. Hricik D, Browning PJ, Kopelman R, *et al.*: Captopril-induced unctional renal insufficiency in patients with bilateral renal-artery stenosis or renal-artery stenosis to a solitary kidney. *N Engl J Med* 1983, 308:373–376.

21. Gifford RW Jr, McCormack LJ, Poutasse EF: The atrophic kidney: its role in hypertension. *Mayo Clin Proc* 1965, 40:834–852.

22. Carman T, Olin JW, Czum J: Noninvasive imaging of renal arteries. *Urol Clin North Am* 2001, 28:815–826.

23. Lawrie GM, Morris GC, Debakey ME: Long-term results of treat-ment of the totally occluded renal artery in 40 patients with reno-vascular hypertension. *Surgery* 1980, 88:753–759.

24. Carman TK, Olin JW: Diagnosis of renal artery stenosis: what is the optimal test? *Curr Interv Cardiol Rep* 2000, 2:111–118.

25. Nally JV: Captopril Renal Flow Scan. *Urol Clin North Am* 1994, 21:232.

26. Nally JV, Clarke HS, Jr, Grecos GP, *et al.*: Effect of captopril on ^{99m}Tc-diethylenetriaminepentaacetic acid renograms in two kidney, one clip hypertension. *Hypertension* 1986, 8:685–693.

27. Nally JV, Barton DP: Contemporary approach to the diagnosis and evaluation of renovascular hypertension. *Urol Clin North Am* 2001, 28:781–91.

28. Black HR, Bourgoignie JJ, Pickering T, *et al.*: Report of the working party group for patient selection and preparation. *Am J Hypertens* 1991, 4:745S–746S.

29. Prigent A, Cosgriff P, Gates GF, *et al.*: Consensus report on quality control of quantitative measurements of renal function obtained from the renogram: International Consensus Committee from the Scientific Committee of Radionuclides in Nephrourology. *Semin Nucl Med* 1991, 29:146–159.

30. Fommei E, Ghione S, Hilson AJW, *et al.*: Captopril radionuclide test in renovascular hypertension: a European multicentre study. *Eur J Nucl Med* 1994, 20:617–623.

31. Geyskes GG, Oei HY, Puylaert CBAJ, *et al.*: Renography with captopril. Changes in a patient with hypertension and unilateral renal artery stenosis. *Arch Intern Med* 1986, 146:1705–1708.

32. Mann SJ, Pickering RG, Sos TA, *et al.*: Captopril renography in the diagnosis of renal artery stenosis: accuracy and limitations. *Am J Med* 1991, 90:30–40.

33. van Jaarsveld BC, Krijnen P, Derkx FH, *et al.*: The place of renal scintigraphy in the diagnosis of renal artery stenosis. Fifteen years of clinical experience. *Arch Intern Med* 1997, 157:1226–1234.

34. Sfakianakis GN, Bourgoignie JJ, Daffe D, *et al.*: Single dose capto-pril scintigraphy in the diagnosis of renovascular hypertension. *J Nucl Med* 1987, 28:1383–1392.

35. Erbsloh-Moller B, Dumas A, Roth E, *et al.*: Furosemide ^{131}I-hippuran renography after angiotensin-converting enzyme inhibition for the diagnosis of renovascular hypertension. *Am J Med* 1991, 90:23–40.

36. Svetkey LP, Kadir S, Dunnick NR, *et al.*: Similar prevalence of renovascular hypertension in selected blacks and whites. *Hypertension* 1991, 17:678–683.

37. Setaro JF, Saddler MC, Chen CC, *et al.*: Simplified captopril renography in diagnosis and treatment of renal artery stenosis. *Hypertension* 1991, 18(3):289–298.

38. Dondi M: Captopril renal scintigraphy with ^{99m}Tc-mercaptoacetyl-triglycine (^{99m}Tc-MAG[3]) for detecting renal artery stenosis. *Am J Hypertens* 1991, 4:737S–740S.

39. Elliott WJ, Martin WB, Murphy MB: Comparison of two noninva-sive screening tests for renovascular hypertension. *Arch Intern Med* 1993, 153:755–764.

40. Mittal BR, Kumar P, Arora P, *et al.*: Role of captopril renography in the diagnosis of renovascular hypertension. *Am J Kidney Dis* 1996, 28:209–213.

41. Miralles M, Covas MI, Martinez ME, *et al.*: Captopril test and renal duplex scanning for the primary screening of renovascular disease. *Am J Hypertens* 1997, 10:1290–1296.

42. Johansson M, Jensen G, Aurell M, *et al.*: Evaluation of duplex ultra-sound and captopril renography for detection of renovascular hypertension. *Kidney Int* 2000, 58:774–782.

43. Olin JW: Role of duplex ultrasonography in screening for signifi-cant renal artery stenosis. *Urol Clin North Am* 1994, 21:215–226.

44. Olin JW, Piedmonte MA, Young JR, *et al.*: Utility of duplex scan-ning of the renal arteries for diagnosing significant renal artery stenosis. *Ann Intern Med* 1995, 122:833–838.

45. Hansen KJ, Tribble RW, Reavis SW, *et al.*: Renal duplex sono-graphy: evaluation of clinical utility. *J Vasc Surg* 1990, 12:227–236.

46. Hudspeth DA, Hansen KJ, Reavis SW, *et al.*: Renal duplex sono-graphy after treatment of renovascular disease. *J Vasc Surg* 1993, 18:381–390.

47. Radermacher J, Clavan A, Bleck J, *et al.*: Use of Doppler ultrasono-graphy to predict the outcome of therapy for renal-artery stenosis. *N Engl J Med* 2001, 344:410–417.

48. Thornton MJ, Thornton F, O'Callaghan J, *et al.*: Evaluation of dynamic gadolinium-enhanced breath-hold MR angiography in the diagnosis of renal artery stenosis. *J Am J Radiol* 1999, 173:1279–1283.

49. Saloner D: Determinants of image appearance in contrast-enhanced magnetic resonance angiography: a review. *Invest Radiol* 1998, 33:488–495.

50. Hahn U, Miller S, Nägele T, *et al.*: Renal MR angiography at 1.0 T: three-dimensional (3D) phase-contrast techniques versus gadolinium-enhanced 3D fast low-angle shot breath-hold imaging. *J Am J Radiol* 1999, 172:1501–1508.

51. Schreier DZ, Weaver FA, Frankhouse J, *et al.*: A prospective study of carbon dioxide-digital subtraction vs. standard contrast arterio-graphy in the evaluation of the renal arteries. *Arch Surg* 1996, 131:503–508.

52. Caridi JG, Hawkins IF Jr: CO_2 digital subtraction angiography: potential complications and their prevention. *J Vasc Interv Radiol* 1997, 8:383–391.

53. Meaney TF, Dustan HP, McCormack LJ: Natural history of renal arterial disease. *Radiology* 1968, 91(5):881–887.

54. Schreiber MJ, Pohl MA, Novick AC: The natural history of athero-sclerotic and fibrous renal artery disease. *Urol Clin North Am* 1984, 11:383–392.

55. Crowley JJ, Santos RM, Peter RH, *et al.*: Progression of renal artery stenosis in patients undergoing cardiac catheterization. *Am Heart J* 1998, 136:913–918.

56. Caps MT, Perissinotto C, Zierler RE *et al.*: Prospective study of atherosclerotic disease progression in the renal artery. *Circulation* 1998, 98:2866–2872.

57. Caps MT, Zierler RE, Polissar NL, *et al.*: Risk of atrophy in kidneys with atherosclerotic renal artery stenosis. *Kidney Int* 1998, 53:735–742.

58. Mallioux LU, Napolitano B, Bellucci AG, *et al.*: Renal vascular disease causing end-stage renal disease, incidence, clinical correlates, and outcomes: a 20-year clinical experience. *Am J Kidney Dis* 1994, 24:622–629.

59. USRDS 1993 Annual Data Report. National Institutes of Diabetes and Digestive Diseases. Bethesda, MD: The National Institutes of Health; 1993.

60. Connolly JO, Higgins RM, Walters HL, *et al.*: Presentation, clinical features and outcome in different patterns of atherosclerotic renovascular disease. *Q J Med* 1994, 87:413–421.

61. Conlon PJ, O'Riordan E, Kalra P: New insights into the epidemio-logic and clinical manifestations of atherosclerotic renovascular disease. *Am J Kid Dis* 2000, 35:573–587.

62. Dorros G, Jaff M, Mathiak L, *et al.*: Four-year follow-up of Palmaz-Schatz stent revascularization as treatment for atherosclerotic renal artery stenosis. *Circulation* 1998, 98:642–647.

63. The sixth report of the Joint National Committee on prevention, detection, evaluation, and treatment of high blood pressure. *Arch Intern Med* 1997, 157:2413–2446.

64. Antiplatelet Trialists' Collaboration: Collaborative meta-analysis of randomized trials of antiplatelet therapy for the prevention of death, myocardial infarction, and stroke in high risk patients. *BMJ* 2002, 324:71–86.

65. The Heart Outcomes Prevention Evaluation Study Investigators: effects of an angiotensin-converting-enzyme inhibitor, ramipril, on cardiovascular events in high-risk patients. *N Engl J Med* 2000, 342:145–153.

66. Jaff MR, Olin JW: Revascularization of atherosclerotic renal artery stenosis: Indications for intervention. *Texas Heart J* 1998, 25:34–39.

67. Pickering TG, Herman L, Devereux RB, *et al.*: Recurrent pulmonary oedema in hypertension due to bilateral renal artery stenosis: treatment by angioplasty or surgical revascularization. *Lancet* 1988, 2:551–552.

68. Van Bockel JH, Van Den Akker PJ, Chang PC, *et al.*: Extracorporeal renal artery reconstruction for renovascular hypertension. *J Vasc Surg* 1991, 13:101–110.

69. Novick AC, Ziegelbaum M, Vidt DG, *et al.*: Trends in surgical revascularization for renal artery disease. *JAMA* 1987, 257:498–501.

70. Libertino JA, Flam TA, Zinman LN, *et al.*: Changing concepts in surgical management of renovascular hypertension. *Arch Intern Med* 1988, 148:357–359.

71. Hansen KJ, Starr SM, Sands E, *et al.*: Contemporary surgical management of renovascular disease. *J Vasc Surg* 1992, 16:319–330.

72. Tarazi RY, Hertzer NR, Beven EG, *et al.*: Simultaneous aortic reconstruction and renal revascularization: risk factors and late results in 89 patients. *J Vasc Surg* 1987, 5:707–714.

73. Brewster DC, Darling RC: Splenorenal arterial anastomosis for renovascular hypertension. *Ann Surg* 1979, 189:353–358.

74. Hallett JW, Fowl R, O'Brien PC, *et al.*: Renovascular operations in patients with chronic renal insufficiency: do the benefits justify the risks? *J Vasc Surg* 1987, 622–627.

75. Bredenberg CE, Sampson LN, Ray FS, *et al.*: Changing patterns in surgery for chronic renal artery occlusive diseases. *J Vasc Surg* 1992, 15:1018–1023.

76. Zinman L, Libertino JA: Revascularization of the chronic totally occluded renal artery with restoration of renal function. *J Urol* 1977, 18:517–521.

77. Olin JW, Young JR, Graor RA: Thrombolytic therapy for renal artery occlusions. *Cleve Clin J Med* 1989, 56:432–438.

78. Kaylor WM, Novick AC, Ziegelbaum M, Vidt DG: Reversal of end stage renal failure with surgical revascularization in patients with atherosclerotic renal artery occlusion. *J Urol* 1989, 141:486–488.

79. Hansen KJ, Thomason RB, Craven TE, *et al.*: Surgical management of dialysis-dependent ischemic nephropathy. *J Vasc Surg* 1995, 21:197–209.

80. Wilms GE, Peene PT, Baert AL, *et al.*: Renal artery stent placement with the use of the Wallstent endoprosthesis. *Radiology* 1991, 179:457–462.

81. Kuhn FP, Kutkuhn B, Torsello G, Modder U: Renal artery stenosis: preliminary results of treatment with the Strecker stent. *Radiology* 1991, 180:367–372.

82. Rees CR, Palmaz JC, Becker GJ, *et al.*: Palmaz stent in atherosclerotic stenosis involving the ostia of the renal arteries: preliminary report of a multicenter study. *Radiology* 1991, 181:507–514.

83. Hennequin LM, Joffre FG, Rousseau HP, *et al.*: Renal artery stent placement: long-term results with the Wallstent endoprosthesis. *Radiology* 1994, 191:713–719.

84. Van de Ven PJ, Kaatee R, Beutler JJ, *et al.*: Arterial stenting and balloon angioplasty in ostial atherosclerotic renovascular disease. A randomised trial. *Lancet* 1999, 353:282–286.

85. Henry M, Amor M, Henry I, *et al.*: Stent placement in the renal artery: three-year experience with the Palmaz stent. *J Vasc Interv Radiol* 1996, 7:343–350.

86. Iannone LA, Underwood PL, Nath A, *et al.*: Effect of primary balloon expandable renal artery stents on long-term patency, renal function and blood pressure in hypertensive and renal insufficient patients with renal artery stenosis. *Cathet Cardiovasc Diagn* 1996, 37:243–250.

87. Blum U, Krumme B, Flugel P, *et al.*: Treatment of ostial renal-artery stenosis with vascular endoprostheses after unsuccessful balloon angioplasty. *N Engl J Med* 1997, 336:459–465.

88. Boisclair C, Therasse E, Oliva VL, *et al.*: Treatment of renal angioplasty failure by percutaneous renal artery stenting with Palmaz stents: midterm technical and clinical results. *Am J Roentgenol* 1997, 168:245–251.

89. Harden PN, MacLeod MJ, Rodger RS, *et al.*: Effect of renal-artery stenting on progression of renovascular renal failure. *Lancet* 1997, 349:1113–1136.

90. White CJ, Ramee SR, Collins TJ, *et al.*: Renal artery stent placement: Utility in lesions difficult to treat with balloon angioplasty. *J Am Coll Cardiol* 1997, 30:1445–1450.

91. Rundback JH, Gray RJ, Rozenblit G, *et al.*: Renal artery stent placement for the management of ischemic nephropathy. *J Vasc Interv Radiol* 1998, 9:413–420.

92. Shannon HM, Gillespie IN, Moss JG: Salvage of the solitary kidney by insertion of a renal artery stent. *Am J Roentgenol* 1998, 171:217–222.

93. Dorros G, Jaff M, Mathiak L, *et al.*: Four-year follow-up of Palmaz-Schatz stent revascularization as treatment for atherosclerotic renal artery stenosis. *Circulation* 1998, 98:642–647.

94. Watson PS, Hadjipetrou P, Cox SV, *et al.*: Effect of renal artery stenting on renal function and size in patients with atherosclerotic renovascular disease. *Circulation* 2000, 102:1671–1677.

95. Leertouwer TC, Gussenhoven EJ, Bosch JL, *et al.*: Stent placement for renal arterial stenosis: where do we stand? A meta-analysis. *Radiology* 2000, 216:78–85.

96. Gray B, Olin JW, Sullivan TM, *et al.*: Renal artery angioplasty with stenting in patients with congestive heart failure. *Vasc Med* 1998, 3:325.

97. Pickering TG, Herman L, Devereux RB, *et al.*: Recurrent pulmonary oedema in hypertension due to bilateral renal artery stenosis: treatment by angioplasty or surgical revascularization. *Lancet* 1988, 2:551–552.

98. Diamond JR: Flash pulmonary edema and the diagnostic suspicion of occult renal artery stenosis. *Am J Kidney Dis* 1993, 21:328–330.

99. Khosla S, White CJ, Collins TJ, *et al.*: Effects of renal artery stent implantation in patients with renovascular hypertension presenting with unstable angina or congestive heart failure. *Am J Cardiol* 1997, 80:363–366.

100. Walker F, Walker DA, Nielson M: Flash pulmonary oedema. *Lancet* 2001, 358:556.

101. Basaria S, Fred HL: Flash pulmonary edema heralding renal artery stenosis. *Circulation* 2002, 105:899.

102. Messina LM, Zelenock GB, Yao KA, Stanley JC: Renal revascularization for recurrent pulmonary edema in patients with poorly controlled hypertension and renal insufficiency: a distinct subgroup of patients with atherosclerotic renal artery occlusive disease. *J Vasc Surg* 1992, 15:73–80.

MESENTERIC VASCULAR DISEASE

CHAPTER 5

Magruder C. Donaldson

The mesenteric circulation is richly endowed with redundant anatomy in the form of collateral channels that connect the beds served by the celiac, superior mesenteric, and inferior mesenteric arteries. Arcades parallel the bowel wall connecting the distal branches of these arteries. Similar redundancy is present in the venous drainage beds. As a result, occlusion of major trunk vessels may be well tolerated, provided the occlusive process is sufficiently gradual to allow compensatory collateral enlargement and the major collaterals are themselves uninvolved. Even without intrinsic mesenteric disease, blood flow is influenced dramatically by physiologic vasoreactivity. This phenomenon comes into play in the face of various severe systemic illnesses associated with hypovolemia and circulatory collapse, and contributes prominently to the pathophysiology of nonocclusive mesenteric ischemia and mesenteric venous occlusion.

Vascular compromise in the mesenteric circulation has profound consequences. Acute arterial or venous occlusion usually results in tissue injury with the release of intracellular contents and byproducts of anaerobic metabolism into the general circulation. Compromised bowel mucosa allows unrestricted influx of toxic material from the bowel lumen with systemic consequences. If serosal surfaces are affected by full-thickness necrosis, bowel perforation and potentially catastrophic peritonitis ensue. The complexity of acute mesenteric insufficiency is all too often compounded by the presence of associated heart disease, systemic atherosclerosis, or life-threatening concurrent illness. In cases of chronic circulatory insufficiency, abdominal pain during eating causes "food fear," leading to reduced caloric intake with poor nutrition and weight loss.

Because acute mesenteric ischemia is so dangerous, early and aggressive diagnostic efforts are imperative. Manifestations may be subtle in patients with severe concurrent illness, although the onset of diffuse abdominal pain, bowel dysfunction, leukocytosis, and systemic effects such as respiratory failure should sound the alert. Endoscopy can provide direct visualization of the mucosal surfaces of the colon and should be considered regardless of the presence or absence of overt gastrointestinal symptoms or blood in the stool. In most circumstances, arteriography is valuable to clarify the status of the major branches of the celiac and mesenteric arteries, to provide information on possible alternative diagnoses, and to allow specific or supportive intra-arterial therapy with vasodilators, anticoagulants, balloon angioplasty, or stenting. Among patients with chronic arterial insufficiency, symptoms may be nonspecific but direct imaging of the vascular anatomy with magnetic resonance angiography, computed tomography, or contrast arteriography is usually sufficiently definitive to be indicated early in the diagnostic evaluation.

Therapy for acute ischemia is simplest and most successful when initiated promptly, since treatment is all too frequently futile after prolonged illness or when perforation and peritonitis have developed. Surgical consultation should be obtained early during the diagnostic evaluation to facilitate prompt exploratory laparotomy with thromboembolectomy and bowel resection when indicated. Surgery is best held in reserve in most cases of nonocclusive arterial insufficiency if aggressive hemodynamic support, antibiotics,

selective intra-arterial vasodilator therapy, and vigorous treatment of concurrent disease can be promptly instituted. It is often not possible to confirm the presence of mesenteric venous occlusion until progressive bowel ischemia forces laparotomy. In all acute situations, treatment of underlying disease is crucial to success, particularly among the majority of patients with concurrent cardiac illness. This comorbidity greatly compounds the severity of the problem and accounts in large measure for the fact that acute mesenteric occlusion is associated with mortality rates of 60% to 100%. In contrast, treatment of chronic mesenteric ischemia by a variety of means usually produces gratifying results.

MESENTERIC VASCULAR ANATOMY

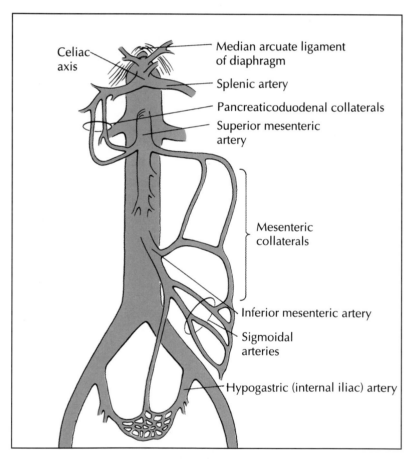

FIGURE 5-1. Diagrammatic representation of the mesenteric arterial anatomy showing the rich collateral network interconnecting celiac, superior mesenteric, inferior mesenteric, and internal iliac vascular beds. Because of these collaterals, gradual occlusion of two or three of the major aortic branches may be well tolerated. (*Adapted from* Stoney and Wylie [1].)

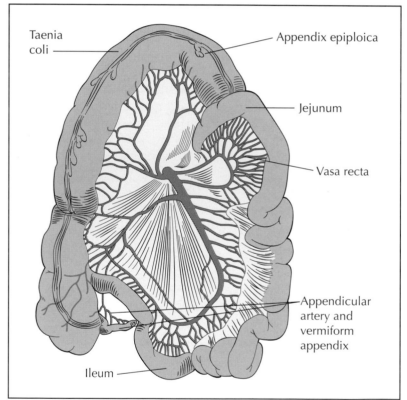

FIGURE 5-2. Anatomy of the small intestinal branches of the superior mesenteric artery. Note the arcades parallel to the bowel interconnecting the adjacent radial branches. (*Adapted from* Grant [2].)

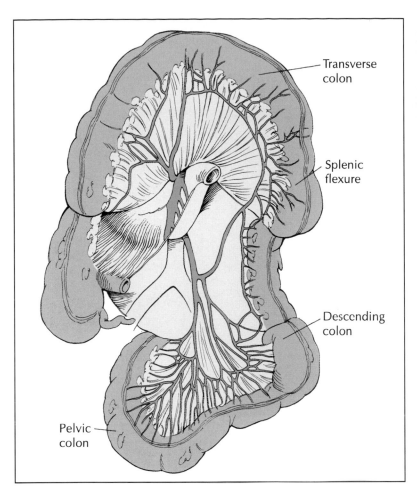

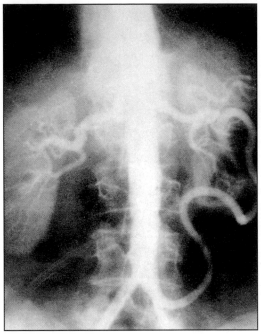

FIGURE 5-4. Large "meandering artery" providing a collateral from the inferior to the superior mesenteric arterial beds in the presence of severe superior mesenteric artery stenosis or occlusion.

FIGURE 5-3. Anatomy of the colonic branches of the superior and inferior mesenteric arteries. Note the anastomotic region between the two arterial beds in the region of the splenic flexure consisting of the ascending left colic branch of the inferior mesenteric artery and the left colic branch (marginal artery) of the middle colic artery. (*Adapted from* Grant [2].)

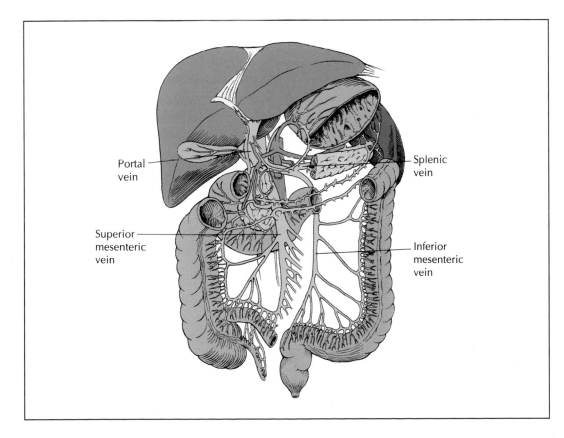

FIGURE 5-5. Anatomy of the mesenteric and portal venous system. Splenic and inferior mesenteric veins can be occluded with little consequence. Superior mesenteric and portal vein occlusion results in significant impairment of venous drainage. Gradual loss of flow generally allows time for collaterals to develop. Acute obstruction may cause stagnation at the capillary level in the bowel wall with consequent tissue damage. (*Adapted from* Sobotta and Figge [3].)

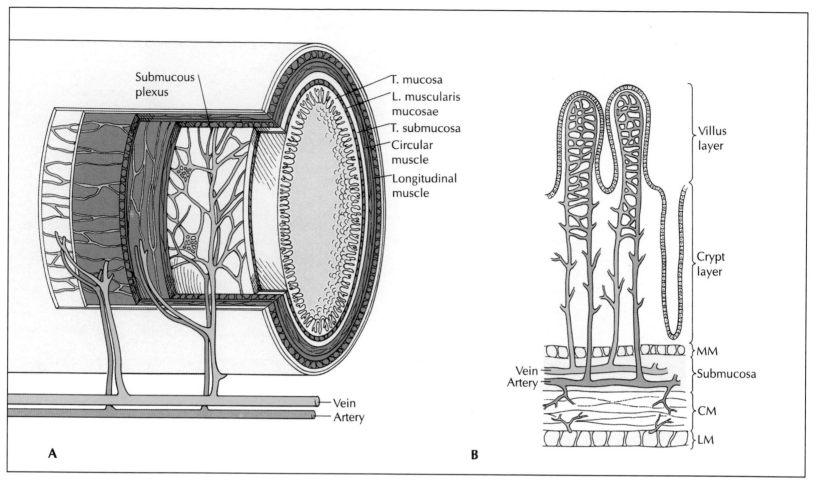

FIGURE 5-6. Vascular anatomy within the bowel wall, demonstrating the rich plexus of vessels in the submucosa supporting the oxygen-dependent mucosal surface. **A,** Cross-section of the bowel. **B,** Magnified view of the blood supply to the bowel mucosa. CM—circular muscle; LM—longitudinal muscle; MM—muscularis mucosa. (*Adapted from* Bloom and Fawcett [4].)

REGULATION OF MESENTERIC BLOOD FLOW

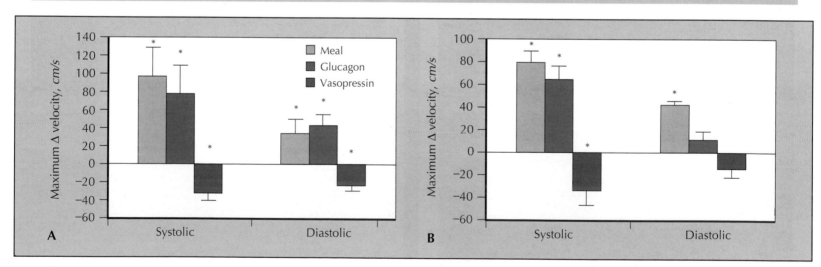

FIGURE 5-7. Measurement of mesenteric blood flow. The mesenteric arterial bed is capable of wide variations in flow in response to various stimuli. These graphs demonstrate maximum flow velocity changes as detected by ultrasound following a test meal and intravenous infusions of glucagon (40 µg/min) and vasopressin (0.2 U/min). **A,** Systolic and diastolic changes in the celiac artery. **B,** Systolic and diastolic changes in the superior mesenteric artery. *Asterisks* indicate values significantly different from control values (*P* < 0.05). *T-bars* indicate SEM. (*Adapted from* Lilly *et al.* [5].)

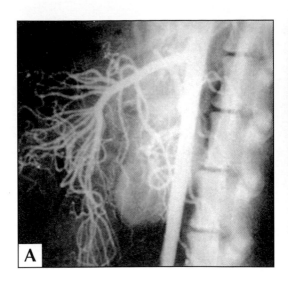
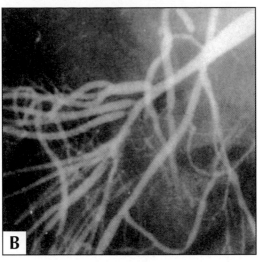

FIGURE 5-8. Vasospasm in the superior mesenteric artery (SMA). Vasospasm is fundamental to the pathophysiology of nonocclusive mesenteric ischemia and often contributes to mesenteric venous thrombosis. **A,** Normal selective arteriogram of the SMA with a smoothly tapering branch anatomy. **B,** Closer view of the SMA after infusion of levarterenol, 5 μg/min, demonstrating arteriographic features of spasm, including pinched origins of branches, interval stenoses, and rapid tapering of the periphery. (*From* Boley *et al.* [6]; with permission.)

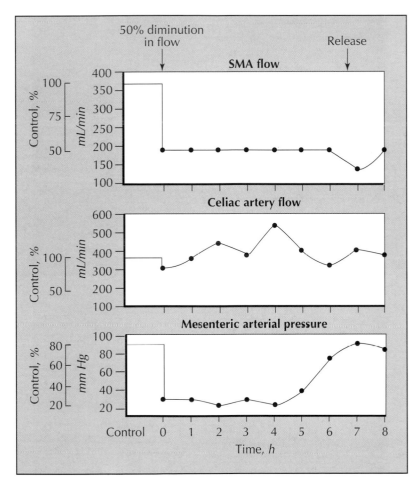

FIGURE 5-9. Vasospasm and bowel ischemia. Vasospasm may prolong bowel ischemia by persisting after relief of temporary proximal arterial occlusion. These graphs demonstrate the normal response to temporary interruption of flow in the canine superior mesenteric artery (SMA). Reduction of SMA flow to 50% of baseline (*top*) results in a reduction in mesenteric pressure, despite increased flow in the celiac artery. After 5 hours of reduced SMA flow, mesenteric pressure begins to increase with vasoconstriction of the mesenteric bed, with a consequent further reduction in SMA flow that persists for 2 hours after release of the SMA obstruction. Persistent SMA flow reduction can be ablated completely by infusions of papaverine into the SMA. (*Adapted from* Boley *et al.* [7].)

PATHOPHYSIOLOGY

RISK FACTORS FOR ACUTE OCCLUSIVE AND NONOCCLUSIVE MESENTERIC ISCHEMIA

Cardiac disease
  Cardiac arrhythmia
  Recent myocardial infarction
  Congestive heart failure
  Digitalis therapy
Previous arterial emboli
Hypercoagulable state
Hypovolemia, circulatory collapse

FIGURE 5-10. Risk factors for acute occlusive and nonocclusive mesenteric ischemia. Mesenteric ischemic frequently is associated with significant cardiac illness and other comorbidity, producing hypercoagulability or generalized circulatory collapse.

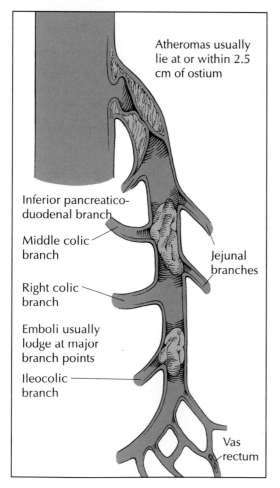

Atheromas usually lie at or within 2.5 cm of ostium

Inferior pancreatico-duodenal branch

Middle colic branch

Jejunal branches

Right colic branch

Emboli usually lodge at major branch points

Ileocolic branch

Vas rectum

FIGURE 5-11. Patterns of superior mesenteric artery (SMA) occlusion. Thrombotic occlusion of chronic atherosclerotic plaque is most often located at the origin of the SMA adjacent to the site of ostial disease, with secondary stasis thrombus deposited to the level of inflow from the chronically enlarged collateral. *Embolic occlusion* most often occurs at a more distal level as the embolus is pushed into the artery to a point where arborization reduces the lumen to a diameter less than that of the embolus. Acute embolic occlusion is generally a more profound and damaging insult than thrombosis at the site of chronic disease because of 1) lack of protection by the enlarged "prepared" collateral from the celiac or inferior mesenteric arteries, 2) occlusion at levels beyond the point of inflow of larger collaterals, and 3) occlusion of multiple branches to adjacent segments at the point of arterial arborization. (*Adapted from* Jackson [8].)

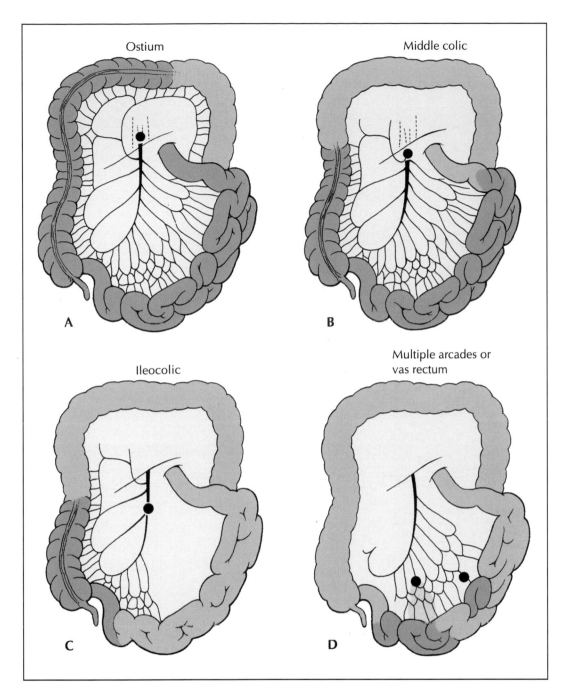

FIGURE 5-12. Patterns of bowel injury caused by isolated acute superior mesenteric artery (SMA) occlusion at various levels. **A,** Occlusion at the ostium of the SMA causes ischemia of the small intestine and the colon up to the transverse colon or splenic flexure when the inferior mesenteric supply is present via the left colic artery. **B,** Occlusion distal to the inferior pancreaticoduodenal and middle colic arteries spares the proximal small intestine and variable portions of the transverse and right colon. **C,D,** More distal occlusion at the ileocolic artery results in segmental distal ileal and cecal injury (*panel C*), and branch or arcade occlusions may cause patches of focal small intestinal ischemia (*panel D*). In many elderly patients, the inferior mesenteric artery is chronically obstructed and an acute proximal SMA occlusion would also cause injury to the left colon with sparing of the most distal colon and rectosigmoid because of the collateral via hemorrhoidal and sigmoid branches fed from the internal iliac arteries. (*Adapted from* Jackson [8].)

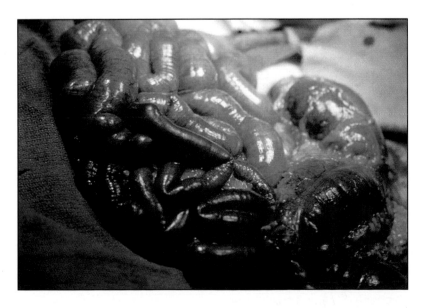

FIGURE 5-13. Gross pathologic specimen of acute small bowel ischemia from the embolus to the superior mesenteric artery. Note patchy areas of partial perfusion of the serosal surfaces. Mucosa typically is completely infarcted despite the presence of flow in some areas of the serosa. (*Courtesy of* Jerrold R. Turner, MD, Brigham and Women's Hospital, Boston, MA.)

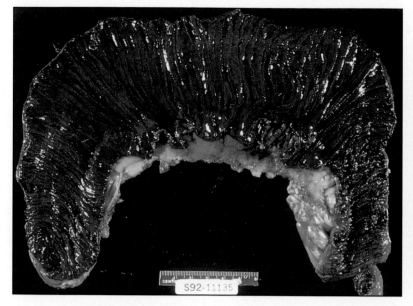

FIGURE 5-14. Gross pathologic specimen of acute small bowel ischemia, opened to reveal total diffuse infarction of the mucosa despite preservation of much of the serosa. (*Courtesy of* Jerrold R. Turner, MD, Brigham and Women's Hospital, Boston, MA.)

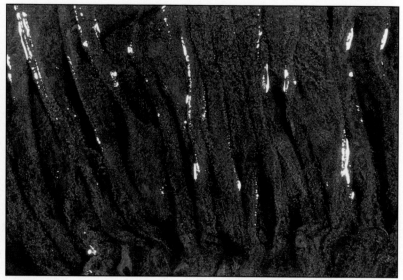

FIGURE 5-15. A closer view of the same specimen as in Fig. 5-14 demonstrating the nonviable, bile-stained mucosal border. (*Courtesy of* Jerrold R. Turner, MD, Brigham and Women's Hospital, Boston, MA)

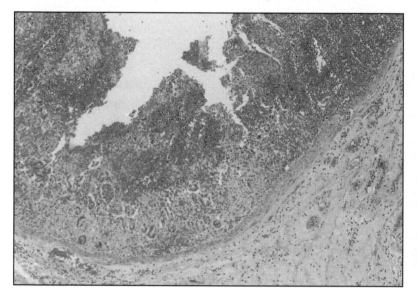

FIGURE 5-16. Micrograph of acute small bowel ischemia demonstrating complete necrosis of the mucosa with hemorrhagic slough in progress, and relatively intact microanatomy of the adjacent serosa. (*Courtesy of* Jerrold R. Turner, MD, Brigham and Women's Hospital, Boston, MA)

CONDITIONS ASSOCIATED WITH MESENTERIC VENOUS THROMBOSIS

Portal hypertension
  Cirrhosis
  Congestive splenomegaly
Inflammation
  Pancreatitis
  Peritonitis
  Inflammatory bowel disease
  Pelvic or intra-abdominal abscess
  Diverticulitis
Postoperative state and trauma
  Splenectomy and other postoperative states
  Blunt abdominal trauma
  Sclerotherapy for esophageal varices
Prothrombotic states
  Neoplasms (colon, pancreas)
  Oral contraceptives
  Pregnancy
  Antithrombin III, protein C/protein S deficiency
  Factor V Leiden
  G20210 prothrombin mutation
  Antiphospholipid syndrome
  Hyperhomocystinemia
  Polycythemia vera
  Thrombocytosis
  Paroxysmal nocturnal hemoglobinuria
Other conditions
  Renal disease (nephrotic syndrome)
  Cardiac disease (congestive heart failure)

FIGURE 5-17. Conditions associated with mesenteric venous thrombosis. Mesenteric venous occlusion results from conditions that produce stasis of flow, local venous injury or inflammation, or hypercoagulability.

PRESENTATION OF ACUTE MESENTERIC ISCHEMIA

Concurrent cardiac or debilitating disease
  Arrhythmia, recent myocardial infarction, valvular
    disease (embolus)
  Congestive heart failure, hemodynamic lability,
    septicemia (acute thrombosis, nonocclusive
    ischemia, venous thrombosis)
Pain out of proportion to tenderness
Abdominal distension, gastrointestinal dysfunction
Guaiac-positive stool

FIGURE 5-18. Presentation of acute mesenteric ischemia. Acute mesenteric ischemia is manifest by the presence of suggestive causative comorbidity, severe visceral pain, and evidence of bowel dysfunction and early mucosal slough.

DIAGNOSIS OF ACUTE MESENTERIC ISCHEMIA

Elevated white cell count (often > 20,000)
Evidence of "third" spacing (oliguria, hemoconcentration)
Metabolic acidosis
Elevated serum enzymes
Bowel distension, wall thickening on plane abdominal radiograph, CT
Endoscopic findings in colon
Specific findings on arteriogram

FIGURE 5-19. Diagnosis of acute mesenteric ischemia. Diagnosis is confirmed by laboratory, endoscopic, and clinical evidence of diffuse inflammation and tissue injury together with arterial occlusion on arteriogram.

PRESENTATION OF MESENTERIC VENOUS THROMBOSIS

Pain (insidious)	81%
Gastrointestinal bleed	19%
Guaiac-positive stool	63%
Anorexia	44%
Previous deep vein thrombosis	44%
Pancreatic cancer	13%
Hepatitis	25%
Thrombocytosis	25%
Increased fibrinogen	13%
Decreased protein C/protein S	50%

FIGURE 5-20. Presentation of mesenteric venous thrombosis. Mesenteric venous thrombosis is manifest by relatively subtle evidence of bowel congestion and stasis injury in association with suggestive comorbidity. (*Adapted from* Harward *et al.* [9].)

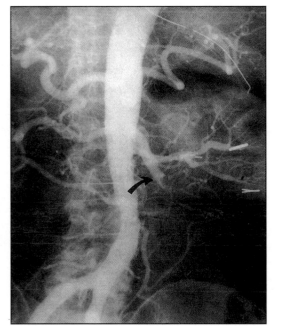

FIGURE 5-21. Anteroposterior aortogram of a patient with atrial fibrillation who presented with acute onset of severe periumbilical abdominal pain and an elevated white blood cell count. Abrupt embolic occlusion of the midsuperior mesenteric artery is evident (*arrow*), with no visible collateral from the normal patent celiac and inferior mesenteric arteries.

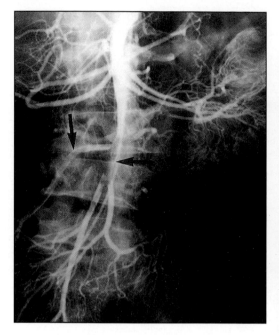

FIGURE 5-22. Anteroposterior aortogram of a patient who presented with acute onset of diffuse abdominal pain demonstrating intraluminal filling defects (*arrows*) in the ileocolic branches of an otherwise normal superior mesenteric artery. This demonstrates a classic pattern of embolic mesenteric occlusion.

RADIOLOGIC FINDINGS IN CLINICAL MESENTERIC VENOUS THROMBOSIS

Plain abdominal radiography (abnormal in 50%–70% of patients)
  Nonspecific ileus
  Ascites
  Small bowel dilatation
  Bowel wall thickening and irregularity
  Air in bowel wall or portal system
Barium studies of small intestine
  Small bowel dilatation
  Bowel wall thickening and irregularity
  Separation of bowel loops
  Focal hemorrhage (pseudotumors, thumbprinting)
Computed tomography
  Delayed venous phase in contrast study of small bowel
Angiographic studies
  Spasm of arteries
  Diminished or absent blood flow in affected bowel wall
  Delayed or absent venous drainage

FIGURE 5-23. Radiologic findings in clinical mesenteric venous thrombosis. Radiologic abnormalities after mesenteric venous thrombosis reflect bowel congestion and dysfunction.

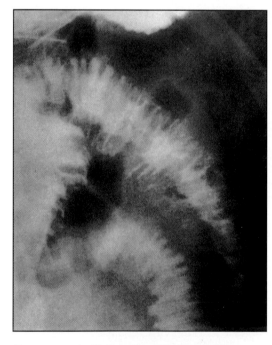

FIGURE 5-24. Delayed washout of dye after selective arterial injection in the presence of significant mesenteric vein obstruction. (*From* Harward and Bergan [10]; with permission.)

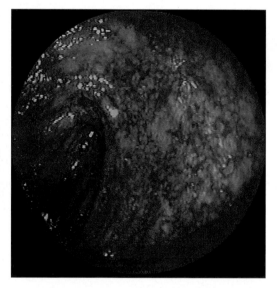

FIGURE 5-25. Colonoscopic view of subacute ischemic colitis of rectosigmoid demonstrating the friable, injected appearance of mucosa. The patient recovered with supportive care. (*Courtesy of* David L. Carr-Locke, MD, Brigham and Women's Hospital, Boston, MA.)

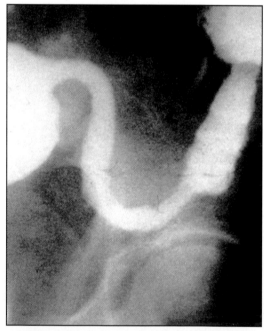

FIGURE 5-26. Healed fibrous stricture of the left colon 18 months after a segmental ischemic insult that recovered without infarction or perforation, a common endpoint of asymptomatic transient local colon ischemia. (*From* Boley *et al.* [6]; with permission.)

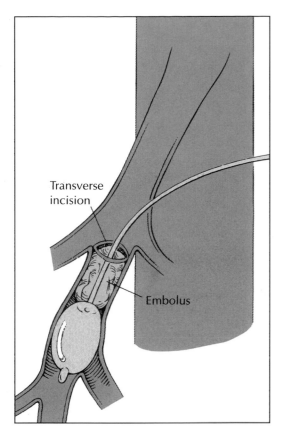

FIGURE 5-27. Thromboembolectomy of the superior mesenteric artery by exposure at the base of the transverse mesocolon. Although a transverse arteriotomy may suffice, it is preferable to open the artery longitudinally in order to afford wider exposure and precise closure with a vein or prosthetic patch angioplasty. This arteriotomy will also provide the point of distal anastomosis for a bypass graft originating from the adjacent aorta, iliac artery, or other source when indicated. (*Adapted from* Jackson [8].)

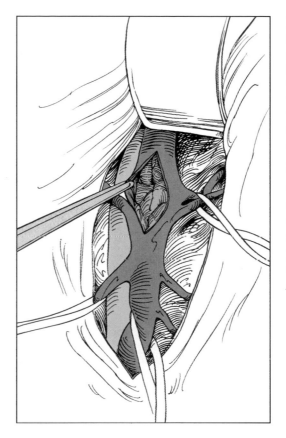

FIGURE 5-28. Surgical exploration for acute mesenteric ischemia. The technique illustrated for transverse opening of the superior mesenteric artery is appropriate for thromboembolectomy only when there is strong clinical evidence of embolization and no intrinsic disease palpable in the artery. (*Adapted from* Yao *et al.* [11].)

SUPPORTIVE MEDICAL THERAPY FOR NONOCCLUSIVE MESENTERIC ISCHEMIA

Aggressive hemodynamic management to obtain optimal cardiac output and reduce peripheral constriction

Specific therapy of underlying cardiac and systemic illness

Selective mesenteric arteriography for early diagnosis and intra-arterial vasodilator therapy

Antibiotics

FIGURE 5-29. Supportive medical therapy for nonocclusive mesenteric ischemia. Initial therapy for nonocclusive mesenteric ischemia emphasizes aggressive support of hemodynamics and treatment of any associated underlying illness.

THERAPY FOR ACUTE MESENTERIC VENOUS OCCLUSION

Aggressive hemodynamic and fluid management

Specific therapy of underlying systemic or peritoneal disease

Anticoagulation when safe

Surgical resection of compromised bowel

FIGURE 5-30. Therapy for acute mesenteric venous occlusion. This therapy emphasizes systemic resuscitation and treatment of associated illness with the judicious use of anticoagulants and surgical exploration.

EXTENT OF OBSTRUCTION IN CHRONIC MESENTERIC ARTERIAL INSUFFICIENCY

Celiac/SMA/IMA	41%–75%
Celiac/SMA	29%–82%
Celiac/IMA	2%
SMA/IMA	5%
Celiac	0%–14%
SMA	1.4%–9%

FIGURE 5-31. Extent of obstruction in chronic mesenteric arterial insufficiency. Although theoretically any one of the three major mesenteric arteries may be sufficient to maintain an adequate blood supply, a variety of patterns of occlusion can be found in studies of symptomatic patients. It is evident that the celiac and superior mesenteric arteries (SMA) are most important and that the inferior mesenteric artery (IMA) is much less important.

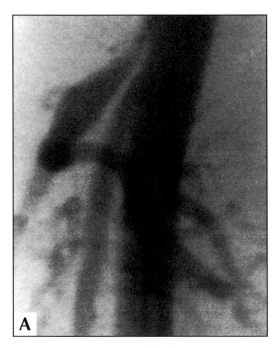
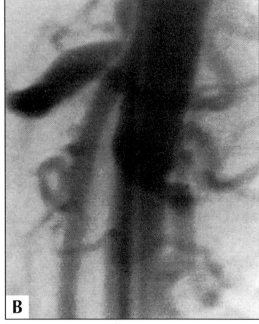

FIGURE 5-32. Median arcuate legament. The median arcuate ligament of the diaphragm frequently impinges upon the celiac artery in asymptomatic subjects. These lateral aortograms filmed during inspiration (**A**) and expiration (**B**) show the classic appearance of median arcuate ligament compression of the celiac axis, which is dramatically enhanced by diaphragmatic contraction during breathing. Although controversy persists, symptoms of vascular and/or neurogenic origin may occur in association with this anatomic finding. The ligament rarely impinges upon both celiac and superior mesenteric arteries. (*From* Reilly *et al.* [12]; with permission.)

SIGNS AND SYMPTOMS OF CHRONIC MESENTERIC ARTERIAL INSUFFICIENCY

SIGN/SYMPTOM	INCIDENCE, %
Pain	100
Weight loss	80–98
Abdominal bruit	68–75
Nausea, vomiting	54–84
Diarrhea	35
Constipation	13–26
Guaiac-positive stool	8

FIGURE 5-33. Signs and symptoms of chronic mesenteric arterial insufficiency. The clinical findings in chronic mesenteric insufficiency reflect postprandial pain, resulting in "food fear" and weight loss due to decreased caloric intake, mild gastrointestinal dysfunction, and, only rarely, evidence of malabsorption or mucosal injury.

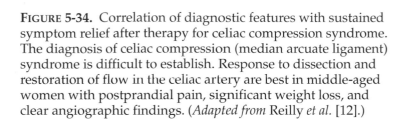

CORRELATION OF DIAGNOSTIC FEATURE WITH SUSTAINED SYMPTOM RELIEF AFTER THERAPY FOR CELIAC COMPRESSION SYNDROME	
FEATURE	CURED, %
Postprandial pain	81
Age 40–60 y	77
Female sex	70
Weight loss > 20 lb	67
Angiogram positive*	64
Atypical pain	43
Psychiatric/alcohol history	40
Age > 60 y	40

*Angiogram with poststenotic dilatation or increased collateral pattern.

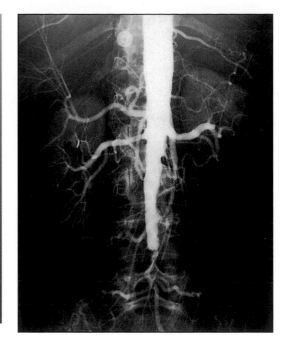

FIGURE 5-35. Anteroposterior aortogram of a patient with chronic abdominal pain and weight loss demonstrating aortic occlusion, severe tapering of the superior mesenteric artery branch anatomy, and apparent occlusion of the inferior mesenteric and splenic arteries.

FIGURE 5-34. Correlation of diagnostic features with sustained symptom relief after therapy for celiac compression syndrome. The diagnosis of celiac compression (median arcuate ligament) syndrome is difficult to establish. Response to dissection and restoration of flow in the celiac artery are best in middle-aged women with postprandial pain, significant weight loss, and clear angiographic findings. (*Adapted from* Reilly *et al.* [12].)

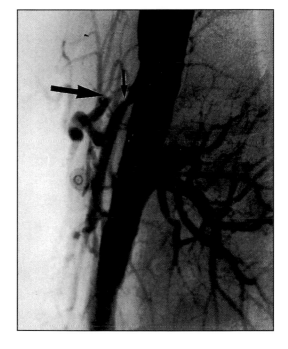

FIGURE 5-36. Lateral aortogram of the same patient as in Figure 5-35 demonstrating virtual total celiac artery occlusion (*large arrow*), superior mesenteric artery stenosis (*small arrow*), and inferior mesenteric occlusion.

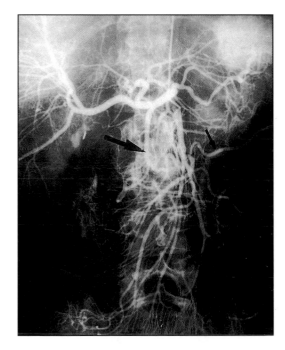

FIGURE 5-37. Selective arteriogram of the superior mesenteric artery (SMA) in the same patient as in Figures 15-35 and 15-36 showing proximal SMA stenosis and celiac occlusion, distal SMA disease, meandering collateral to left colic bed (*small arrow*), and retrograde reconstitution of the celiac artery branches via the pancreaticoduodenal and gastroduodenal arteries (*large arrow*).

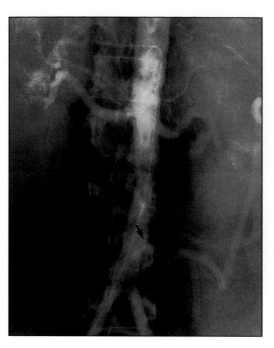

FIGURE 5-38. Anteroposterior aortogram of a patient with chronic postprandial pain demonstrating occlusion of the celiac and superior mesenteric arteries, with a large inferior mesenteric artery (*arrow*) giving rise to a retrograde collateral via the meandering artery. (*Courtesy of* C.J. Grassi, MD, and R.P. Chaturvedi, MD, Brigham and Women's Hospital, Boston, MA.)

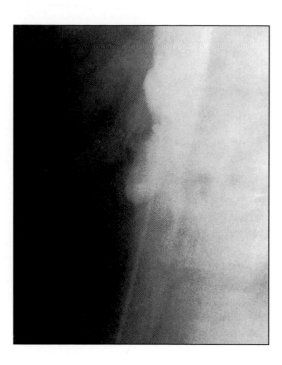

FIGURE 5-39. Lateral aortogram of the same patient as in Figure 5-38 demonstrating occlusion of the celiac and superior mesenteric arteries at their origins. Surgical exploration revealed a low median arcuate ligament impinging upon both arteries, and a thrombus was found in the arterial orifices and lining the adjacent aorta on aortotomy. Arteries otherwise appeared normal. (*Courtesy of* C.J. Grassi, MD, and R.P. Chaturvedi, MD, Brigham and Women's Hospital, Boston, MA.)

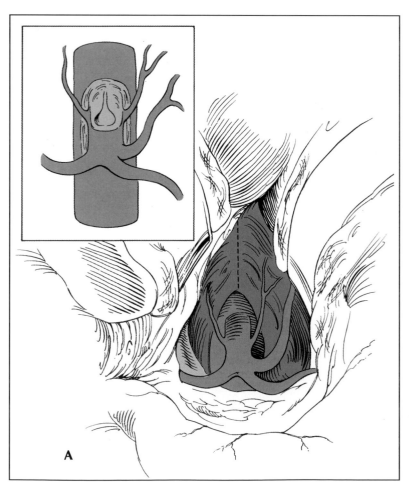

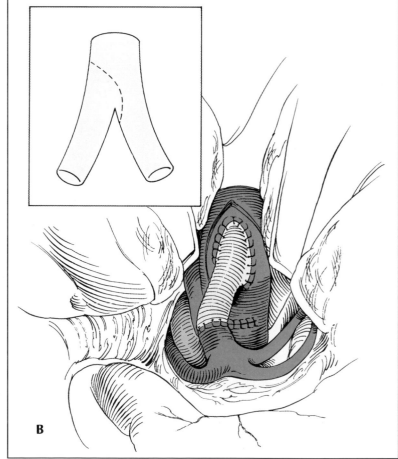

FIGURE 5-40. Therapy for chronic mesenteric ischemia. Treatment usually requires surgical bypass or endarterectomy of the involved arteries. **A,** Supraceliac exposure of the aorta through the gastrohepatic ligament for prosthetic bypass of the diseased celiac artery. **B,** Completion of a Dacron bypass using a tailored bifurcation prosthesis to create a conduit between the supraceliac aorta and celiac artery. (*Adapted from* Wylie *et al.* [13].)

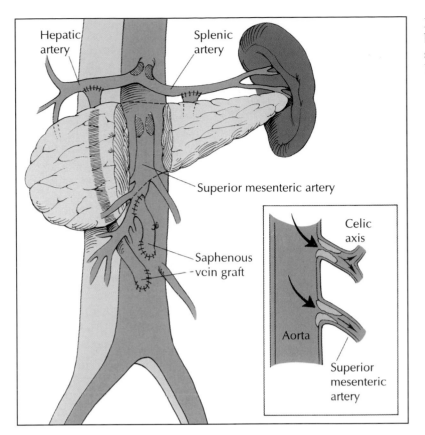

FIGURE 5-41. Some options for autogenous saphenous vein bypass from the aorta to the visceral arteries using hepatic or splenic branches to revascularize the celiac axis. (*Adapted from* Bergan and Yao [14].)

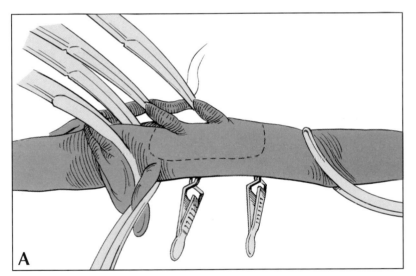

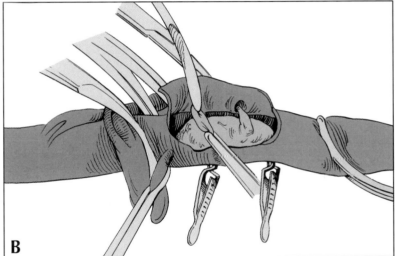

FIGURE 5-42. Transaortic endarterectomy of the celiac and superior mesenteric arteries is often the simplest and most direct means of revascularization for chronic mesenteric insufficiency. The visceral abdominal aorta has been exposed through the left retroperitoneum with medial visceral rotation to the right. The aorta and the celiac, superior mesenteric, and renal arteries have been occluded temporarily after heparinization. **A,** A "trap door" incision has been made in the aorta adjacent to the celiac and mesenteric arteries, with initiation of aortic endarterectomy. **B,** Aortomesenteric endarterectomy is completed by gently teasing out extensions of the aortic plaque that protrude into the orifices of the visceral arteries. (*Adapted from* Wylie *et al.* [13].)

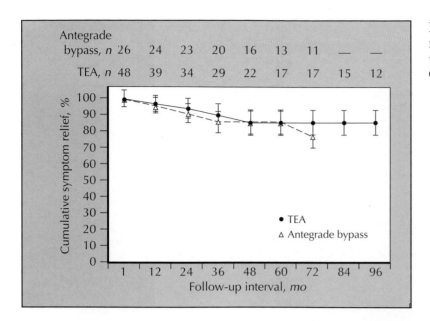

Antegrade bypass, n	26	24	23	20	16	13	11	—	—
TEA, n	48	39	34	29	22	17	17	15	12

FIGURE 5-43. Cumulative life table representation of symptom relief provided by antegrade bypass and transaortic endarterectomy (TEA) for chronic mesenteric insufficiency. (*Adapted from* Cunningham *et al.* [15].)

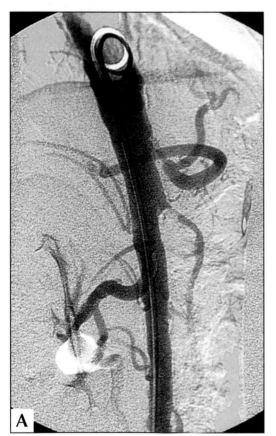

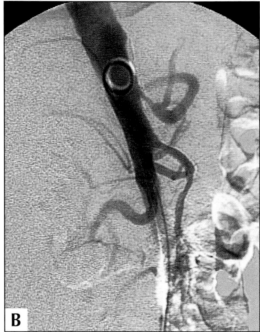

FIGURE 5-44. A, Lateral aortogram demonstrating stenosis of both celiac and superior mesenteric (SMA) arteries in a patient with chronic mesenteric ischemia. Note that the celiac stenosis is mainly extrinsic due to compression by the median arcuate ligament, making this artery an unfavorable target for catheter-based percutaneous intervention. In distinction, the SMA stenosis is nonostial in nature with no likely extrinsic component, making it a favorable target for percutaneous intervention with balloon angioplasty or stent. **B,** Favorable appearance of SMA after placement of a stent across the stenosis. Although percutaneous mesenteric angioplasty/stent procedures are appealing because of low procedural morbidity experienced in most series, they appear to be less durable than surgical therapy.

REFERENCES

1. Stoney RJ, Wylie EJ: Surgery of celiac and mesenteric arteries. In *Vascular Surgery: Principles and Techniques*. Edited by Haimovici H. New York: McGraw-Hill Book Company; 1976:668–679.

2. Grant JCB: *An Atlas of Anatomy*, edn 5. Baltimore: Williams & Wilkins; 1962.

3. Sobotta J, Figge FHJ: *Atlas of Human Anatomy*, vol 2. Baltimore: Urban & Schwarzenberg; 1977:115.

4. Bloom W, Fawcett DW: *A Textbook of Histology*. Philadelphia: WB Saunders; 1982:454.

5. Lilly MP, Harward TRS, Flinn WR, *et al.*: Duplex ultrasound measurement of changes in mesenteric flow velocity with pharmacologic and physiologic alteration of intestinal blood flow in man. *J Vasc Surg* 1989, 9:18–25.

6. Boley SJ, Brandt LJ, Veith FJ: Ischemic disorders of the intestines. In *Current Problems in Surgery*, vol XV, no 4. Chicago: Year Book Medical Publishers, Inc.; 1978:21.

7. Boley SJ, Regan JA, Tunick PA, *et al.*: Persistent vasoconstriction: a major factor in non-occlusive mesenteric ischemia. *Curr Top Surg Res* 1971, 3:425.

8. Jackson BB: *Occlusion of the Superior Mesenteric Artery*. Springfield, IL: C.C. Thomas; 1963.

9. Harward TRS, Green D, Bergan JJ, *et al.*: Mesenteric venous thrombosis. *J Vasc Surg* 1989, 9:328–333.

10. Harward TRS, Bergan JJ: Mesenteric venous thrombosis. In *Vascular Surgery*, edn 3. Edited by Rutherford RB. Philadelphia: W.B. Saunders; 1989:1113–1115.

11. Yao JST, Bergan JJ, Pearce WH, *et al.*: Operative procedures in visceral ischemia. In *Techniques in Arterial Surgery*. Edited by Bergan JJ, Yao JST. Philadelphia: W.B. Saunders; 1990:284–293.

12. Reilly LM, Ammar AD, Stoney RJ, *et al.*: Late results following operative repair for celiac artery compression syndrome. *J Vasc Surg* 1985, 2:79–91.

13. Wylie EJ, Stoney RJ, Ehrenfeld WK: *Manual of Vascular Surgery*, vol I. New York: Springer-Verlag; 1980.

14. Bergan JJ, Yao JST: Chronic intestinal ischemia. In *Vascular Surgery*, edn 3. Edited by Rutherford RB. Philadelphia: W.B. Saunders; 1989:1097–1103.

15. Cunningham CG, Reilly LM, Rapp JH, *et al.*: Chronic visceral ischemia: three decades of progress. *Ann Surg* 1991, 214:276–288.

6
CHAPTER

CEREBROVASCULAR DISEASE

Frances E. Jensen and Mark A. Creager

Stroke remains the third leading cause of death in the United States, with approximately 500,000 new stroke cases reported each year [1]. The term stroke encompasses both hypoxic/ischemic brain infarction as well as a variety of hemorrhagic conditions, including hypertensive intracerebral hemorrhage, subarachnoid hemorrhage, and hemorrhage related to arteriovenous malformation rupture.

Cerebrovascular disease can be classified broadly into several categories. The most common form is atherothrombotic stroke, which includes large- and small-vessel (lacunar) disease and accounts for approximately 60% of all strokes. Transient ischemic attacks occur almost as frequently, followed by cerebral embolism. Hemorrhagic disease, including intracerebral and subarachnoid hemorrhage, accounts for the majority of the remainder of cases. The differential diagnosis of stroke includes other causes of focal neurologic deficit or alteration of consciousness, including syncope, seizure, classic migraine, brain tumor, metabolic encephalopathy, vestibular vertigo, drug intoxication, or conversion reaction.

This chapter emphasizes cerebrovascular disorders that are encountered frequently by specialists in cardiovascular disease, including carotid stenosis, vertebrobasilar disease, and cerebral embolism from a cardiac source. The clinical presentation and diagnostic tests used to diagnose carotid stenosis are reviewed. These tests include duplex ultrasonography, magnetic resonance imaging, and contrast angiography. Therapeutic options ranging from platelet inhibitors to carotid endarterectomy are also discussed, with commentary on recent clinical trials. Also presented are cerebrovascular syndromes resulting from occlusive disease in the posterior cerebral circulation, such as those caused by vertebral and basilar artery atherosclerosis and those occurring after lacunar infarctions. Since stroke resulting from cardiac embolism is a treatable form of cerebrovascular disease, clinical trials that have assessed the prophylactic use of warfarin for cerebral embolism resulting from atrial fibrillation are reviewed.

CAUSES OF CEREBROVASCULAR ISCHEMIA AND INFARCTION

Atherosclerosis
Thrombosis
Lacunar disease
Embolism
Vasculitis
Vasospasm
Dissection
Venous thrombosis

FIGURE 6-1. Causes of cerebrovascular ischemia and infarction. Cerebrovascular ischemia and infarction can be classified into several major categories according to pathogenesis. Disorders of extracranial and intracranial arteries constitute the most common causes of cerebrovascular ischemia or infarction, and include atherosclerosis and thrombosis as well as microvascular occlusions and lacunar disease. The next most common causes are cerebral embolic events. Rarer causes of cerebral infarction include vasculitis, vasospasm (migraine), dissection, coagulopathies, and venous occlusive disease.

CEREBROVASCULAR DISEASE: CLINICAL PRESENTATION

Asymptomatic
TIA
RIND
Stroke

FIGURE 6-2. Clinical presentation of cerebrovascular ischemia secondary to carotid artery stenosis. Patients with carotid artery stenosis may have asymptomatic carotid bruits or may present with transient or fixed neurologic deficits. Transient cerebrovascular ischemia (transient ischemic attack [TIA]) causes symptoms that last from several minutes to 24 hours. TIAs are more commonly caused by intrinsic vessel disease than by cardioembolic events. Symptom complexes include transient monocular blindness and/or transient hemispheric attacks with hemiparesis, hemianesthesia, or aphasia. If untreated, TIAs carry a significant risk of stroke, approximately 5% to 6% per year. Reversible ischemic neurologic deficit (RIND) is a term that has been used to designate neurologic symptoms that improve within 24 to 36 hours, except for a mild residual neurologic deficit. A stroke in the carotid artery territory is a fixed neurologic deficit such as hemiparesis, hemianesthesia, and aphasia.

NATURAL HISTORY OF CAROTID STENOSIS

ANNUAL PERCENTAGE RATE OF VASCULAR EVENTS

DEGREE OF STENOSIS	TIA, %	STROKE, %	CARDIAC EVENT, %	VASCULAR DEATH, %
< 50% (mild)	1.0	1.3	2.7	1.8
50%–75% (moderate)	3.0	1.3	6.6	3.3
> 75% (severe)	7.2	3.3	8.3	6.5

FIGURE 6-3. Natural history of carotid stenosis. The risks of stroke, myocardial ischemia, and vascular death were determined by Norris *et al.* [2] using duplex ultrasonography in a cohort of 696 patients with asymptomatic carotid stenosis. Subjects were followed for an average of 44 months. The annual stroke rate was 1.3% in patients with carotid stenosis less than 75%, and 3.3% in patients with carotid stenosis greater than 75%. With stenosis of greater than 75% the combined transient ischemic attack (TIA) and stroke rate was 10.5%. Seventy-five percent of the events were ipsilateral to the stenosed artery. The annual cardiac event rate was 8.3% and the death rate in patients with greater than 75% carotid stenosis was 6.5%. (*Adapted from* Norris *et al.* [2].)

CAROTID ARTERY DISEASE: TIA

Transient hemispheric ischemia
  Duration < 24 h, usually < 15 min
  Symptoms: motor and sensory
    dysfunction of contralateral limbs
    (arm > leg)
  Pure sensory dysfunction
  Isolated dysphasia

Transient monocular blindness
  Duration < 30 min, usually < 10 min
  Symptoms: monocular visual
    obscuration, "blur, fog, shade, bright
    lights"

FIGURE 6-4. Carotid artery disease: transient ischemic attacks (TIAs). TIAs affecting the cerebral territory in the distribution of the carotid artery must, by definition, last less than 24 hours. The vast majority of TIAs last for less than 15 minutes. The clinical presentation may include motor and/or sensory deficits affecting the contralateral side of the face and limbs. Cognitive deficits, such as aphasia or apraxia, may also develop with cerebral cortical ischemia. Transient monocular blindness refers to a monocular alteration or loss of vision due to retinal ischemia. Retinal arterial occlusion is thought to result from platelet/fibrin plaques; classic Hollenhorst plaques are less common. Because the episodes are usually extremely short, occlusions are very rarely visualized by ophthalmoscopic examination. It is important to recognize that while the complaint of a "shade" lowering across the monocular field is a common presentation, other less well-defined symptoms can also be experienced, such as blurred or foggy vision, or bright flashes or lights.

CAROTID ARTERY DISEASE: STROKE

Territory
  Anterior cerebral artery
  Middle cerebral artery
Mechanisms
  Proximal stenosis/occlusion
  Artery-to-artery embolism
Clinical presentation
  Contralateral weakness
  Contralateral sensory deficit
  Aphasia, apraxia
  Visual deficits

FIGURE 6-5. Carotid artery disease: stroke. Stroke caused by carotid artery disease usually affects the middle and/or anterior cerebral artery divisions of the internal carotid artery. The posterior cerebral artery distribution is often spared because it is supplied from the posterior vertebrobasilar circulation. The major mechanisms of ischemic injury in the carotid territory are reduced distal flow secondary to a proximal stenosis, and artery-to-artery embolization from a proximal atherosclerotic plaque. Regardless of the cause, transient ischemic attacks often precede stroke. Clinical deficits are often less severe in patients with distal arterial insufficiency compared with deficits occurring as a result of cerebral embolism. The most commonly occurring symptoms are contralateral weakness, apraxia, numbness and tingling, and homonomous hemifield visual deficits. Cognitive deficits include aphasia, confusional episodes, and difficulty reading or writing. Ocular infarction is uncommon, and can take the form of either central retinal artery occlusion or ischemic optic neuropathy. Patients presenting with central retinal artery occlusion, visible as retinal pallor on funduscopic examination, have a high incidence (50% to 70% of cases) of concurrent carotid disease. These patients present with the complaint of monocular blindness or scotoma.

DIAGNOSTIC TESTS

DIAGNOSTIC TESTS FOR CAROTID STENOSIS AND STROKE

CAROTID STENOSIS

Duplex ultrasonography
MR angiography
Contrast angiography

STROKE

CT
MR imaging

FIGURE 6-6. Diagnostic tests. A variety of diagnostic tests can be used to evaluate patients for carotid artery stenosis and stroke. Duplex ultrasonography is a noninvasive diagnostic test for carotid stenosis that combines gray scale imaging and pulsed Doppler analysis to localize a stenosis and assess its severity. The positive predictive value for duplex carotid ultrasonography to detect a hemodynamically significant stenosis is more than 95%. Magnetic resonance (MR) angiography is also noninvasive and is utilized often as an effective method to demonstrate cerebrovascular stenoses. Contrast angiography is invasive but remains the gold standard for diagnosis of carotid and other cerebrovascular stenoses and occlusions. In many centers, duplex ultrasonography, often combined with MR angiography, has replaced the need for most contrast angiograms in patients with carotid artery disease. Tests used to confirm stroke and precisely localize the affected part of the brain include computed tomography (CT) and MR imaging.

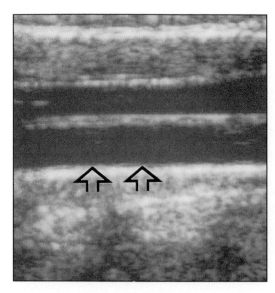

FIGURE 6-7. B-scan imaging. Ultrasonic examination of the carotid artery uses instruments that combine real-time B-mode imaging and Doppler ultrasound, and is referred to as *duplex ultrasonography*. High-resolution B-scan imaging can identify the boundaries between different layers of the arterial wall in normal individuals. Shown is an example of a B-scan image of a normal carotid artery. Typically, with a longitudinal view of the carotid artery, the layers appear as two parallel echogenic lines separated by a hypoechoic space. The lines represent the intima-media and the media-adventitia interfaces; the echolucent space is the media. In this normal artery, the intima-media interface is visible as a thin echodense line (*arrows*). There is no plaque formation and the lumen is unobstructed.

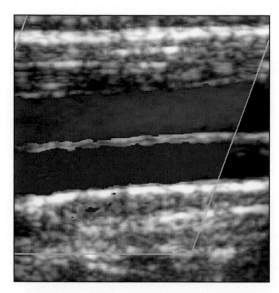

FIGURE 6-8. Color-assisted duplex ultrasonography. The color-assisted duplex ultrasound processes the Doppler ultrasound signal in real time to assess the velocity of blood in the artery over the entire field that is being imaged. This information is superimposed on the grayscale (B-scan) image to provide a composite real-time display of both anatomy and flow. This example of a color-assisted duplex ultrasound examination of a normal carotid artery (*red*) demonstrates normal laminar blood flow within a vessel. The internal jugular vein (*blue*) can be seen anterior to the carotid artery.

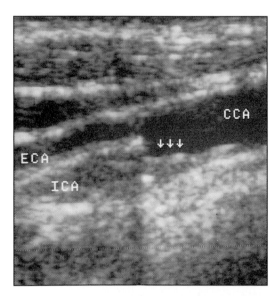

FIGURE 6-9. Duplex ultrasonography. Ultrasound imaging techniques are capable of demonstrating atherosclerotic plaque, but Doppler techniques are necessary to assess the severity of more advanced stenoses. In this example of a duplex ultrasound examination of a carotid artery, there is significant atherosclerotic plaque causing a stenosis of 90%. The thickened intima and media interface is evident (*arrows*). Plaque formation has encroached upon the lumen, creating a stenosis. The severity of stenosis was determined by measuring the Doppler velocity, which increases as the severity of stenosis increases. CCA—common carotid artery; ECA—external carotid artery; ICA—internal carotid artery.

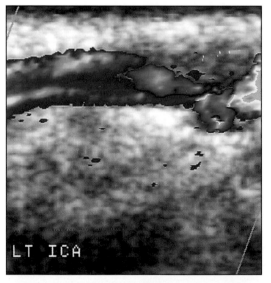

FIGURE 6-10. Color-assisted duplex ultrasound examination of a stenotic left internal carotid artery (LT ICA). In this vessel, blood flow accelerates through the stenosis. Flow becomes turbulent at the site of the stenosis, which is depicted by the color examination showing both dropout of color at the site of the plaque as well as turbulence of flow (red to blue).

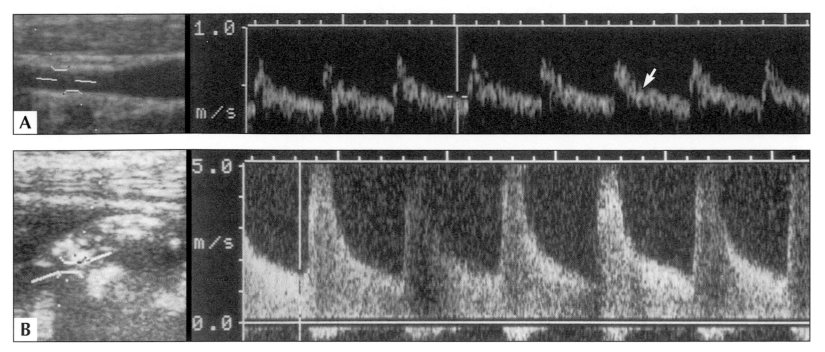

FIGURE 6-11. Pulse-wave Doppler velocity. The pulsed-wave Doppler component of the carotid ultrasound examination enables the examiner to interrogate the blood velocity within the lumen of the vessel. In a normal vessel, flow accelerates during systole. Most red cells move at a similar rate of speed, accounting for the envelope (*arrow*) that defines the velocity profile.

A, Normally, the pulsed-wave Doppler velocity is less than 1 m/s (< 100 cm/s). **B,** In the presence of a significant stenosis, however, the velocity accelerates through the stenotic lesion. In this example, the velocity has increased to 4 m/s (400 cm/s). Furthermore, cells are no longer moving at the same rate of speed, accounting for substantial broadening of the Doppler display.

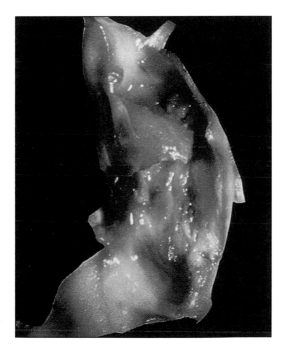

FIGURE 6-12. Gross pathologic specimen of a carotid atherosclerotic plaque, showing near occlusion of the lumen. Atherosclerotic plaques can be complicated by ulceration, the production of microemboli from plaque fragmentation, and plaque hemorrhage.

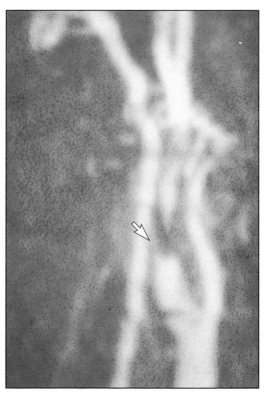

FIGURE 6-13. Magnetic resonance (MR) angiogram of extracranial arteries, showing high-grade stenosis of the internal carotid artery (*arrow*). Recent advances in MR angiography technology have produced high-quality imaging of the neck and proximal intracranial vessels. The technique is noninvasive, and its accuracy approaches that of duplex ultrasonography.

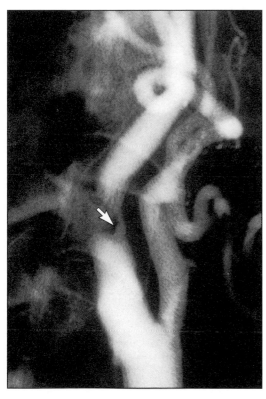

FIGURE 6-14. Conventional contrast angiogram of the carotid arteries from the patient in Fig. 6-13, demonstrating a high-grade stenosis in the proximal carotid artery (*arrow*). Standard arteriography is still the preferred method when magnetic resonance angiography and ultrasound have yielded ambiguous results regarding the status of extracranial carotid arteries, or when information regarding the status of the intracranial vasculature is required.

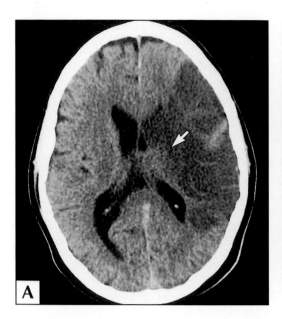

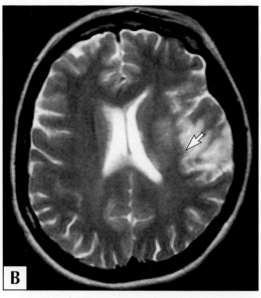

FIGURE 6-15. Computed tomography scan and magnetic resonance image of a cortical infarct. **A,** Computed tomography of a cortical infarct in the distribution of the left middle cerebral artery. This scan was obtained in a patient 3 days after a stroke who presented with sudden onset of aphasia, right hemiparesis, right-sided sensory deficit, and right homonomous hemianopsia. It shows a large low-density lesion (*arrow*) in the left middle cerebral artery distribution. **B,** A T$_2$-weighted magnetic resonance image of the same lesion. The infarction is visible as a hyperintense area (*arrow*). This image was obtained 2 weeks after the stroke. (*From* Jensen [3]; with permission.)

TREATMENT OF CEREBRAL ATHEROTHROMBOSIS

TREATMENT OF CEREBRAL ATHEROTHROMBOSIS

Platelet inhibitors
　Aspirin
　Aspirin with dipyridamole
　Clopidogrel/ticlopidine
Anticoagulants
　Heparin
　Warfarin
Lipid lowering drugs
　Statins
Carotid endarterectomy
Carotid artery stent

FIGURE 6-16. Multiple therapeutic options for the treatment of cerebral atherothrombosis. Surgical endarterectomy is recommended for both symptomatic and asymptomatic high-grade lesions (> 70%) of the internal carotid artery. For patients with lower-grade lesions, antiplatelet agents are the first line of therapy. Anticoagulants are reserved for patients who have failed antiplatelet therapy and do not have high-grade occlusion.

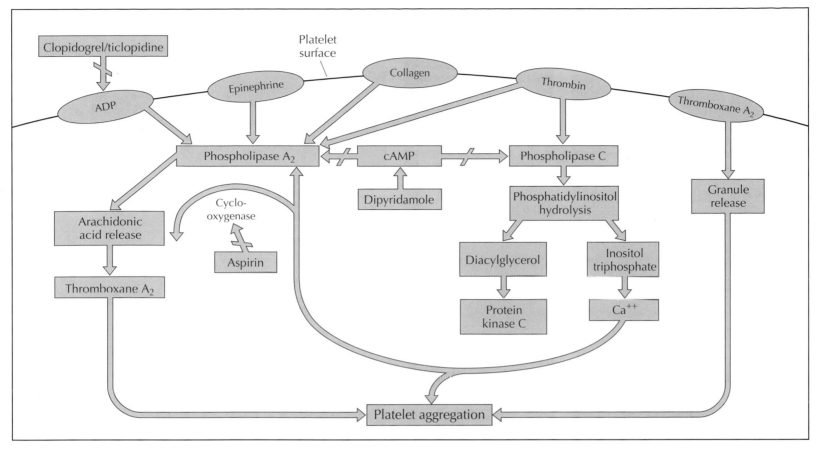

FIGURE 6-17. Platelet activation. Platelet activation is a key step in the development of cerebral ischemia due to atherosclerosis, and antiplatelet agents have proven useful therapeutic agents. Aspirin (usually in doses of 81 to 325 mg/d) alone or in combination with dipyridamole (400 mg/d) and the thienopyridine derivatives, ticlopidine (250 mg twice daily) or clopidogrel (75 mg/d), have been shown to have clinical efficacy in large multicenter trials [4–8]. These drugs can prevent transient ischemic attacks and stroke due to atherosclerosis. The mechanism of action of aspirin is to reduce platelet aggregation by inhibiting platelet cyclo-oxygenase and preventing the formation of thromboxane A_2. Ticlopidine and clopidogrel inhibit ADP-dependent platelet-fibrinogen binding and subsequent platelet-platelet interactions. Dipyridamole inhibits phosphodiesterase and increases cAMP, which inhibits phospholipase A_2 and phospholipase C.

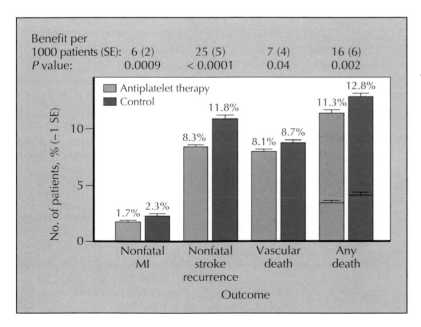

FIGURE 6-18. The effect of antiplatelet therapy on stroke, myocardial infarction, or vascular death in patients with cerebrovascular disease: the Antithrombotic Trialists' Collaboration [4]. A meta-analysis evaluating the effect of antiplatelet therapy in all trials conducted up to 1997 was performed. Data for more than 18,000 patients with a prior history of stroke or transient ischemic attack who were followed for a mean duration of 29 months were analyzed. There was a 22% relative reduction in the risk of either stroke, myocardial infarction, or cardiovascular death in patients randomized to active treatment with antiplatelet drugs as compared with control patients. Among these patients, there was a significant reduction in nonfatal stroke (25 per 1000), nonfatal myocardial infarction (6 per 1000), and vascular deaths (7 per 1000). *T-bars* indicate standard error. (*Adapted from* [4].)

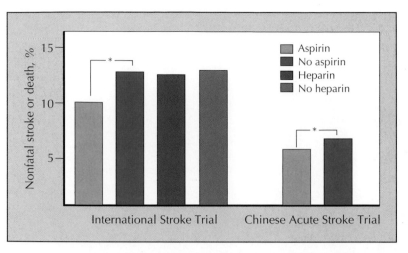

FIGURE 6-19. Efficacy and safety of aspirin and heparin in patients with acute ischemic strokes. The International Stroke Trial

randomized 19,435 patients with acute ischemic stroke to unfractionated heparin (5000 units or 12,500 units twice daily), aspirin (300 mg/d), or both heparin and aspirin. Among the patients treated with aspirin, there were 2.8% recurrent ischemic strokes within 14 days compared with 3.9% in the groups not receiving aspirin and no excess of hemorrhagic strokes. At 14 days, there was a 9% relative risk reduction in death or any nonfatal recurrent stroke in the aspirin-treated group (11.3% vs 12.4%). Among the heparin-treated patients, there were 2.9% recurrent ischemic strokes within 14 days compared with 3.8% in the group not receiving heparin, but there were more hemorrhagic strokes in the patients receiving heparin (1.2% vs 0.4%). At 14 days there was no difference in the risk of death or nonfatal stroke between heparin and no heparin treatment (11.7% vs 12.0%, respectively). The Chinese Acute Stroke Trial studied the effect of aspirin (160 mg/d) versus placebo in 21,106 patients with acute ischemic stroke. At 4 weeks, there was a 12% reduction (5.3% vs 5.9%) in the risk of death or nonfatal stroke. (*Adapted from* [7,8].)

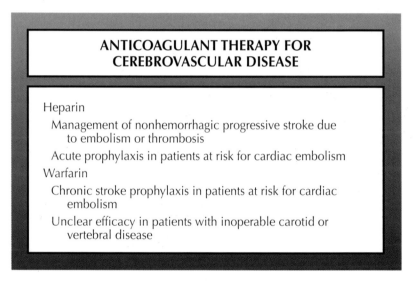

FIGURE 6-20. Anticoagulant therapy for cerebrovascular disease. Heparin inhibits activation of factor Xa and catalyzes the inhibition of factors IXa, XIa, and XIIa by antithrombin III. It is indicated for both acute management of nonhemorrhagic progressive embolic or thrombotic stroke and acute stroke prophylaxis in patients with cardioembolic risk factors, *ie*, atrial fibrillation.

Warfarin inhibits vitamin K–induced hepatic synthesis of factors II, VII, IX, and X, and proteins S and C. It is indicated for chronic stroke prophylaxis in patients at risk for emboli from a cardiac source. Its efficacy in patients with inoperable carotid or vertebral disease and in those with symptoms refractory to antiplatelet therapy due to large-vessel disease is not known.

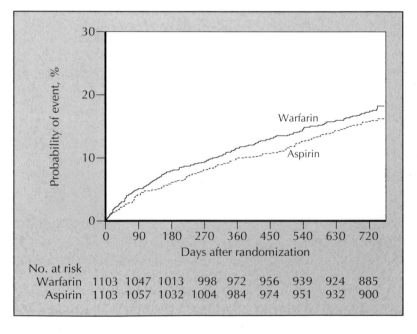

FIGURE 6-21. Efficacy of warfarin versus aspirin for the prevention of recurrent ischemic stroke. In a multicenter, double-blind, randomized trial, the effect of warfarin (dose-adjusted for an international normalized ratio of 1.4 to 2.8) was compared with that of aspirin (325 mg/d) on the combined primary endpoint of recurrent ischemic stroke or death from any cause. The primary endpoint was reached by 17.8% of patients assigned to warfarin (196 of 1103 patients) and 16% of those assigned to aspirin (176 of 1103 patients). There was no significant treatment-related difference between the two groups in the frequency or time to recurrent ischemic stroke or death. The rates of major hemorrhage were 2.22 per 100 patient-years in the warfarin group and 1.49 per 100 patient-years in the aspirin group. The results of this study indicate that both aspirin and warfarin are reasonable therapies to prevent recurrent ischemic stroke. (*Adapted from* Mohr *et al.* [6].)

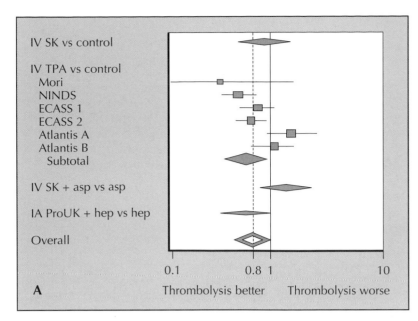

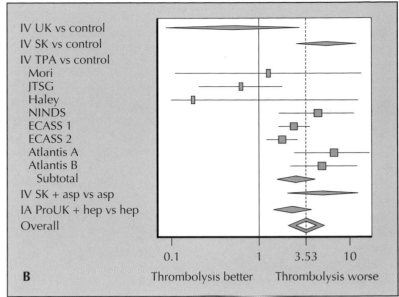

A Thrombolysis better   Thrombolysis worse

B Thrombolysis better   Thrombolysis worse

FIGURE 6-22. Efficacy of thrombolytic therapy following ischemic stroke. A meta-analysis of 17 completed randomized control trials of thrombolytic therapy versus control in 5216 patients determined the effect of thrombolytic therapy after an ischemic stroke on death, intracranial hemorrhage, and poor functional outcome within the first 7–10 days after treatment (**A**) and symptomatic intracranial hemorrhage at long-term follow-up (**B**). There was a reduction in poor functional outcome, *ie*, death or dependency with thrombolysis treatment at the end of follow-up (odds ratio, 0.83) and an increase of symptomatic intracranial

hemorrhage with thrombolytic therapy (odds ratio, 3.53). In the subgroup of patients treated within 3 hours of symptom onset, there was an even greater reduction in poor functional outcome with thrombolysis (odds ratio, 0.58). Asp—aspirin; ECASS—European Cooperative Acute Stroke Study; hep—heparin; IA—intra-arterial; IV—intravenous; JTSG—Japanese Thrombolysis Study Group; NINDS—National Institute of Neurological Disorders and Stroke; ProUK—prourokinase; SK—streptokinase; TPA—tissue plasminogen activator; UK—urokinase.(*Adapted from* Wardlaw *et al.* [9].)

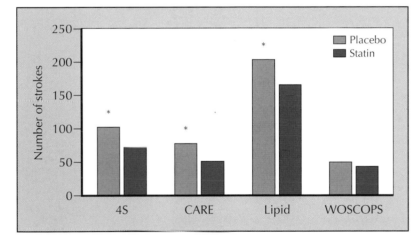

FIGURE 6-23. Efficacy of statins in reducing the incidence of stroke. Lipid lowering therapy with statins has been shown to reduce the incidence of stroke in secondary prevention trials of patients with coronary artery disease and hypercholesterolemia. The Scandinavian Simvastatin Survival Study (4S) found that simvastatin compared with placebo resulted in a 30% reduction in the incidence of ischemic stroke and transient ischemic attack. The Cholesterol and Recurrent Events (CARE) trial found that pravastatin compared with placebo resulted in a 32% reduction in the incidence of stroke. In the Long-term Intervention with Pravastatin in Ischemic Disease (LIPID) study, pravastatin resulted in a 19% reduction in the incidence of stroke. In the West of Scotland Coronary Prevention Study (WOSCOPS), a primary prevention study, pravastatin reduced the incidence of stroke by 11%. (*Adapted from* Mohler *et al.* [10].)

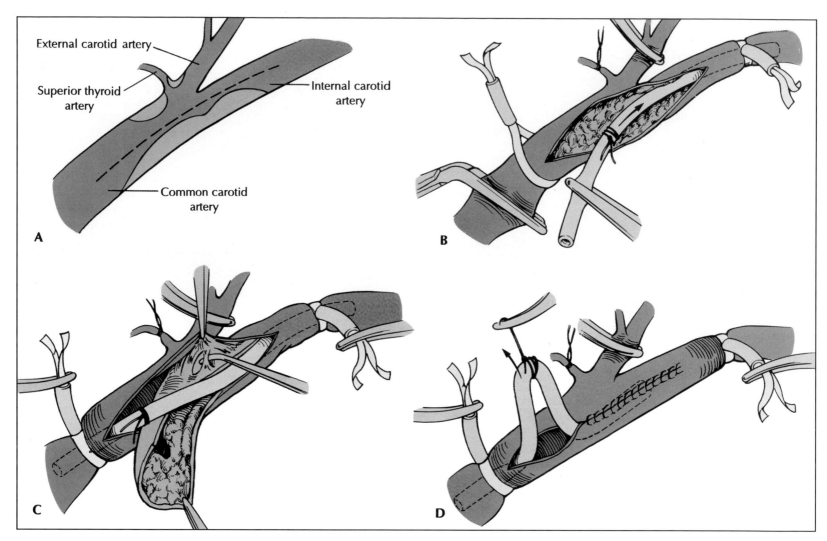

Labels in figure A:
External carotid artery
Superior thyroid artery
Internal carotid artery
Common carotid artery

FIGURE 6-24. Carotid endarterectomy. Carotid endarterectomy was shown to reduce the risk of stroke in patients with symptomatic high-grade stenosis in three randomized studies [11–13]. **A,** A longitudinal arteriotomy is initiated in the distal common carotid artery and is extended through the atheromatous plaque into the internal carotid artery. **B,** An indwelling shunt is inserted if there is deterioration of the electroencephalographic tracing. **C,** The atheroma is separated from the underlying residual media with a spatula and removed. **D,** The endarterectomy is carried out and the shunt is removed just prior to completion of the closure. (*Adapted from* Whittemore and Mannick [14].)

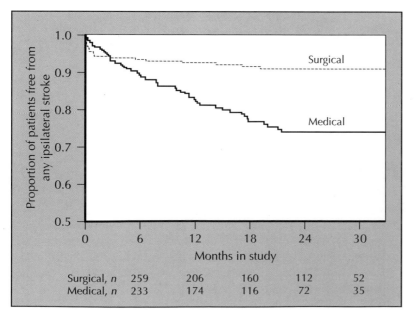

| Surgical, n | 259 | 206 | 160 | 112 | 52 |
| Medical, n | 233 | 174 | 116 | 72 | 35 |

FIGURE 6-25. The effect of carotid endarterectomy in symptomatic patients with high-grade carotid stenosis: North American Symptomatic Carotid Endarterectomy Trial (NASCET) [11]. In this trial, patients with carotid artery stenosis of 70% to 99% who had transient hemispheric symptoms, amaurosis fugax, or a nondisabling stroke were randomized to carotid endarterectomy or optimal medical care, including antiplatelet therapy. The cumulative risk of any ipsilateral stroke at 2 years was 26% in the medical care group and 9% in the surgical group, resulting in an absolute risk reduction of 17%. Carotid endarterectomy was also found to be beneficial when all strokes and deaths were included in the analysis. (*Adapted from* [11].)

INCIDENCE OF IPSILATERAL STROKE

STENOSIS, %	MEDICAL, %	SURGICAL, %	ABSOLUTE RISK REDUCTION, %
90–99	34.6	8.5	26±8.1
80–89	28.5	10.6	18±6.2
70–79	19.9	7.4	12±4.8

FIGURE 6-26. Incidence of ipsilateral stroke. In the North American Symptomatic Carotid Endarterectomy Trial, the greatest reduction in stroke risk was in patients with stenoses greater than 90%. The absolute risk reduction for all ipsilateral strokes at 2 years among patients with stenoses greater than 90% was 26%. In patients with stenoses of 80% to 89%, there was a clinically significant risk reduction of 18%; in patients with stenoses of 70% to 79%, there was a risk reduction of 12%. (*Adapted from* [11].)

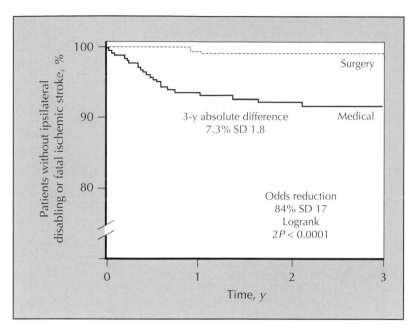

FIGURE 6-27. The effect of carotid endarterectomy on disabling or fatal ipsilateral stroke in patients with symptomatic severe carotid stenoses: Medical Research Council (MRC) European Carotid Surgery Trial [12]. This trial also demonstrated a beneficial effect of carotid endarterectomy in patients with carotid stenoses of 70% to 99% who have had either transient ischemic attacks, a retinal infarct, or a nondisabling ischemic stroke. Patients were randomized to medical treatment, including aspirin, or carotid endarterectomy. After 3 years of follow-up, carotid endarterectomy resulted in an eightfold reduction in ipsilateral ischemic strokes compared with medical therapy.

In the same study, patients with carotid stenoses (< 30%) and symptoms of a transient ischemic attack, retinal infarct, or a nondisabling ischemic stroke were randomized to medical therapy, including aspirin, or carotid endarterectomy. At the end of 3 years of follow-up, only one ipsilateral ischemic stroke occurred in patients randomized to surgery, and none occurred in patients randomized to medical therapy. These findings indicate that surgical therapy for symptomatic patients whose carotid stenosis is less than 30% is not helpful in reducing the incidence of stroke. (*Adapted from* [12].)

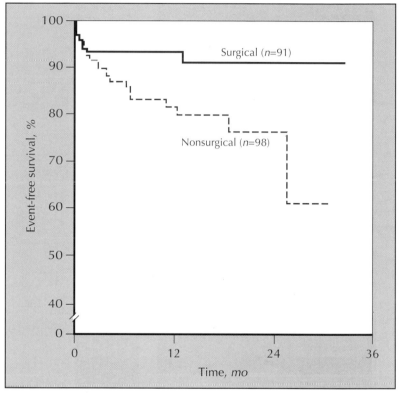

FIGURE 6-28. The effect of carotid endarterectomy on prevention of stroke and survival in patients with significant carotid stenosis: Veterans Affairs Cooperative Studies Program [13]. Patients with symptoms of transient ischemic attacks (TIAs), amaurosis fugax, or nondisabling strokes with carotid stenoses greater than 50% were randomized to either the best medical care or the best medical care plus carotid endarterectomy. After approximately 1 year of treatment there were event rates (death, stroke, crescendo TIAs) of approximately 19.4% in medically treated patients and 7.7% in surgically treated patients, resulting in an absolute risk reduction of 11.7%. In patients with an internal carotid artery stenosis greater than 70%, surgery resulted in an absolute risk reduction of 17.7%. (*Adapted from* Mayberg *et al.* [13].)

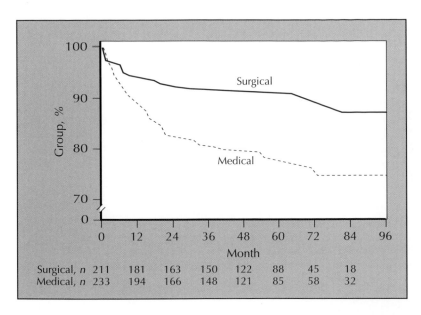

FIGURE 6-29. The effect of carotid endarterectomy on patients with asymptomatic carotid stenosis: Veterans Affairs Cooperative Studies Program [13]. In this trial, patients with asymptomatic carotid stenosis greater than 50% were randomized to either medical therapy, including platelet inhibitors, or surgical therapy. The primary endpoint comprised transient ischemic attacks (TIAs) and stroke. In patients randomized to medical treatment, 21% experienced either TIAs, transient monocular blindness, or stroke versus 8% in those randomized to surgery (*P* < 0.01). (*Adapted from* Mayberg *et al.* [13].)

ASYMPTOMATIC CAROTID STENOSIS: VA STUDY INCIDENCE OF EVENTS

ENDPOINT	INCIDENCE IN SURGICAL GROUP (*n*=211), *n* (%)	INCIDENCE IN MEDICAL GROUP (*n*=233), *n* (%)
TIA	6 (2.8)	15 (6.4)
Transient monocular blindness	1 (0.5)	11 (4.7)
Stroke (nonfatal and fatal)	10 (4.7)	22 (9.4)
All* (*P* < 0.01)	17 (8.0)	48 (20.6)

* Indicates *P* < 0.001 between groups.

FIGURE 6-30. The effect of carotid endarterectomy on patients with asymptomatic carotid stenosis: Veterans Affairs (VA) Cooperative Study Group [15]. In patients randomized to medical treatment, 11.1% experienced either transient ischemic attacks (TIAs) or transient monocular blindness, versus 3.3% in patients randomized to surgery. Stroke occurred in 9.4% of medically treated patients and in 4.7% of surgically treated patients. These differences were not significant, most likely because of inadequate statistical power. However, the combined endpoints of TIA and stroke occurred less frequently in the group treated with carotid endarterectomy. (*Adapted from* Hobson *et al.* [15].)

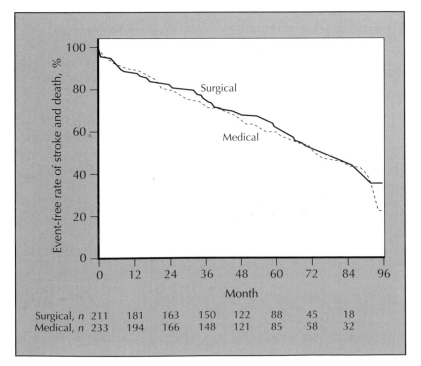

FIGURE 6-31. Surgical treatment of asymptomatic carotid stenosis. Surgery did not affect the combined endpoint of stroke and death in the Veterans Affairs Cooperative Study Group [15]. In the surgical group, 41% of the participants experienced stroke or death versus 44% in the medical group (*P* = NS). Death from cardiac causes occurred in 21% of patients in the surgical group and in 20% of patients in the medical group. This underscores the prevalence of co-existing cardiac disease in patients with carotid artery stenosis. (*Adapted from* Hobson *et al.* [15].)

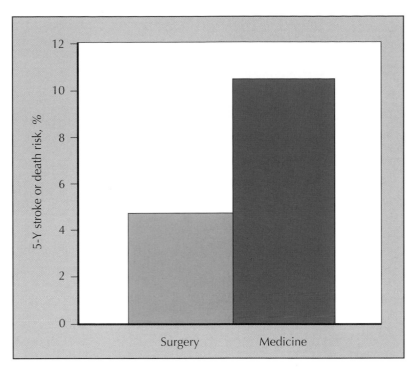

FIGURE 6-32. Surgery versus nonsurgical therapy for carotid stenosis. The Asymptomatic Carotid Atherosclerosis Study was a multicenter randomized controlled clinical trial that examined the effect of carotid endarterectomy versus nonsurgical therapy in patients with asymptomatic carotid artery stenoses of greater than 60%. Of the 1662 eligible patients who participated in this trial, 828 were randomized to receive surgery and 834 to medical management. The median follow-up was 2.7 years. The risk of stroke or death was 4.8% in the patients randomized to surgery and 10.6% in those randomized to medical treatment. The relative risk reduction conferred by surgery was 55% ($P = 0.004$) [16].

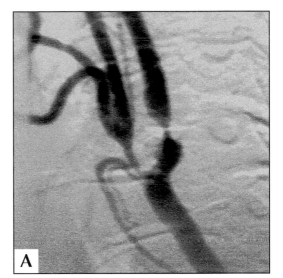

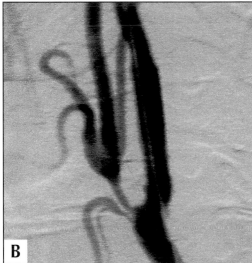

FIGURE 6-33. Carotid artery stenting. Carotid artery stenting is being used in selected centers to treat carotid artery stenosis. **A**, A contrast arteriogram demonstrates a 95% stenosis of the internal carotid artery. The stenosis was successfully treated by percutaneous placement of a stent. **B**, There is no residual stenosis.

A. THIRTY-DAY OUTCOME FOLLOWING CAROTID ARTERY STENTING

EVENT	HEMISPHERES ($n = 604$) (%)	PATIENTS ($n = 528$) (%)
Minor nonfatal strokes	29* (4.8)	29* (5.5)
Major nonfatal strokes	6 (1.0)	6 (1.0)
Fatal strokes		3 (0.6)
Non-neurologic deaths		5 (1.0)
Major nonfatal stroke and all deaths	14 (2.6)	14 (2.6)
All nonfatal strokes and all deaths	43 (7.4)	43 (8.1)

*One retinal artery embolus 2 weeks after procedure.

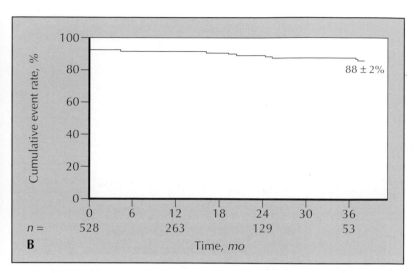

FIGURE 6-34. Carotid artery stenting. A 5-year prospective study evaluated the immediate and late clinical outcomes of carotid artery stenting in patients with symptomatic and asymptomatic carotid artery stenosis. **A**, Of 528 consecutive patients undergoing carotid stenting, 5.5% had a minor nonfatal stroke, 1% had a major nonfatal stroke, and 1% died from non-neurologic causes. **B**, The 3-year freedom from all fatal and nonfatal strokes was 88 ± 2%. (*Adapted from* Roubin *et al.* [17].)

VERTEBROBASILAR DISEASE

VERTEBROBASILAR DISEASE

Atherosclerosis
Thrombosis in situ
Embolism
Lacunar disease
Dissection
Vasculitis

FIGURE 6-35. Vertebrobasilar disease. Strokes and transient ischemic attacks in the distribution of the vertebral and basilar arteries can be caused by atherosclerosis, thrombosis, embolism, lacunar disease, dissection, and vasculitis (*ie*, granulomatous arteritis, polyarteritis nodosa).

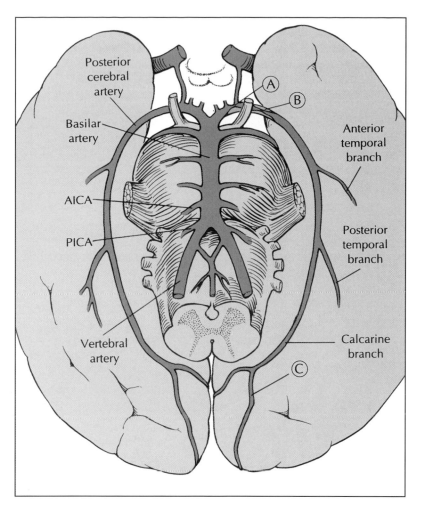

FIGURE 6-36. Anatomy of the vertebrobasilar circulation. The left and right vertebral arteries coalesce to form the basilar artery, which bisects the pons. Major branches of the basilar artery are the left and right posterior cerebral arteries and the anterior (AICA) and posterior (PICA) inferior cerebellar arteries. Stenosis of the proximal posterior cerebral artery (**A**), stenosis of the ambient cisternal portion (**B**), and occlusion of its calcarine artery branch (**C**) are common causes of vertebrobasilar ischemia and infarction. (*Adapted from* Caplan [18].)

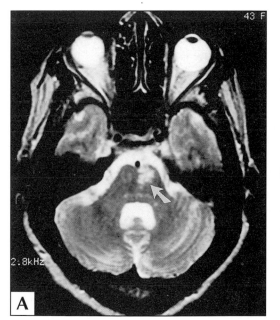 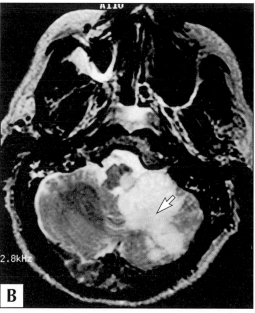 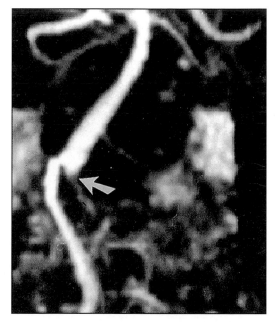

FIGURE 6-37. Common sites of infarction. The most common sites of infarction in the vertebral circulation are the pons, cerebellum, and lateral medulla. **A,** A pontine infarction, in which a T_2-weighted magnetic resonance (MR) image reveals a left medial pontine infarct (*arrow*). Lesions in this region of the pons result in ataxia, paresis of rightward gaze, and right hemiparesis without a sensory deficit. **B,** A T_2-weighted MR image of a lateral medullary and cerebellar infarction. In this case, occlusion of the posterior-inferior cerebellar artery results in the lateral medullary syndrome (Wallenberg syndrome), which is a distinct constellation of symptoms occurring as a result of medullary ischemia, including vertigo, nystagmus, ataxia, ipsilateral Horner's syndrome, facial numbness and mild weakness, contralateral pain and temperature loss, and hoarseness and dysarthria due to ipsilateral weakness of the vocal cords and palate. The ipsilateral cerebellum was also affected (*arrow*), contributing to the ataxia. (*Panel A from* Jensen [3]; with permission.)

FIGURE 6-38. Magnetic resonance (MR) angiography. The resolution of MR angiography is adequate to isolate lesions in the vertebrobasilar circulation. In this example, MR angiography reveals an occlusion of the left vertebral artery as it joins the basilar artery (*arrow*). The remainder of the vertebrobasilar circulation is intact, suggesting embolic occlusion of this vessel from a proximal source.

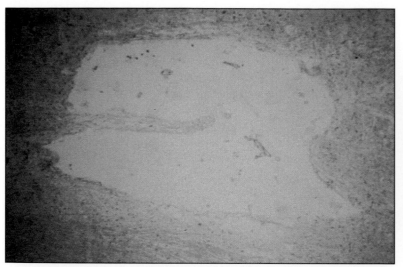

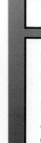

FIGURE 6-39. Photomicrograph of a lacunar lesion in the cerebral white matter. Lacunar infarcts range from 0.2 to 15 mm in diameter. They are caused by occlusions in blood vessels of 100 to 400 μm. The area in the center of the lacune shows decreased myelin staining. These vessels contain microatheroma and lipohyalinosis, and will develop fibrinoid necrosis. The major risk factors for lacunar disease are hypertension and diabetes. No controlled trials have been performed to evaluate the role of antiplatelet agents in this state, and treatment of the underlying condition (*ie*, hypertension or diabetes) is the mainstay of therapy.

FIGURE 6-40. Common lacunar syndromes. The clinical manifestations of lacunar infarction in the vertebrobasilar territory are dependent upon the specific vessels involved and the subsequent area of brainstem or internal capsule affected. The common lacunar syndromes include dysarthria–clumsy hand, pure motor hemiplegia, pure hemisensory deficit, ataxic hemiparesis, contralateral motor and sensory deficit, and lateral medullary syndrome.

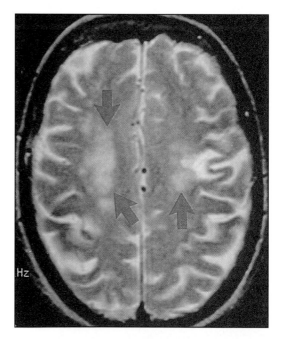

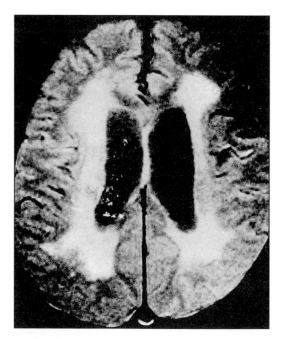

FIGURE 6-41. T$_2$-weighted magnetic resonance image of multiple hemispheric lacunes. Multiple hyperdense lesions (*arrows*) can be seen bilaterally in the subcortical white matter. The risk of small-vessel disease increases with age, hypertension, diabetes, smoking, hypercoagulable states, and hyperlipidemia. This patient was hypertensive and diabetic, and had a history of multiple discrete episodes of weakness and sensory deficits.

FIGURE 6-42. Pathologic example of Binswanger's disease, or leukoariosis, demonstrating multifocal, periventricular demyelinated lesions. The pathophysiology has been thought to be due to chronic arterial hypertension and its effect on small penetrating vessels. Chronic hypertension is the main risk factor for this disease. Clinically, the more extensive lesions are associated with dementia, and leukoariosis can occur simultaneously with dementia due to a multi-infarct or multi-lacune state. No specific treatment has been suggested for leukoariosis other than control of hypertension.

VASCULITIS

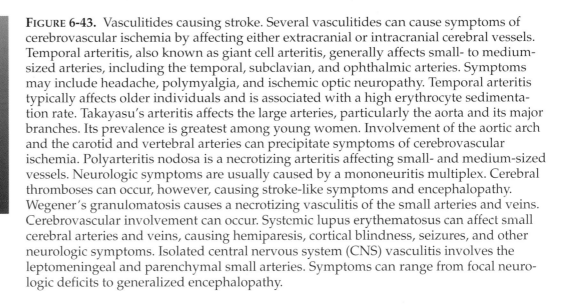

FIGURE 6-43. Vasculitides causing stroke. Several vasculitides can cause symptoms of cerebrovascular ischemia by affecting either extracranial or intracranial cerebral vessels. Temporal arteritis, also known as giant cell arteritis, generally affects small- to medium-sized arteries, including the temporal, subclavian, and ophthalmic arteries. Symptoms may include headache, polymyalgia, and ischemic optic neuropathy. Temporal arteritis typically affects older individuals and is associated with a high erythrocyte sedimentation rate. Takayasu's arteritis affects the large arteries, particularly the aorta and its major branches. Its prevalence is greatest among young women. Involvement of the aortic arch and the carotid and vertebral arteries can precipitate symptoms of cerebrovascular ischemia. Polyarteritis nodosa is a necrotizing arteritis affecting small- and medium-sized vessels. Neurologic symptoms are usually caused by a mononeuritis multiplex. Cerebral thromboses can occur, however, causing stroke-like symptoms and encephalopathy. Wegener's granulomatosis causes a necrotizing vasculitis of the small arteries and veins. Cerebrovascular involvement can occur. Systemic lupus erythematosus can affect small cerebral arteries and veins, causing hemiparesis, cortical blindness, seizures, and other neurologic symptoms. Isolated central nervous system (CNS) vasculitis involves the leptomeningeal and parenchymal small arteries. Symptoms can range from focal neurologic deficits to generalized encephalopathy.

VASCULITIDES CAUSING STROKE

Temporal arteritis
Takayasu's arteritis
Polyarteritis nodosa
Wegener's granulomatosis
Systemic lupus erythematosus
Isolated CNS vasculitis

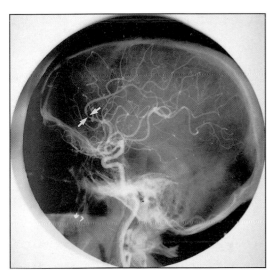

FIGURE 6-44. Angiogram of arteritic vessels demonstrating areas of focal arterial narrowing (*arrows*). This patient with cerebral vasculitis presented with recurrent episodes of encephalopathy and multifocal strokes.

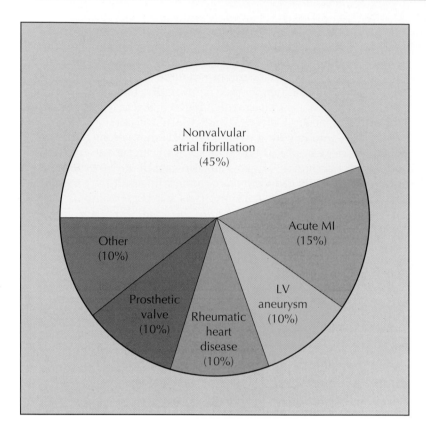

FIGURE 6-45. Cardiac causes of cerebral embolism. Strokes due to cerebral embolism can be artery-to-artery or can originate from a cardiac source. In general, cardiac embolic strokes are larger than those due to atherosclerosis, and produce significant deficits when they occur in the cerebral hemispheres or brainstem. Cardiac conditions associated with cerebral emboli have been described by the Cerebral Embolism Task Force [19]. These include atrial fibrillation, acute myocardial infarction (MI), left ventricular (LV) aneurysm, rheumatic heart disease, a prosthetic valve, cardiomyopathy, atrial myxoma, and paradoxic emboli from venous thrombosis via a patent foramen ovale, or atrial or ventricular septal defect. (*Adapted from* [19].)

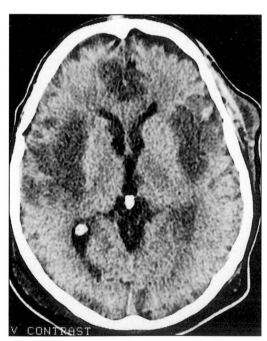

FIGURE 6-46. Computed tomogram of multiple embolic hemispheric strokes resulting from a cardiac embolism. Typically, embolic infarcts involve cortical structures and can extend to the cortical surface. (*From* Jensen [3]; with permission.)

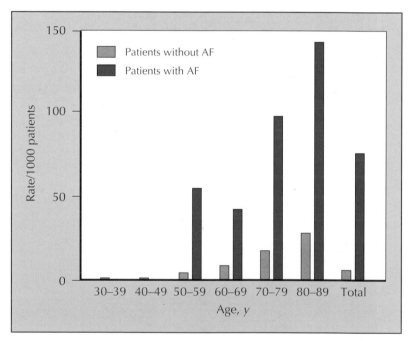

FIGURE 6-47. Atrial fibrillation (AF) and stroke. The effect of AF on the risk of stroke was studied in 5184 men and women participating in the Framingham Heart Study over a 30-year period. The age-specific incidence of stroke in patients with AF was significantly greater than in those without AF. During the course of this study, 14% of patients with AF developed stroke. (*Adapted from* Wolf *et al.* [20].)

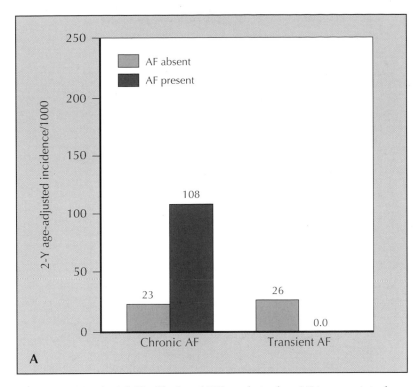

A

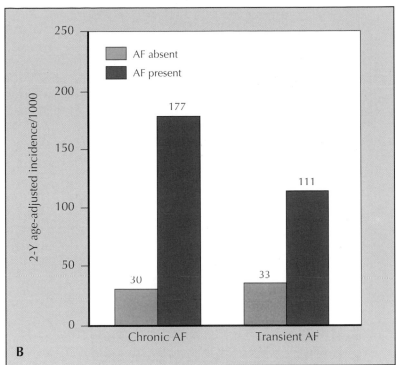

B

Figure 6-48. Atrial fibrillation (AF) and stroke. AF is associated with an increased risk of stroke. The age-adjusted incidence of stroke in men (**A**) and women (**B**) followed in the Framingham Heart Study in relation to chronic and transient AF is illustrated. In men with chronic AF, the relative risk of developing a stroke is 4.7; in women with chronic AF it is 5.9. The relative risk of stroke with transient AF was not affected significantly in either men (in whom it appears to be lower) or women (in whom it appears to be higher). (*Adapted from* Kannel *et al.* [21].)

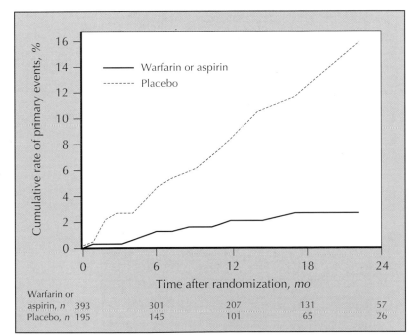

| Warfarin or aspirin, n | 393 | | 301 | | 207 | | 131 | | 57 |
| Placebo, n | 195 | | 145 | | 101 | | 65 | | 26 |

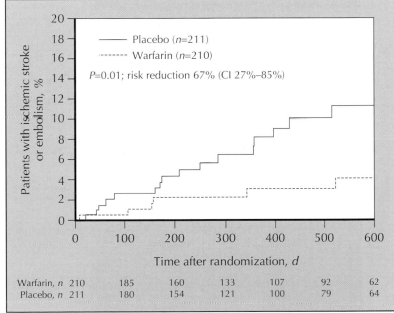

| Warfarin, n | 210 | 185 | 160 | 133 | 107 | 92 | 62 |
| Placebo, n | 211 | 180 | 154 | 121 | 100 | 79 | 64 |

Figure 6-49. The Stroke Prevention in Atrial Fibrillation study (SPAF). This study examined the effect of anticoagulant and antiplatelet treatment on 1244 patients followed for a mean of 1.3 years [22]. Compared with the group randomized to placebo treatment, the group randomized to either warfarin or aspirin had a substantial reduction in the rate of ischemic stroke and systemic embolism. The event rates were 1.6% per year in the 393 patients comprising the active treatment arms (warfarin or aspirin), compared with 8.3% per year in the 195 patients comprising the placebo arm. The beneficial effect of aspirin was confined to those patients younger than 75 years of age. (*Adapted from* [22].)

Figure 6-50. The effect of warfarin as shown by the Stroke Prevention in Atrial Fibrillation (SPAF) study. In the subgroup of participating warfarin-eligible patients, warfarin significantly reduced the risk of ischemic stroke and systemic embolus by 67% (warfarin vs placebo, 2.3% vs 7.4% per year; *P* = 0.01). The risk of a primary event or death was reduced by 58% in the group of individuals assigned to warfarin (*P* = 0.01). (*Adapted from* [23].)

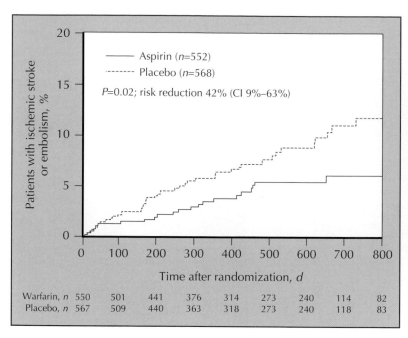

FIGURE 6-51. Effects of aspirin as shown by The Stroke Prevention in Atrial Fibrillation (SPAF) study. Aspirin reduced the risk of ischemic stroke and systemic embolus by 42% (aspirin vs placebo, 3.6% vs 6.2%; $P = 0.02$). The reduction in primary events (ischemic stroke or systemic embolism) or death was 32% in the group of patients assigned to aspirin ($P = 0.02$). (*Adapted from* [23].)

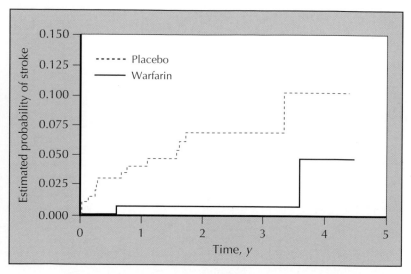

FIGURE 6-52. Effects of warfarin in patients with nonrheumatic atrial fibrillation. The Boston Area Anticoagulation Trial studied the effect of low-dose warfarin on the risk of stroke in patients with nonrheumatic atrial fibrillation. A total of 420 patients (212 in the warfarin group and 208 in the control group) were followed for an average of 2.2 years. There were only two strokes in the warfarin group (incidence, 0.41% per year) compared with 13 in the control group (incidence, 2.98% per year). The death rate was also significantly lower in the warfarin group than in the control group. The warfarin group had a higher rate of minor hemorrhage than the control group, but fatal hemorrhage was rare, occurring in only one subject in each group. (*Adapted from* [24].)

EMBOLIC COMPLICATIONS IN THE AFASAK STUDY

COMPLICATIONS	WARFARIN, n	ASPIRIN, n	PLACEBO, n
Cerebral emboli			
TIA	0	2	3
Minor stroke	0	1	2
Nondisabling stroke	0	7	3
Disabling stroke	4	4	7
Fatal stroke	1	3	4
Visceral emboli	0	2	2
Emboli in extremities	0	1	0
Total	5	20	21

FIGURE 6-53. Embolic complications in the Atrial Fibrillation, Aspirin, Anticoagulant (AFASAK) study. The Copenhagen AFASAK study evaluated the effect of warfarin in patients with chronic rheumatic atrial fibrillation. The trial involved 1007 individuals: 335 randomized to warfarin, 336 randomized to aspirin (75 mg/d), and 336 randomized to placebo. The incidence of thromboembolism was lower in the warfarin group than in the aspirin or placebo group. More patients in the warfarin group had nonfatal bleeding complications than in the aspirin or placebo group. The aspirin and placebo groups did not differ from each other. TIA—transient ischemic attack. (*Adapted from* Peterson *et al.* [25].)

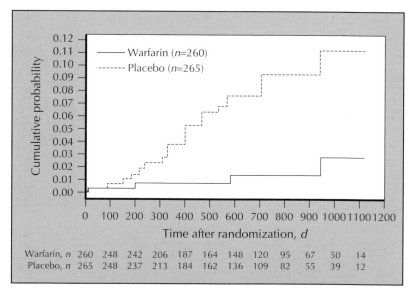

FIGURE 6-54. Warfarin versus placebo in patients with nonrheumatic atrial fibrillation. A Veterans Administration study (Veterans Affairs Stroke Prevention in Nonrheumatic Atrial Fibrillation) examined the efficacy of warfarin versus placebo in preventing stroke in patients with nonrheumatic atrial fibrillation. Warfarin significantly reduced the probability of stroke, which occurred in 19 of 265 patients taking placebo and in four of 260 patients taking warfarin ($P < 0.001$), accounting for a relative risk reduction of 79%. (*Adapted from* Ezekowitz *et al.* [26].)

COMPARISON OF STUDIES OF ANTITHROMBOTIC PROPHYLAXIS IN ATRIAL FIBRILLATION

	AFASAK	SPAF	BAATAF	VA
Age, *y*	74	67	68	67
Type of AF	Chronic	Chronic/paroxysmal	Chronic/paroxysmal	Chronic
Aspirin dose, *mg/d*	75	325	—	—
Intracerebral hemorrhage	Primary endpoint	Side effect	Side effect	Secondary endpoint
Aspirin effect	No	Yes, in patients ≤ 75 y	—	—
Warfarin therapeutic interval (INR)	4.2–2.8	3.5–2.0	2.7–1.5	1.4–2.8
Multicenter study	No	Yes	Yes	Yes
Warfarin effect on mortality	No	No	Yes	Yes

FIGURE 6-55. Comparison of four prospective studies of antithrombotic prophylaxis in atrial fibrillation (AF) [22–26]. Whereas each study showed that warfarin reduced the probability of stroke or systemic embolism, the studies differed in the reported efficacy of aspirin. AFASAK—Atrial Fibrillation, Aspirin, Anticoagulation Study; BAATAF—Boston Area Anticoagulation Trial for Atrial Fibrillation; INR—international normalized ratio; SPAF—Stroke Prevention in Atrial Fibrillation; VA—Veterans Administration. (*Adapted from* Petersen [27].)

REFERENCES

1. American Heart Association: *2001 Heart and Stroke Statistical Update.* Dallas, TX: American Heart Association; 2001.

2. Norris JW, Zhu CZ, Bornstein NM, Chambers BR: Vascular risks of asymptomatic carotid stenosis. *Stroke* 1991, 22:1485–1490.

3. Jensen FE: *Cerebrovascular disease.* In *Textbook of Vascular Medicine,* edn 2. Edited by Loscalzo J, Creager MA, Dzau VJ. Boston: Little, Brown; 1996:781–795.

4. Collaborative meta-analysis of randomised trials of antiplatelet therapy for prevention of death, myocardial infarction, and stroke in high risk patients. *BMJ* 2002, 324:71–86.

5. Albers GW, Amarenco P, Easton JD, *et al.*: Antithrombotic and thrombolytic therapy for ischemic stroke. *Chest* 2001, 119:300S–320S.

6. Mohr JP, Thompson JLP, Lazar RM, *et al.*: A comparison of warfarin and aspirin for the prevention of recurrent ischemic stroke. *N Engl J Med* 2001, 345:1444–1451.

7. The International Stroke Trial (IST): a randomised trial of aspirin, subcutaneous heparin, both, or neither among 19435 patients with acute ischaemic stroke. International Stroke Trial Collaborative Group. *Lancet* 1997, 349:1569–1581.

8. CAST: randomised placebo-controlled trial of early aspirin use in 20,000 patients with acute ischaemic stroke. CAST (Chinese Acute Stroke Trial) Collaborative Group. *Lancet* 1997, 349:1641–1649

9. Wardlaw JM: Overview of Cochrane thrombolysis meta-analysis. *Neurology* 2001, 57:S69–S76.

10. Mohler ER III, Delanty N, Rader DJ, Raps EC: Statins and cerebrovascular disease: plaque attack to prevent brain attack. *Vasc Med* 1999, 4:269–272.

11. Beneficial effect of carotid endarterectomy in symptomatic patients with high-grade carotid stenosis. *N Engl J Med* 1991, 325:445–453.

12. MRC European Carotid Surgery Trial: interim results from symptomatic patients with severe (70–99%) or mild (0–29%) carotid stenosis. *Lancet* 1991, 337:1235–1243.

13. Mayberg MR, Wilson SE, Yatsu F, *et al.*, for the Veterans Affairs Cooperative Studies Program 309 Trialist Group: Carotid endarterectomy and prevention of cerebral ischemia in symptomatic carotid stenosis. *JAMA* 1991, 266:3289–3294.

14. Whittemore AD, Mannick JA: Principles of vascular surgery. In *Textbook of Vascular Medicine,* edn 2. Edited by Loscalzo J, Creager MA, Dzau VJ. Boston: Little, Brown and Co.; 1996:675–702.

15. Hobson RW, Weiss DG, Fields WS, *et al.*: Efficacy of carotid endarterectomy for asymptomatic carotid stenosis. *N Engl J Med* 1991, 328:221–227.

16. Endarterectomy for asymptomatic carotid artery stenosis. Executive Committee for the Asymptomatic Carotid Atherosclerosis Study. *JAMA* 1995, 273:1421–1428.

17. Roubin GS, New G, Iyer SS, *et al.*: Immediate and late clinical outcomes of carotid artery stenting in patients with symptomatic and asymptomatic carotid artery stenosis: a 5-year prospective analysis. *Circulation* 2001, 103:532–537.

18. Caplan LR: Vertebrobasilar system syndromes. In *Handbook of Clinical Neurology,* vol 53, *Vascular Diseases.* Part I. Edited by Toole JF. Amsterdam: Elsevier; 1988:371–408.

19. Cardiogenic brain embolism. Cerebral Embolism Task Force. *Arch Neurol* 1986, 43:71–84.

20. Wolf PA, Abbott RD, Kannel WB: Atrial fibrillation: a major contributor to stroke in the elderly: the Framingham Study. *Arch Intern Med* 1987, 147:1561–1564.

21. Kannel WB, Abbott RD, Savage DD, et al.: Coronary heart disease and atrial fibrillation. *Am Heart J* 1983, 106:389–396.

22. Preliminary report of the Stroke Prevention in Atrial Fibrillation study. *N Engl J Med* 1990, 322:863–868.

23. Stroke Prevention in Atrial Fibrillation study: final results. *Circulation* 1991, 84:527–539.

24. The effect of low-dose warfarin on the risk of stroke in patients with nonrheumatic atrial fibrillation. The Boston Area Anticoagulation Trial for Atrial Fibrillation Investigators. *N Engl J Med* 1990, 323:1505–1511.

25. Petersen P, Boysen G, Godtfredsen J, *et al.*: Placebo-controlled, randomised trial of warfarin and aspirin for prevention of thromboembolic complications in chronic atrial fibrillation: the Copenhagen AFASAK Study. *Lancet* 1989, 1:175–179.

26. Ezekowitz MD, Bridgers SL, James KE, *et al.*: Warfarin in the prevention of stroke associated with nonrheumatic atrial fibrillation. *N Engl J Med* 1992, 327:1406–1412.

27. Petersen P: Anticoagulant therapy for atrial fibrillation. In *Atrial Fibrillation: Mechanisms and Management.* Edited by Falk RH, Podrid PJ. New York: Raven Press; 1992:307–319.

EVALUATION AND MEDICAL MANAGEMENT OF THE VASCULAR SURGERY PATIENT

CHAPTER 7

Khether E. Raby

Patients with peripheral vascular disease have a high prevalence of coronary artery disease. Coronary artery disease is often occult, and its activity is difficult to measure by conventional means. For these reasons, coronary artery disease is by far the most important factor contributing to morbidity and mortality in vascular surgery patients.

Preoperative assessment strategies for vascular surgery patients have been well established. The majority of patients could have their risk assessed preoperatively by a thorough history, physical examination, and electrocardiogram. This clinical assessment accurately predicts the majority of patients at low and high risk for postoperative cardiac events. Patients believed to be at intermediate or indeterminate risk by clinical assessment are most likely to benefit from further noninvasive cardiac testing. Of the noninvasive testing strategies that have been employed in this patient population, exercise testing is very useful in those who can exercise, with exercise capacity and ST depression both predicting perioperative and long-term outcome. Among patients who cannot exercise, dipyridamole-thallium-201/^{99m}Tc-sestamibi SPECT imaging and dobutamine stress echocardiography have emerged as the most widely used modalities to assess preoperative risk. While there is sample data to support their use, some argue their routine use is not cost efficient, given the dropping cardiac risk among vascular surgery patients.

While it is clear that patients identified to be at low risk by clinical and noninvasive means have an excellent perioperative prognosis and can proceed to vascular surgery, the approach to high-risk patients remains controversial. Studies that cite an excellent prognosis after elective surgery among patients who have had prior coronary revascularization advocate prophylactic coronary revascularization in all high-risk patients undergoing vascular surgery. To date, no randomized trial has been performed to address the merit of prophylactic coronary revascularization, taking into account the potentially high morbidity and mortality of coronary revascularization in vascular surgery patients. Until such data is available, the most prudent approach is to recommend coronary angiography and revascularization to vascular surgery patients who have an indication for such an approach, independent of elective surgery. New data support the use of perioperative β-adrenergic blockade as prophylaxis against myocardial ischemia to lower both perioperative and long-term risk among all vascular surgery patients. Randomized control trials currently underway should help to address the relative merits of coronary revascularization and medical therapy in this population group.

CARDIOVASCULAR MORTALITY IN PATIENTS WITH VASCULAR DISEASE

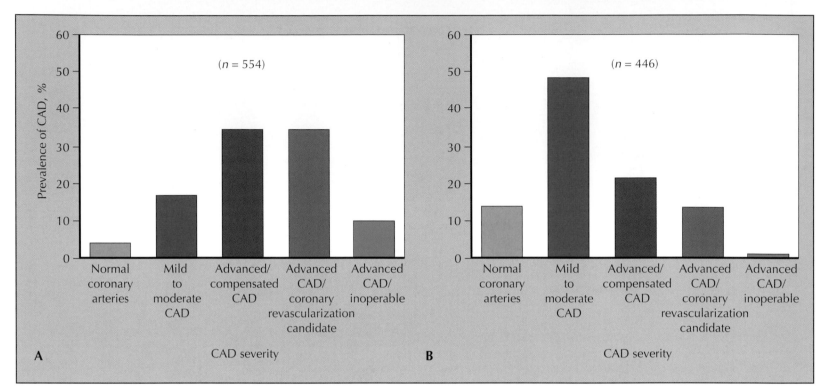

FIGURE 7-1. Prevalence of coronary artery disease (CAD) among patients with peripheral vascular disease. In a large, comprehensive study, Hertzer *et al.* [1] performed coronary angiography in 1000 patients undergoing elective peripheral vascular surgery over a 5-year period. The coronary anatomy was delineated among 554 patients with suspected CAD (including prior history of myocardial infarction, angina pectoris, or abnormal electrocardiogram) (**A**) and 446 patients without suspected CAD (**B**). In addition to defining the coronary anatomy, patients were classified according to the severity of CAD. The classification categories included the following: those with normal coronary arteries; those with mild to moderate CAD (< 70% stenosis of a major coronary artery); and those with advanced or compensated CAD (> 70% stenosis of a major coronary artery but with adequate collateralization or with a supplied

area of myocardium already replaced by scar), advanced CAD suitable for coronary revascularization (> 70% stenosis of a major coronary artery without the benefit of collaterals while supplying a viable area of myocardium), and advanced CAD that is not suitable for revascularization (> 70% stenosis of at least one coronary artery but with diffuse distal disease or generalized ventricular impairment making the risk of coronary artery surgery prohibitively high).

The data are summarized for patients with (*A*) or without (*B*) suspected CAD. It can be seen that the prevalence of CAD is extremely high regardless of prior suspicion. While advanced CAD is more prevalent among patients with a historical suspicion of CAD, the prevalence of advanced CAD remains quite significant even among patients without suspected CAD. (*Adapted from* Hertzer *et al.* [1].)

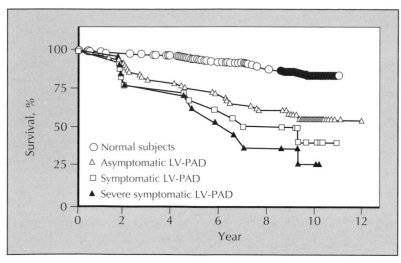

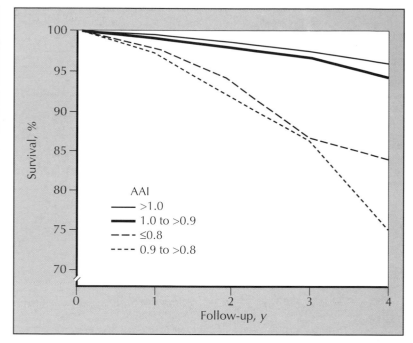

FIGURE 7-2. Kaplan-Meier survival curves from all causes of death among normal subjects as well as subjects with large-vessel peripheral arterial disease (LV-PAD). The study considered a population of men and women who participated in a Lipids Research Clinics protocol and who agreed to be evaluated noninvasively for LV-PAD. All patients underwent systolic blood pressure measurements in the arms and legs and had flow velocities measured in their legs by Doppler ultrasound. Based on these studies as well as on a questionnaire to determine the symptoms of intermittent claudication, patients were divided into four groups: normal subjects (*n* = 408); patients without symptoms of intermittent claudication but with LV-PAD documented by abnormal leg-to-arm blood pressure ratio (asymptomatic LV-PAD; *n* = 49); patients with symptoms of intermittent claudication and LV-PAD documented by abnormal leg-to-arm blood pressure ratios (symptomatic LV-PAD; *n* = 18); and patients with symptoms of intermittent claudication and LV-PAD documented by both abnormal leg-to-arm blood pressure measurements more severe than among patients with symptomatic LV-PAD and abnormal Doppler flow measurements (severe symptomatic LV-PAD; *n* = 13). The presence of LV-PAD, with or without symptoms, predicted a high risk of death, mostly from cardiac causes. The severity of LV-PAD further predicted poor survival. (*Adapted from* Criqui *et al.* [2].)

FIGURE 7-3. Survival curves comparing mortality among elderly women with normal and abnormal ankle-arm blood pressure indices (AAI; a reliable test for infra-inguinal arterial vascular disease). More than 1600 women over age 65 years (who were initially enrolled in a study for osteoporosis) agreed to participate in this study by having systolic blood pressure measured in the arms and ankles. The average systolic blood pressure of both feet was divided by the average systolic pressure of both arms to arrive at the AAI. These women were then subdivided into four distinct groups stratified by their AAI: women with an AAI of higher than 1 were considered normal; women with an AAI of 1 to 0.9 were considered to have mild lower extremity arterial occlusive disease; women with an AAI of 0.8 to 0.9 were considered to have mild to moderate disease; and finally, women with an AAI of 0.8 or less were considered to have the most severe lower extremity arterial occlusive disease. Mortality was substantially higher among the two groups with the more severe lower extremity arterial occlusive disease at 3 years of follow-up. (*Adapted from* Vogt *et al.* [3].)

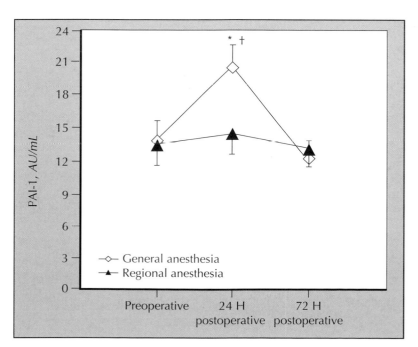

FIGURE 7-4. Plasminogen activator inhibitor-1 (PAI-1) levels for patients undergoing vascular surgery with general and regional anesthesia. Among factors contributing to alterations in myocardial oxygen supply in the postoperative period is the hypercoagulable state associated with general anesthesia, which can cause coronary thrombosis. General anesthesia appears to result in increased PAI-1 levels 24 hours postoperatively (values are mean ± SEM). *Asterisk* indicates *P* = 0.05 general compared with regional anesthesia; *dagger* indicates *P* < 0.001 compared with the preoperative and 72-hour postoperative values. AU—activity units. (*Adapted from* Rosenfeld *et al.* [4].)

TREATMENT CHARACTERISTICS

	THROMBOSIS (n = 22)	NO THROMBOSIS (n = 73)	P VALUE
Surgical procedure, n (%)			
Femoral-proximal	10 (46)	31 (42.5)	0.80
Femoral-popliteal	8 (36)	31 (42.5)	0.61
Femoral-distal	2 (9)	7 (9.6)	0.94
Other*	2 (9)	4 (5.4)	0.54
Blood administered, U	0.41±0.67	0.19±0.57	0.18
Estimated blood loss, mL	470±689	458±521	0.94
Hypotension SICU, h	0.77±1.5	0.81±2.1	0.94
Type of anesthesia			0.01
General	17 (77)	35 (48)	
Regional	5 (23)	38 (52)	

*Femoral-femoral bypass and popliteal artery aneurysm repair.

FIGURE 7-5. Treatment characteristics of vascular surgery patients who experienced major thrombotic events postoperatively (including, but not exclusively, cardiac events) compared with those in vascular surgery patients who did not experience thrombosis. Postoperative thrombosis appears associated with the use of general anesthesia in this patient population. Values are mean + SD. SICU—surgical intensive care unit. (*Adapted from* Rosenfeld *et al.* [4].)

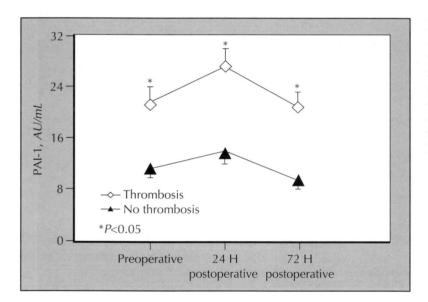

FIGURE 7-6. Plasminogen activator inhibitor-1 (PAI-1) levels among patients who experienced postoperative thrombotic events after vascular surgery and those who did not (values are mean ± SEM). PAI-1 levels are higher in the 24-hour period after surgery among patients who experienced clinical thrombotic events. This study indirectly suggests that the use of regional anesthesia may be helpful in postoperative risk reduction in vascular surgery patients. AU—activity units. (*Adapted from* Rosenfeld *et al.* [4].)

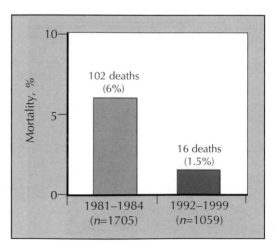

FIGURE 7-7. Perioperative cardiac mortality as a percentage of all patients undergoing vascular surgery. Despite increased risks for suffering cardiac events after vascular surgery, the cardiac risk from all vascular surgeries appears to be decreasing. The first bar includes 1705 patients pooled from three large studies published from 1981 to 1984 [5–7], and represents an overall perioperative mortality from cardiac causes of 6%, which is reflective of the accepted cardiac risk from vascular surgery in the early 1980s. The second bar represents 1059 patients pooled from four studies published between 1990 and 1999 [8–11], all of which were performed at medical centers that routinely employ preoperative medical evaluation and risk reduction of all vascular surgery patients. The overall mortality from cardiac causes was 1.5%, which illustrates a trend toward decreasing cardiac risk among vascular surgery patients.

CARDIAC RISK INDEX

VARIABLE	POINTS
Coronary artery disease (angina)	5–10
Congestive heart failure	10–20
Valvular heart disease (aortic stenosis)	20
Arrhythmia	5
Poor general condition	5
Age > 70 y	5
Emergency surgery	10

FIGURE 7-8. Cardiac risk index. In the 1970s several large studies developed multifactorial cardiac risk indices that attempted to quantify historical information, physical examination, and basic laboratory findings by assigning them weighted scores based on their ability to predict cardiac risk prior to noncardiac surgery. A large series of patients undergoing noncardiac surgery had extensive, well-documented histories, physical examinations, and baseline electrocardiographic (ECG) studies. Factors that predicted postoperative cardiac events were identified retrospectively by multivariate analysis. These factors were subsequently given numerical weight based on their predictive ability, and the overall predictive ability of a risk score was tested and validated by prospective analysis. The multifactorial cardiac risk index was subsequently modified for a population with a high preoperative likelihood of coronary artery disease, such as patients with peripheral vascular disease, and this modified index is shown here. Risk indices demonstrate the importance of medical history, physical examination, and baseline ECG in accurately establishing risk in the majority of patients undergoing vascular surgery. (*Adapted from* Detsky *et al.* [12].)

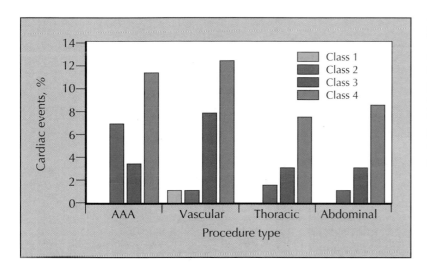

FIGURE 7-9. Adverse cardiac events and the cardiac risk index. This recently revalidated cardiac risk index depicts risk of perioperative cardiac events among low-risk (class 1), intermediate-risk (classes 2 and 3), and high-risk patients (class 4) undergoing noncardiac surgery. Note that the risk index correctly stratifies patients undergoing abdominal aortic aneurysm (AAA) and other vascular surgeries, with class 4 patients undergoing vascular surgery having highest risks (approximately 11% to 13%) when compared with other surgeries and other risk groups. (*Adapted from* Lee *et al.* [13].)

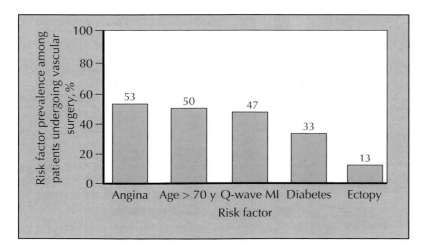

FIGURE 7-10. Risk factors in vascular surgery patients. More recently, an approach similar to that of multifactorial cardiac risk indices has been employed to better identify preoperative risk exclusively among vascular surgery patients. Eagle *et al.* [14] identified the prevalence of five clinical markers among vascular surgery patients undergoing dipyridamole-thallium-201 imaging that were retrospectively found by multivariate analysis to be helpful in stratifying preoperative cardiac risk. These factors include a history of significant angina, age greater than 70 years, a history of prior Q-wave myocardial infarction (MI), a history of diabetes, and a history of ventricular ectopic activity on baseline electrocardiogram or prior treatment for ventricular ectopy. Using such a clinical approach, patients at very low risk (no clinical markers) and patients at very high risk (three to five clinical markers) required no further stratification with noninvasive testing, since the results were unlikely to affect further therapy. By contrast, patients at intermediate risk (one or two clinical markers) were most likely to benefit from further testing. (*Adapted from* Eagle *et al.* [14].)

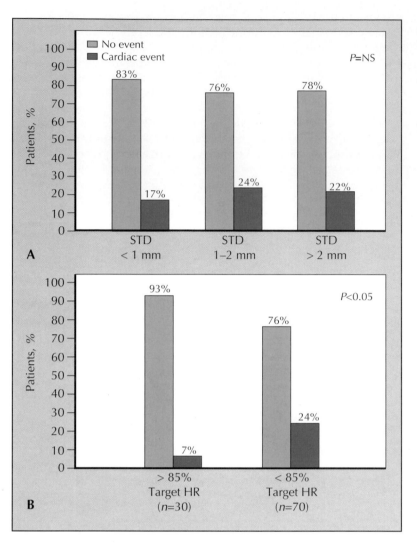

FIGURE 7-11. Exercise testing in vascular surgery patients as a predictor of risk. This study by McPhail *et al.* [15] revealed that the degree of ST-segment depression (STD) (**A**) does not predict postoperative cardiac events, whereas the inability to reach 85% of the target heart rate (HR), regardless of exercise test outcome, was highly predictive of postoperative cardiac events (**B**). (*Adapted from* McPhail *et al.* [15].)

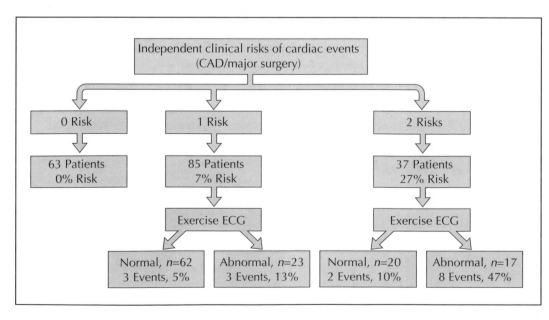

FIGURE 7-12. Preoperative exercise stress testing and risk assessment among high-risk patients undergoing noncardiac surgery. Patients were divided into three groups: no risk (those without evidence of coronary artery disease [CAD] undergoing nonmajor surgery); one risk (those with CAD *or* who are undergoing major surgery); and three risks (those with CAD who are undergoing major surgery). A positive exercise test was defined as 0.1 mV of ST depression in otherwise normal baseline leads. Stress testing successfully predicted events among intermediate and high-risk groups. ECG—electrocardiogram. (*Adapted from* Gauss *et al.* [16].)

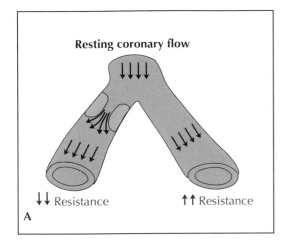

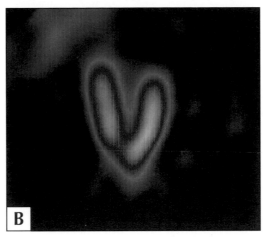

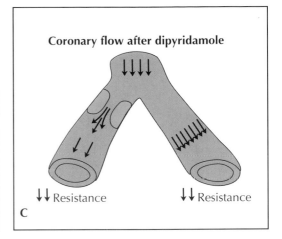

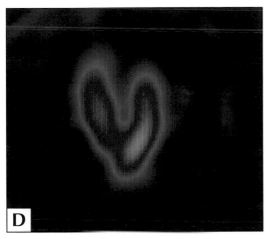

FIGURE 7-13. Representative model of coronary flow in a normal vessel and in a vessel with stenosis at rest and after intravenous dipyridamole administration. **A,** Under resting conditions, distal coronary resistance drops in the stenosed vessel, maintaining normal coronary flow compared with a vessel without stenosis. **B,** Hence, thallium-201/^{99m}Tc-sestamibi SPECT imaging reveals uniform distribution throughout the myocardium. **C,** Intravenous dipyridamole causes equalization of the resistance of coronary vessels both with stenoses and without stenoses. Hence, coronary autoregulation of flow is impeded, and blood flow pre-ferentially flows down the normal coronary artery. **D,** This results in hypoperfusion of the area supplied by the stenosed coronary artery and redistribution of thallium-201/sestamibi in the direction of myocardium with normal flow. This represents the basis behind the use of intravenous dipyridamole in lieu of exercise for thallium-201/^{99m}Tc-sestamibi SPECT imaging in vascular surgery patients. (*Panels A,C adapted from* [17]; *panels B,D from* [17]; with permission.)

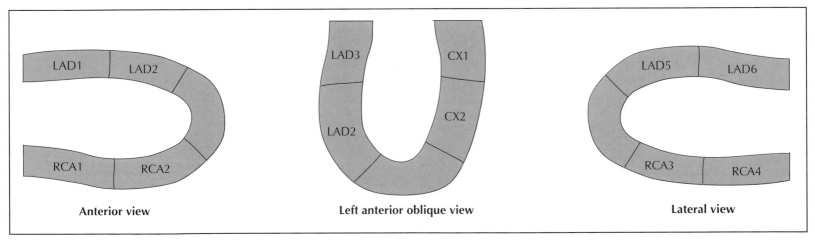

FIGURE 7-14. Quantitative analysis of dipyridamole-thallium-201 redistribution imaging to improve risk stratification of vascular surgery patients undergoing preoperative testing. In this approach, three separate views of thallium imaging—anterior, left anterior oblique, and lateral—are subdivided into segments corre-sponding to the coronary artery supplying that area. In these schematic views, the left anterior descending (LAD) has six segments of distribution in three different views, the circumflex (CX) has two segments, and the right coronary artery (RCA) has four segments. (*Adapted from* Levinson *et al.* [18].)

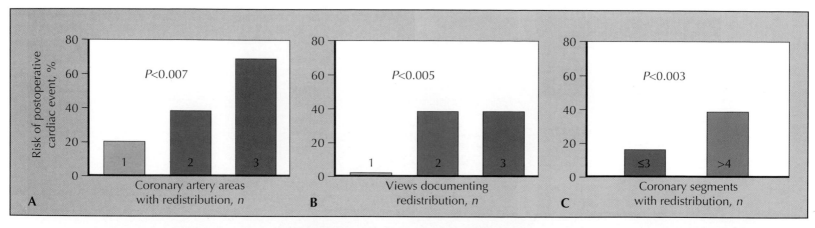

FIGURE 7-15. Results of a study of 62 patients undergoing preoperative dipyridamole-thallium-201 imaging. **A,** As suggested by imaging, the risk of postoperative cardiac events rose with the number of coronary arteries involved. **B,** In addition, the risk of postoperative cardiac events was only high when redistribution was seen in at least two views. **C,** Finally, postoperative risk was higher when more than four segments showed redistribution. (*Adapted from* Levinson *et al.* [18].)

PREOPERATIVE CORRELATES OF A CARDIAC ISCHEMIC EVENT AFTER PERIPHERAL VASCULAR SURGERY

	CARDIAC ISCHEMIC EVENT, *n (%)*		
	YES (*n* = 8)	NO (*n* = 40)	*P* VALUE
Age (mean±SD), *y*	63±5	62±7	NS
Patients, *n*	8 (100)	34 (85)	NS
History of chest pain	6 (75)	20 (50)	NS
Previous myocardial infarction	4 (50)	24 (60)	NS
Intra-abdominal procedure	4 (50)	23 (58)	NS
Abnormal thallium scan	8 (100)	20 (50)	< 0.05
Persistent thallium defect only	0 (0)	12 (30)	NS
Thallium redistribution	8 (100)	8 (20)	< 0.0001
Chest pain with dipyridamole	3 (38)	8 (20)	NS
ST depression with dipyridamole	2 (25)	3 (8)	NS

FIGURE 7-16. Data from 48 selected patients undergoing vascular surgery who were referred for preoperative dipyridamole-thallium-201 imaging. All eight patients who suffered a postoperative cardiac event had abnormal thallium redistribution-while only eight of 40 patients who were event-free had defects. Dipyridamole-thallium-201 imaging was the only factor considered that predicted risk. NS—not significant (*Adapted from* Boucher *et al.* [19].)

UNIVARIATE AND MULTIVARIATE ANALYSIS OF 86 PATIENTS WITH CARDIAC COMPLICATIONS

	PATIENTS WITH ADVERSE CARDIAC OUTCOME AND VARIABLE/PATIENTS	ODDS RATIO (95% CI)	
PREOPERATIVE VARIABLE	WITH VARIABLE, *n/n*	UNIVARIATE ANALYSIS	MULTIVARIATE ANALYSIS
Age > 65 y	52/202	2.3 (1.4–3.6)*	2.3 (1.4–3.6)*
Abdominal aortic aneurysm	51/252	1.2 (0.8–2.0)	
Previous myocardial infarction	22/73	2.2 (1.2–3.9)†	
History of angina	25/87	2.0 (1.2–3.5)†	
Ischemic ST-T abnormalities	18/71	1.6 (0.9–2.9)	
Definite coronary artery disease	47/163	2.6 (1.6–4.3)†	2.7 (1.7–4.4)†
Previous coronary artery graft	5/17	1.8 (0.6–5.5)	
Previous left ventricular failure	4/13	2.0 (0.6–6.7)	
Hypertension	50/218	1.7 (1.0–2.7)‡	
Rhythm other than sinus	3/12	1.5 (0.4–5.6)	
Ejection fraction < 50%	22/75	2.1 (1.2–3.7)†	1.7 (0.9–3.2)§
Fixed thallium defect	23/94	1.5 (0.9–2.7)	1.1 (0.6–2.2)§
Thallium redistribution	31/160	1.1 (0.6–1.7)	1.1 (0.6–2.0)§
Type 1 diabetes	1/6	0.9 (0.1–7.8)	
Type 2 diabetes	3/34	0.4 (0.1–1.4)	

*P<0.001.

†P<0.01.

‡P<0.05.

§Indicates the value of the adjusted odds ratio when the thallium scintigraphic data and ejection fraction were inserted into the model in order to obtain the best estimate of the predictive power of these variables that are not identified as significant predictors in the logistic regression.

FIGURE 7-17. Data from 457 consecutive unselected patients undergoing surgery for aortic aneurysms who also had preoperative dipyridamole-thallium-201 imaging and gated radionuclide angiography. Neither dipyridamole-thallium-201 imaging nor radionuclide angiography were predictors of cardiac risk. Results of multivariate analysis of the 86 patients with cardiac complications are shown only for predictive variables, thallium scintigraphic data, and ejection fraction. CI—confidence internal. (*Adapted from* Baron *et al.* [20].)

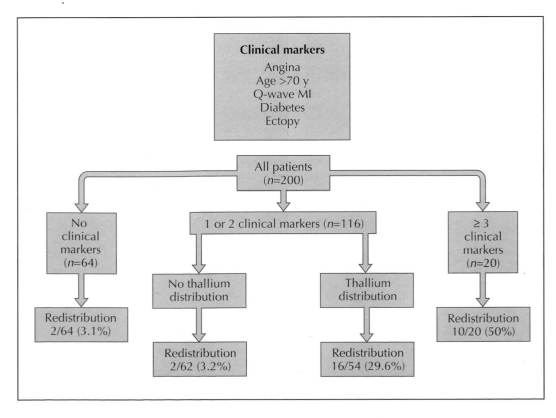

FIGURE 7-18. The interaction of clinical evaluation and dipyridamole-thallium-201 imaging for optimal preoperative assessment of vascular surgery patients. Based on clinical markers previously identified by Eagle *et al.* [14] (*see* Fig. 7-10), 200 patients were divided into a low-risk group (0 markers; *n* = 64), an intermediate-risk group (1 or 2 markers; *n* = 116), and a high-risk group (3 or more markers; *n* = 20). Redistribution of thallium uptake on imaging was most helpful in further stratifying the intermediate-risk group (3.2% risk with no redistribution defects vs a 29.6% risk with redistribution defects). In the high-risk group the postoperative risk remains exceedingly high, even in the absence of redistribution defects. Finally, in the low-risk group, while the presence of a redistribution defect is predictive of a slightly higher postoperative risk, the low prevalence of serious postoperative cardiac events makes uniform dipyridamole-thallium-201 testing in this group of questionable value. MI—myocardial infarction. (*Adapted from* Eagle *et al.* [14].)

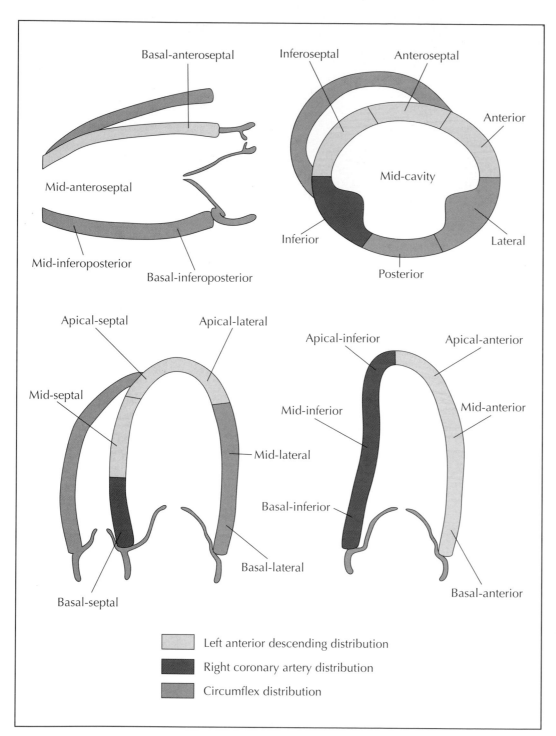

Basal-anteroseptal

Inferoseptal   Anteroseptal

Anterior

Mid-anteroseptal

Mid-cavity

Mid-inferoposterior

Inferior   Lateral

Basal-inferoposterior

Posterior

Apical-septal   Apical-lateral

Apical-inferior   Apical-anterior

Mid-septal

Mid-inferior   Mid-anterior

Mid-lateral

Basal-inferior

Basal-lateral

Basal-anterior

Basal-septal

Left anterior descending distribution

Right coronary artery distribution

Circumflex distribution

FIGURE 7-19. Echocardiography under pharmacologic stress (*eg*, dobutamine, dipyridamole, adenosine) prior to vascular surgery as a predictor of risk. This diagram of a 16-segment model depicts distribution of coronary artery territories as demonstrated by 2-dimensional echocardiography. Stress-induced abnormalities in wall motion corresponding to these territories correlate closely with distribution of coronary artery disease as shown. Depicted clockwise from the left are parasternal long- and short-axis, and two- and four-chamber views. (*Adapted from* Marcovitz and Armstrong [21].)

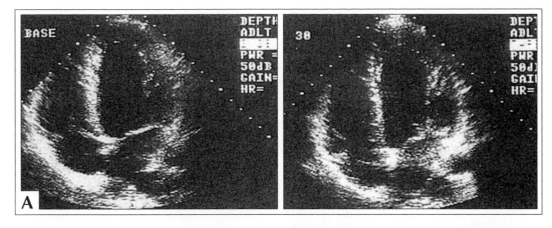

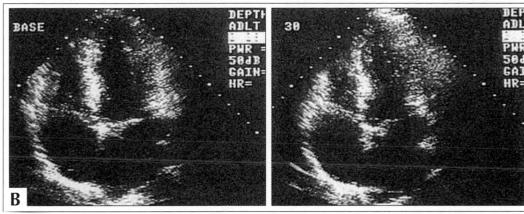

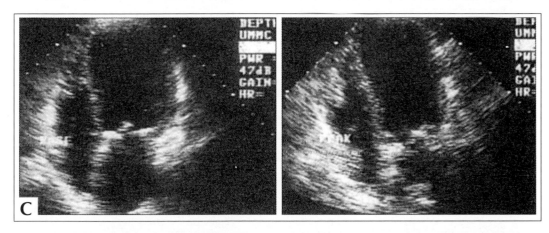

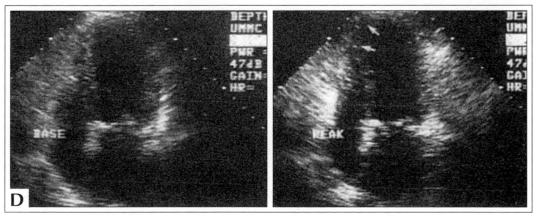

Figure 7-20. Dobutamine stress echocardiography. Two-dimensional echocardiographic images are obtained in various views to document diastolic and systolic dimensions of the left ventricular (LV) chamber and hence overall LV function and wall motion at baseline. Dobutamine, a potent intravenous inotrope that can exacerbate myocardial ischemia among patients with coronary artery disease, is infused at high doses over minutes. Patients with significant coronary artery disease will develop new LV systolic wall motion abnormalities that will be detected by repeat 2-dimensional echocardiography.

A series of 2-dimensional echocardiography images of the LV in the apical four-chamber view is shown. Diastolic (**A**) and systolic (**B**) echocardiograms at baseline and during peak dobutamine infusion in a patient with normal wall motion at rest and normal hyperdynamic response to dobutamine are shown. During systole all segments thicken normally and exhibit normal motion. Diastolic (**C**) and systolic (**D**) echocardiograms at baseline and during peak dobutamine infusion are also shown in the left anterior descending coronary artery distribution in a patient with significant coronary artery disease. In this patient, all segments contract normally at baseline. At peak dose the distal septum and apex become dyskinetic. This illustrates the mechanism by which dobutamine stress echocardiography can identify significant coronary artery disease and LV dysfunction, hence accurately assessing cardiac risk prior to noncardiac surgery. (*From* Marcovitz and Armstrong [21]; with permission.)

CARDIAC RISK ASSESSMENT USING DOBUTAMINE STRESS TESTING

	UNIVARIATE ODDS RATIO
Age > 70 y	2.3*
History of angina	5.1
History of infarction	4.0
Diabetes	3.5
Wall motion abnormality at rest	2.9
New wall motion abnormality during test	72*

*Independent predictors.

FIGURE 7-21. Important predictors of perioperative risk among patients who undergo major vascular surgery and have dobutamine stress echocardiography as a preoperative test. The historical factors of age, angina, prior infarction, and diabetes have been well documented in past studies. In this study, the findings of age and a new wall motion abnormality on echocardiography under the stress of dobutamine was a significant independent predictor of perioperative risk. (*Adapted from* Poldermans *et al.* [22].)

HOLTER (AMBULATORY) ECG MONITORING

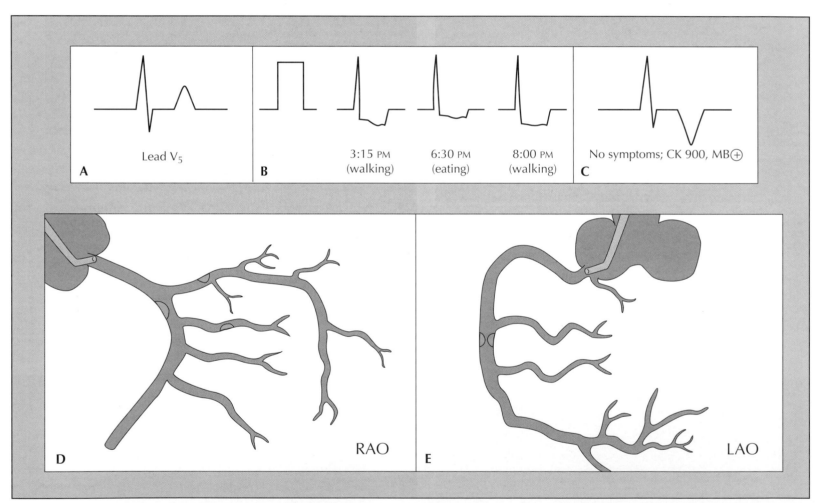

FIGURE 7-22. Use of Holter (ambulatory) electrocardiographic monitoring for asymptomatic ischemia for preoperative risk assessment among vascular surgery patients. Asymptomatic ischemia detected by Holter monitoring has long been known to predict cardiac risk in a variety of settings. Patients with a high prevalence of coronary artery disease often exhibit episodes of asymptomatic ST-segment depression corresponding to myocardial ischemia with heart rates far below those expected during exercise testing or pharmacologic interventions. These episodes of asymptomatic ST depression appear to predict cardiac risk among vascular surgery patients.

This diagram shows the history and clinical course of a 70-year-old diabetic woman with no clinical coronary artery disease who was about to undergo vascular surgery. Diabetes and age placed her at intermediate risk for postoperative cardiac events. **A,** Baseline electrocardiogram (ECG) was within normal limits. **B,** Preoperative Holter monitoring documented three separate episodes of asymptomatic ST-segment depression, occurring during a variety of activities. These episodes occurred at heart rates below those usually obtained with exercise or stress. **C,** On the first postoperative day she had an asymptomatic non–Q-wave myocardial infarction. **D** and **E,** On the third postoperative day she developed unstable angina. Three-vessel coronary artery disease was subsequently documented by coronary angiography. This case illustrates the potential use of preoperative Holter monitoring to predict cardiac risk in vascular surgery patients. CK—creatine kinase; LAO—left anterior oblique; MB—myocardial creatine kinase; RAO—right anterior oblique.

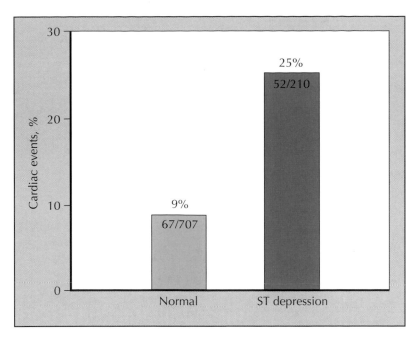

Figure 7-23. Pooled analysis of all studies that use preoperative Holter monitoring for ST-segment depression to predict postoperative cardiac events (death, myocardial infarction, unstable angina, pulmonary edema) in vascular surgery patients [23–26], including a study that did not show an independent association [24]. ST depression on Holter monitoring has an overall 25% positive predictive value and a 92% negative predictive value.

CORRELATION OF PREOPERATIVE ISCHEMIA WITH POSTOPERATIVE CARDIAC EVENTS

	ISCHEMIA PRESENT (n = 35)	ISCHEMIA ABSENT (n = 173)
Postoperative cardiac event, n (%)	13 (37%)	2 (1%)
Event type		
Fatal MI	1	0
Nonfatal MI	4	1
Unstable angina	4	0
Pulmonary edema	4	1

Figure 7-24. Correlation of preoperative ischemia detected by Holter monitoring with postoperative cardiac events among 208 consecutive patients undergoing vascular surgery. While 13 of 35 patients (37%) with myocardial ischemia had a postoperative cardiac event, a summary of the events revealed that only one event was fatal and only five were irreversible (death or myocardial infarction [MI]). The majority of postoperative cardiac events are transient unstable angina or pulmonary edema. In addition, the majority of patients with preoperative myocardial ischemia were able to undergo vascular surgery uneventfully. These observations represent the basis to support conservative medical management of perioperative high risk among vascular surgery patients. (*Adapted from* Raby *et al.* [23,27].)

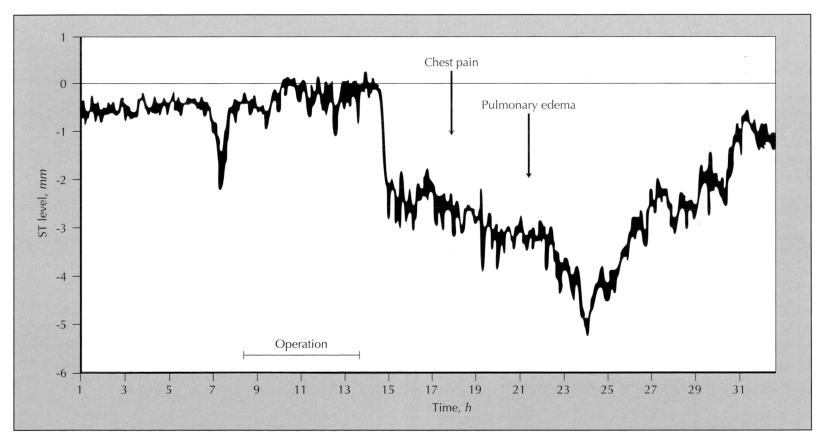

Figure 7-25. ST-segment trend plot of a typical patient undergoing vascular surgery while wearing a Holter monitor. An episode of ST-segment depression to 2.5 mm is evident preoperatively. The ST segment at baseline is essentially normal during surgery, reflecting the low prevalence of intraoperative ischemia usually noted in these patients. Postoperative ischemia, with ST-segment depressions of up to 6 mm, is evident shortly after operation. The clinical events of chest pain and pulmonary edema are clearly preceded by asymptomatic ischemia, detected as ST depression lasting at least 1 hour. This illustrates the typical pattern that is reported in the literature when describing the relationship of preoperative, intraoperative, and postoperative ischemia with cardiac events in vascular surgery patients. Postoperative ischemia precedes clinical events, and its detection may be useful for future treatment of myocardial ischemia in this patient population. (*Adapted from* Landesberg *et al.* [28].)

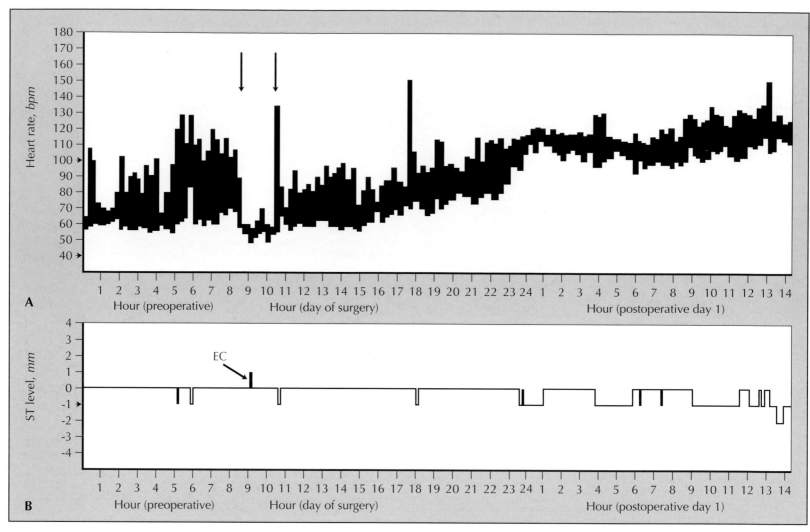

FIGURE 7-26. Heart rate (**A**) and ST level (**B**) histograms measured over time in a patient wearing a Holter monitor prior to, during, and after vascular surgery. The record begins at midnight on the day of surgery and ends at 2 PM on postoperative day 1. The arrows over the heart rate histogram represent the time period of the operation. Prior to surgery, heart rate is variable over a wide range (*panel A*), and episodes of high heart rate are associated with two episodes of myocardial ischemia (*panel B*). During surgery the heart rate is strictly controlled and below 70 bpm at all times. There is no associated myocardial ischemia (*EC* represents an electrocautery artifact). Immediately after surgery, there is a surge in heart rate (*panel A*) associated with an episode of myocardial ischemia (*panel B*). Over the next 48 hours, there are relatively few surges in heart rate that are abrupt, but the overall trend is upward. While tachycardia is not often achieved in the absolute sense (*eg*, heart rates greater than 110 bpm), an acceleration in heart rate relative to the intraoperative and postoperative periods does occur. This increase in heart rate is associated with multiple episodes of ischemia (*panel B*). The low prevalence of myocardial ischemia in the intraoperative setting (where maximal control of heart rate, blood pressure, and analgesia is achieved) is demonstrated. More importantly, this example also demonstrates the high prevalence of postoperative ischemia and its association with the gradual increase in heart rate that is noted over the first 48 hours. The *orange area* area is depicted under the minimum heart rate curve for computer integration purposes. (*Adapted from* McCann and Clements [29].)

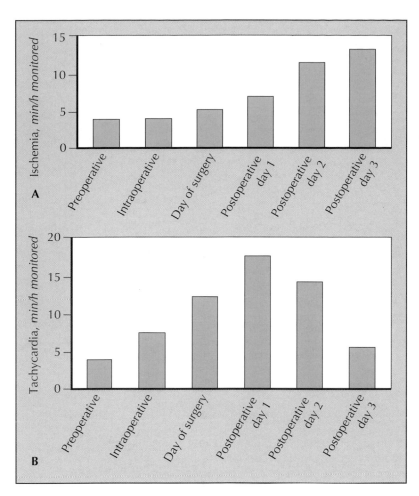

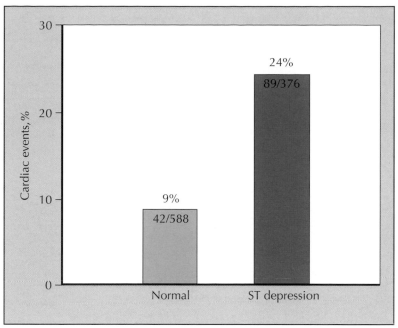

FIGURE 7-27. The prevalence of preoperative, intraoperative, and postoperative ischemia (defined as minutes of ST depression per hour monitored in a group of patients with and without preoperative ischemia undergoing vascular surgery. **A,** While the prevalence of preoperative and intraoperative ischemia is relatively low, the prevalence of postoperative ischemia is higher, particularly in the first 48 hours after surgery. This is the same time period in which the prevalence of tachycardia (defined as minutes of heart rate being more than 100 bpm per hour monitored) is highest (**B**). Ischemia occurs more often in patients with preoperative ischemia. (*Adapted from* McCann and Clements [29].)

FIGURE 7-28. Accuracy of postoperative Holter monitoring in predicting cardiac risk in vascular surgery patients. Many studies have shown that postoperative ischemia detected by Holter monitoring is an even stronger predictor of cardiac risk than preoperative ischemia in vascular surgery patients [24,25,27,28,30]. Pooled data, however, suggest that pre- and postoperative ischemia are comparable. Postoperative ischemia detected by Holter monitoring has a positive predictive value of 24% and a negative predictive value of 91%. A strong association of postoperative ischemia with postoperative cardiac events makes postoperative ischemia an excellent marker for measuring the effect of medical management on high-risk patients.

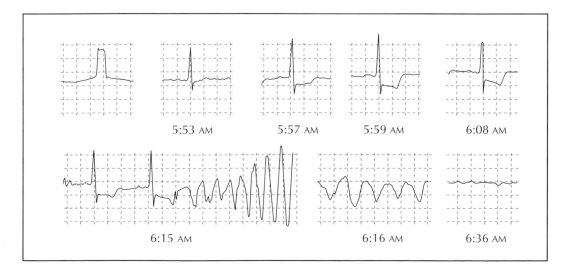

FIGURE 7-29. Graphic summary of Holter electrocardiographic data from an elderly man with carotid stenosis and known coronary artery disease who was felt to be at high risk by preoperative clinical and Holter markers. On the first postoperative day after carotid endarterectomy, he developed profound ST-segment depression several minutes prior to ventricular tachycardia, fibrillation, and cardiac arrest. This case illustrates the potential value of postoperative Holter monitoring in detecting silent ischemia that precedes a catastrophic cardiac event, thereby making pre-emptive therapy possible. (*Adapted from* Ganz *et al.* [31].)

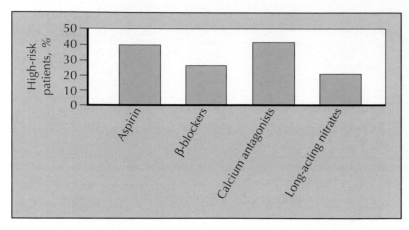

FIGURE 7-30. The proportion of 78 high-risk vascular surgery patients who received aspirin, β-blocker, calcium antagonist, or long-acting nitrate therapy at any time in the perioperative period. Despite the knowledge that such patients are at high risk, clinicians placed fewer than 50% of patients on any one of these well-accepted therapies for myocardial ischemia. This documents a significant under-utilization of medical therapy for myocardial ischemia in vascular surgery patients. In particular, the low rate of aspirin and β-blocker therapy is especially noteworthy, since both drugs are well known to reduce long-term risk attributable to myocardial ischemia [28,32].

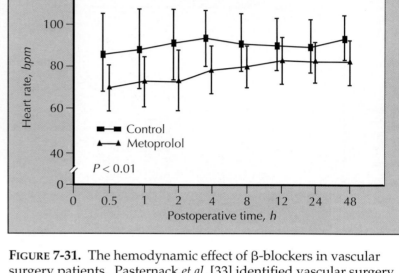

FIGURE 7-31. The hemodynamic effect of β-blockers in vascular surgery patients. Pasternack *et al.* [33] identified vascular surgery patients who had received postoperative metoprolol for 48 hours and compared their overall heart rate and ultimate outcome with a similar group of vascular surgery patients who did not receive any β-blocker therapy. Depicted are differences in heart rate between vascular surgery patients who received metoprolol during the postoperative period versus vascular surgery patients who served as controls. β-blocker therapy significantly reduced average heart rate over the first 48 hours postoperatively. (*Adapted from* Pasternack *et al.* [33].)

FIGURE 7-32. The effect of metoprolol therapy given to patients undergoing vascular surgery in the postoperative setting compared with similar patients receiving no therapy (same study as Fig. 7-31). The metoprolol group (group 1) experienced significantly fewer perioperative myocardial infarctions (MI) than did controls (group 2). These preliminary data suggest that β-blocker therapy in the postoperative setting effectively controls heart rate and results in lower cardiac risk ($P < 0.05$). (*Adapted from* Pasternack *et al.* [33].)

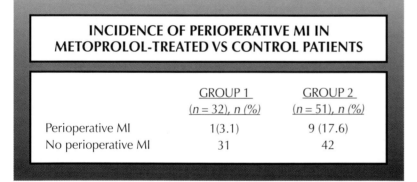

INCIDENCE OF PERIOPERATIVE MI IN METOPROLOL-TREATED VS CONTROL PATIENTS

	GROUP 1 ($n = 32$), n (%)	GROUP 2 ($n = 51$), n (%)
Perioperative MI	1(3.1)	9 (17.6)
No perioperative MI	31	42

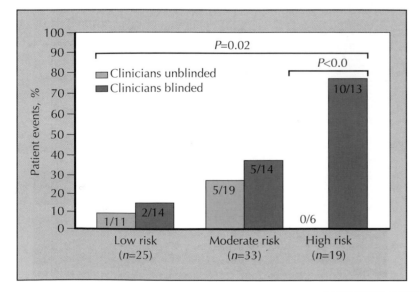

FIGURE 7-33. Perioperative cardiac outcomes among vascular surgery patients who had demonstrated myocardial ischemia and whose clinicians were unblinded to Holter monitor results compared with vascular surgery patients who had demonstrated myocardial ischemia and whose clinicians were blinded to equivalent Holter results (all 77 patients in this trial had myocardial ischemia preoperatively). When patients were stratified into low-, moderate-, and high-risk groups by clinical criteria alone (*see* Eagle's criteria, Fig. 7-10), the effect of unblinding clinicians to the presence of preoperative myocardial ischemia had a large impact on risk reduction among the high-risk group. Preoperative testing may best alter medical management in the postoperative setting. This may result in protection of the high-risk patients. (*Adapted from* Andrews *et al.* [32].)

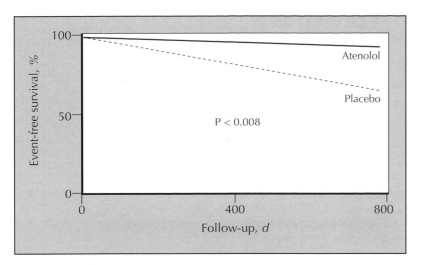

FIGURE 7-34. Effect of atenolol on long-term prognosis after noncardiac surgery. The first trial of β-adrenergic blockade in noncardiac surgery randomized 201 consecutive patients, many of whom had coronary artery disease or underwent vascular surgery, to atenolol versus placebo prior to major surgery. Kaplan-Meier analysis showed that patients randomized to β-blockers had significantly lower perioperative event rates and longer cardiac event rates, even if atenolol were discontinued at hospital discharge. Researchers attribute the latter phenomenon to avoiding postoperative ischemia, which they speculate contributes to longer-term cardiac morbidity. (*Adapted from* Mangano *et al.* [34].)

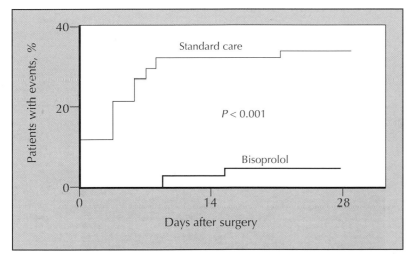

ATENOLOL AND POSTOPERATIVE MYOCARDIAL ISCHEMIA

	ATENOLOL (*n* = 99)	PLACEBO
Preoperative	13	12
Operative	12	18
Postoperative day 0–7	24	39
Postoperative day 0–2	17	34*

*$P < 0.008$.

FIGURE 7-35. Atenolol and postoperative myocardial ischemia. Analysis of Holter monitors to detect postoperative ischemia in patients randomized to atenolol versus placebo while undergoing major surgery showed that when compared with placebo, atenolol significantly reduced silent ischemia during the high prevalence postoperative periods. (*Adapted from* Wallace *et al.* [35].)

FIGURE 7-36. Effect of bisoprolol on perioperative risk. Patients were randomized to receive bisoprolol versus placebo following a positive dobutamine echocardiogram in preparation for major or vascular surgery. Bisoprolol significantly reduced cardiac risk or perioperative events among a very high-risk population, and was associated with significantly lowered postoperative heart rates during the highest risk postoperative period. (*Adapted from* Poldermans *et al.* [36].)

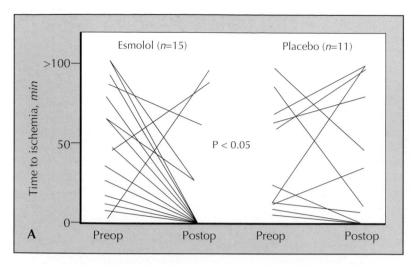

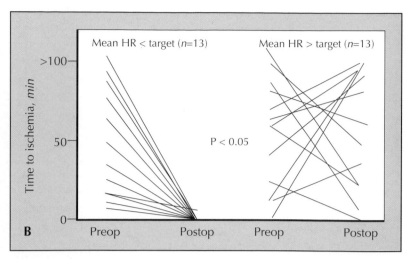

FIGURE 7-37. Heart rate control and myocardial ischemia. Comparison of preoperative and postoperative ischemic episodes among patients with preoperative ischemia undergoing vascular surgery who were then randomized to postoperative esmolol versus placebo. **A,** Esmolol significantly reduced or eliminated most postoperative ischemia in this high-risk group. **B,** This secondary analysis shows that if the heart rate is maintained below a target threshold (established as that level below which no preoperative ischemias occurred), postoperative ischemia was virtually eliminated. (*Adapted from* Raby *et al.* [37].)

EFFECT OF CORONARY ARTERY BYPASS SURGERY ON CARDIAC RISK

OUTCOMES OF NONCARDIAC SURGERY AFTER CORONARY REVASCULARIZATION

	AFTER CABG (*n* = 538)	AFTER PTCA (*n* = 511)
Death (%)	5 (0.9)	6 (1.2)
MI (%)	2 (0.4)	2 (0.4)

FIGURE 7-38. Outcomes of noncardiac surgery after coronary revascularization. This figure shows the incidence of death, nonfatal myocardial infarction (MI), and average length of stay among 501 patients randomized to receive either coronary artery bypass grafting (CABG) or percutaneous transluminal coronary angioplasty (PTCA), who went on to have noncardiac surgery. After noncardiac surgery, length of stay was comparably short and adverse cardiac events were low and comparable in angioplasty and coronary surgery arms. These data suggest that if coronary revascularization was undertaken prior to noncardiac surgery, patents were at low risk. Since this analysis does not take into account the morbidity and mortality of the coronary revascularization, it does not justify prophylactic coronary revascularization in patients undergoing vascular surgery. (*Adapted from* Hassan *et al.* [38].)

COST ANALYSIS OF AAA REPAIR AMONG 201 PATIENTS

DIAGNOSTIC MODALITY (*n*)	COST PER PATIENT, $*	TOTAL STUDY COST, $*
Selective nuclear test (58)	567	32,886
Catheterization (18)	9200	27,600
PTCA (2)	21,760	43,520
CABG (11)	44,200	486,200

In 1996 US dollars.

FIGURE 7-39. Cost analysis among 201 patients undergoing abdominal aortic aneurysm (AAA) repair who underwent risk assessment via a history, physical examination, and electrocardiogram. Those judged at high risk were subjected to dipyridamole-thallium-201 scintigraphy and, if positive, coronary angiography and where appropriate, coronary revascularization. In this consecutive series of patients, the overall perioperative mortality was low (0.5%); therefore, using this conventional approach appears unjustified on a cost basis. Preoperative testing and prophylactic revascularization are only warranted when dealing with a very high-risk cohort of patients. CABG—coronary artery bypass grafting; PTCA—percutaneous transluminal coronary angioplasty. (*Adapted from* Bartels *et al.* [11].)

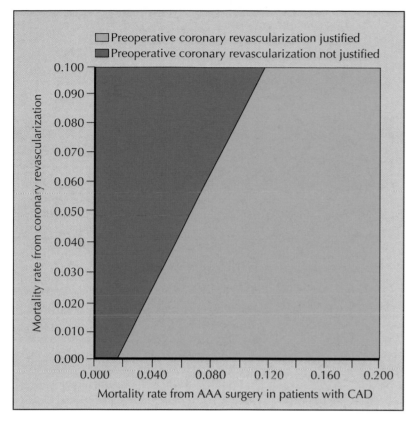

FIGURE 7-40. Two-way sensitivity analysis of mortality from abdominal aortic aneurysm (AAA) surgery in patients with coronary artery disease (CAD) versus mortality from coronary revascularization prior to AAA repair in the same patients. In this study, Fleisher *et al.* [39] determined the following from the literature: 1) mortality estimates for AAA surgery without the benefit of coronary bypass surgery in patients with CAD; and 2) mortality esti-mates among the same patients if they undergo coronary revascularization prior to AAA repair. Using decision analytic techniques, the mortality from AAA repair alone is plotted against the mortality from coronary revascularization prior to AAA repair. The lower the risk of preoperative coronary revascularization and/or the higher the risk of AAA repair without prophylactic coronary revascularization, the more justified an approach of preoperative prophylactic coronary revascularization becomes. By contrast, the higher the risk of coronary revascularization among AAA patients and/or the lower the risk of AAA surgery without prior coronary revascularization, the less justified preoperative prophylactic coronary revascularization becomes. More specifically, if cardiac mortality from AAA surgery in patients with CAD is less than 2%, prophylactic coronary revascularization would never be justified (*blue area*). By contrast, if cardiac mortality from AAA surgery in CAD patients approaches 12%, prophylactic coronary revascularization would always be justified, provided cardiac mortality from coronary revascularization does not exceed 10% (*pink area*).

This study illustrates how a strategy to employ preoperative prophylactic coronary revascularization among vascular surgery patients is heavily dependent on how dangerous coronary revascularization is *and* how safe vascular surgery alone is in this patient population. Using best estimates from the literature and assuming a 5% cardiac mortality from vascular surgery without prior revascularization, preoperative coronary revascularization is justified only if the *overall* mortality of coronary revascularization is *less* than 2%. Assuming a 10% mortality from vascular surgery alone, preoperative coronary revascularization would be justified only if the overall mortality from coronary revascularization was less than 8%. Given that the estimates of mortality from coronary revascularization among vascular surgery patients are thought to exceed these levels, prophylactic coronary revascularization appears unjustified for most patients. (*Adapted from* Fleisher *et al.* [39].)

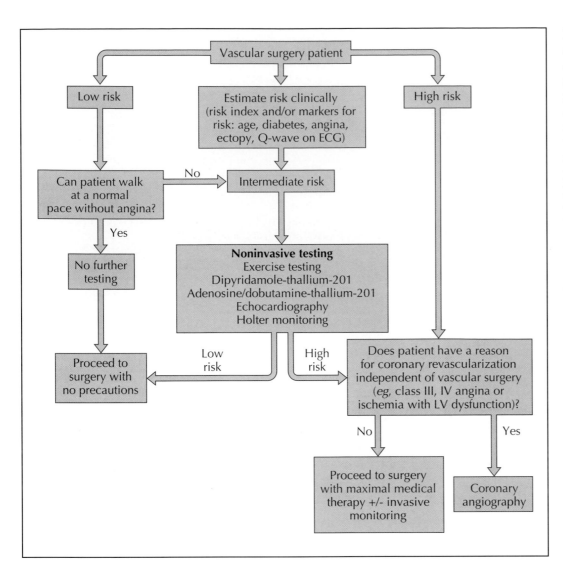

FIGURE 7-41. Algorithm suggesting a reasonable approach to the diagnostic evaluation and medical management of vascular surgery patients. The cardiac risk is first estimated by history, physical examination, and electrocardiographic (ECG) findings. The majority of patients will be at low risk, and if they are asymptomatic despite normal activities (such as walking two blocks at a normal pace), they will require no further testing to proceed with surgery without precautions. Patients felt to be at high risk as indicated by clinical grounds require no further noninvasive testing to confirm this. Patients at intermediate risk are the most likely to benefit from noninvasive testing. Exercise testing is still the optimal choice in patients who can exercise. In patients who cannot exercise, dipyridamole-thallium-201 is the most widely accepted alternative method. Adenosine/dobutamine-thallium-201 have also shown promise as has dobutamine stress echocardiography and Holter monitoring in selected patient subsets. Patients at low risk by noninvasive testing may proceed to surgery without precautions. Patients at high risk by noninvasive testing or by clinical criteria should have coronary angiography with an eye toward myocardial revascularization *only* if there is an indication for myocardial revascularization independent of vascular surgery (such as class III or IV angina pectoris or ischemia with left ventricular [LV] dysfunction). If there is no such indication, many high-risk patients can proceed to surgery but with maximal medical therapy plus the consideration of invasive monitoring. (*Adapted from* Wong and Detsky [40].)

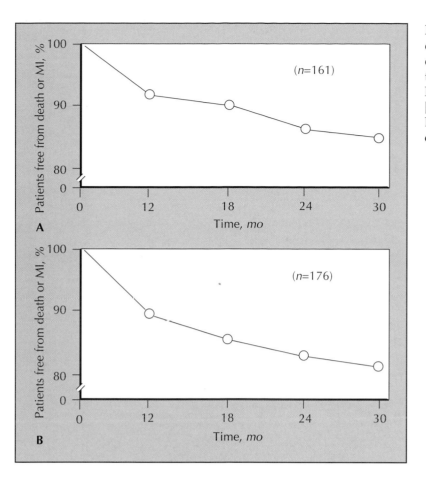

A

B

FIGURE 7-42. Kaplan-Meier curves demonstrating the percentage of patients free from fatal or nonfatal myocardial infarction (MI) on long-term follow up after vascular surgery. **A,** Of 161 consecutive patients studied in 1982 [5], less than 90% remained free from MI at 30 months. **B,** Of 176 consecutive patients studied in 1990 [41], less than 90% of patients were free from MI at 30 months. Despite advances in perioperative risk management, long-term cardiac risk appears not to have changed over that time period.

REFERENCES

1. Hertzer NR, Beven EG, Young JR, *et al*.: Coronary artery disease in peripheral vascular patients: a classification of 1000 coronary angiograms and results of surgical management. *Ann Surg* 1984, 199:223–233.

2. Criqui MH, Langer RD, Fronek A, *et al*.: Mortality over a period of 10 years in patients with peripheral arterial disease. *N Engl J Med* 1992, 329:381–386.

3. Vogt MT, Cauley JA, Newman AB, *et al*.: Decreased ankle/brachial blood pressure index and mortality in elderly women. *JAMA* 1993, 270:465–469.

4. Rosenfeld BA, Beattie C, Christopherson R, *et al*.: The effects of different anesthetic regimens on fibrinolysis and the development of postoperative arterial thrombosis. *Anesthesiology* 1993, 79:435–443.

5. Jamieson WI, Janusz MT, Miyagishima RT, Gerein AN: Influence of ischemic heart disease on early and late mortality after surgery for peripheral occlusive vascular disease. *Circulation* 1982, 66:I-92–I-98.

6. Hertzer NR: The natural history of peripheral vascular disease. *Circulation* 1991, 83:I-12–I-19.

7. Hollier LH, Plate G, O'Brien PC, *et al*.: Late survival after abdominal aortic aneurysm repair: influence of coronary artery disease. *J Vasc Surg* 1984, 1:290–299.

8. Golden MA, Whittemore AD, Donaldson MC, Mannick JA: Selective evaluation and management of coronary artery disease in patients undergoing repair of abdominal aortic aneurysms. *Ann Surg* 1990, 212:415–423.

9. Donaldson MC, Mannick JA, Whittemore AD: Femoral-distal bypass with in situ greater saphenous vein: long-term results using the Mills valvulotome. *Ann Surg* 1991, 213:457–465.

10. Bunt TJ: The role of a defined protocol for cardiac risk assessment in decreasing perioperative myocardial infarction in vascular surgery. *J Vasc Surg* 1992, 15:626–634.

11. Bartels JF, Bechtell M, Hossmann V, Svante H: Cardiac risk stratification for high-risk surgery. *J Vasc Surg* 1992, 15:626–634.

12. Detsky AS, Abrams HB, McLaughlin JR, *et al*.: Predicting cardiac complications in patients undergoing noncardiac surgery. *J Gen Intern Med* 1981, 141:1631–1634.

13. Lee TH, Marcantonio ER, Mangione CM, *et al*.: Derivation and prospective validation of a simple index for prediction of cardiac risk in major noncardiac surgery. *Circulation* 1999, 100:1043–1049.

14. Eagle KA, Coley CM, Newell JB, *et al*.: Combining clinical and thallium data optimizes preoperative assessment of cardiac risk for major vascular surgery. *Ann Intern Med* 1989, 110:859–866.

15. McPhail N, Calvin JE, Shariatmadar A, *et al*.: The use of preoperative exercise testing to predict cardiac complications after arterial reconstruction. *J Vasc Surg* 1988, 7:60–68.

16. Gauss A, Rohm HJ, Schauffelen A, *et al*.: Electrocardiographic exercise stress testing for cardiac risk assessment in patients undergoing noncardiac surgery. *Anesthesiology* 2001, 94:38–46.

17. IV Persantine, Physician's Guide. Billerica, MA: Dupont-Merck Pharmaceuticals. Serial #MF-100/8362; pp. 4–5.

18. Levinson JR, Boucher CA, Coley CM, *et al*.: Usefulness of semi-quantitative analysis of dipyridamole-thallium 201 redistribution for improving risk stratification before vascular surgery. *Am J Cardiol* 1990, 66:406–410.

19. Boucher CA, Brewster DC, Darling RC, *et al*.: Determination of cardiac risk by dipyridamole-thallium imaging before peripheral vascular surgery. *N Engl J Med* 1985, 312:389–394.

20. Baron JF, Mundler O, Bertrand M, *et al.*: Dypridamole-thallium scintigraphy and gated radionuclide angiography to assess cardiac risk before abdominal aortic surgery. *N Engl J Med* 1994, 330:663–996.

21. Marcovitz PA, Armstrong WF: Accuracy of dobutamine stress echocardiography in detecting coronary artery disease. *Am J Cardiol* 1992, 69:1269–1273.

22. Poldermans D, Fioretti PM, Forster T, *et al.*: Dobutamine stress echocardiography for assessment of perioperative cardiac risk in patients undergoing major vascular surgery. *Circulation* 1993, 87:1506–1512.

23. Raby KE, Goldman L, Creager MA, *et al.*: Correlation between preoperative ischemia and major cardiac events after peripheral vascular surgery. *N Engl J Med* 1989, 321:1296–1300.

24. Mangano DT, Browner WS, Hollenberg M, *et al.*: Association of perioperative myocardial ischemia with cardiac morbidity and mortality in men undergoing noncardiac surgery. *N Engl J Med* 1990, 323:1781.

25. Pasternack PF, Grossi EA, Baumann FG, *et al.*: Silent myocardial ischemia monitoring predicts late as well as perioperative cardiac events in patients undergoing vascular surgery. *J Vasc Surg* 1992, 16:171–180.

26. Fleisher LA, Rosenbaum SH, Nelson AH, Barash PG: The predictive value of preoperative silent ischemia for postoperative ischemic cardiac events in vascular and nonvascular surgery patients. *Am Heart J* 1991, 122:980–985.

27. Raby KE, Barry J, Creager MA, *et al.*: Detection and significance of intraoperative and postoperative ischemia in peripheral vascular surgery. *JAMA* 1992, 268:222–227.

28. Landesberg G, Luria MH, Cotev S, *et al.*: Importance of long-duration postoperative ST-segment depression in cardiac morbidity after vascular surgery. *Lancet* 1993, 341:715–719.

29. McCann RL, Clements FN: Silent myocardial ischemia in patients undergoing peripheral vascular surgery: incidence and association with perioperative cardiac morbidity and mortality. *J Vasc Surg* 1989, 9:583–587.

30. Ouyang P, Gerstenblith G, Furman WI, *et al.*: Frequency and significance of early postoperative silent myocardial ischemia in patients having peripheral vascular surgery. *Am J Cardiol* 1989, 64:1113.

31. Ganz L, Andrews TC, Barry J, Raby KE: Silent ischemia preceding sudden cardiac death in a patient after vascular surgery. *Am Heart J* 1994, 127:1652–1654.

32. Andrews TC, Goldman L, Creager MA, *et al.*: Identification and treatment of perioperative myocardial ischemia in patients undergoing peripheral vascular surgery. *J Vasc Med Biol* 1994, 5:8–15.

33. Pasternack PF, Imparato AM, Baumann FG, *et al.*: The hemodynamics of beta-blockade in patients undergoing abdominal aortic aneurysm repair. *Circulation* 1987, 76:III1–III7.

34. Mangano DT, Layug EL, Wallace A, Tateo I: Effect of atenolol on mortality and cardiovascular morbidity after noncardiac surgery. Multicenter Study of Perioperative Ischemia Research Group. *N Engl J Med* 1996, 335(23):1713–1720.

35. Wallace A, Layug B, Tateo I, *et al.*: Prophylactic atenolol reduces postoperative myocardial ischemia. McSPI Research Group. *Anesthesiology* 1998, 88(1):7–17.

36. Poldermans D, Boersma E, Bax JJ, *et al.*: The effect of bisoprolol on perioperative mortality and myocardial infarction in high-risk patients undergoing vascular surgery. Dutch Echocardiographic Cardiac Risk Evaluation Applying Stress Echocardiography Study Group. *N Engl J Med* 1999, 341(24):1789–1794.

37. Raby KE, Brull SJ, Timimi F, *et al.*: The effect of heart rate control on myocardial ischemia among high-risk patients after vascular surgery. *Anesth Analg* 1999, 88(3):477–482.

38. Hassan SA, Hlatky MA, Boothroyd DB, *et al.*: Outcomes of noncardiac surgery after coronary bypass surgery or coronary angioplasty in the Bypass Angioplasty Revascularization Investigation (BARI). *Am J Med* 2001, 110(4):260–266.

39. Fleisher LA, Skolnick ED, Holroyd KJ, Lehmann HP: Coronary artery revascularization before abdominal aortic aneurysm surgery: a decision analytic approach. *Anesth Analg* 1994, 79:661–669.

40. Wong T, Detsky AS: Preoperative cardiac risk assessment for patients having peripheral vascular surgery. *Ann Intern Med* 1992, 116:743–753.

41. Raby KE, Goldman L, Cook EF, *et al.*: Long-term prognosis of myocardial ischemia detected by Holter monitoring in peripheral vascular disease. *Am J Cardiol* 1990, 66:1309–1313.

8
CHAPTER

RAYNAUD'S PHENOMENON AND OTHER VASOSPASTIC DISORDERS

Marie Gerhard-Herman and Mark A. Creager

Raynaud's phenomenon is defined as episodic digital vasospasm characterized by well-demarcated pallor or cyanosis that occurs in the digits during exposure to cold. This chapter reviews the pathophysiology, associated disorders, and treatment of Raynaud's phenomenon. The mechanisms proposed to explain this phenomenon include increased sympathetic nervous system activity, local vascular hyperreactivity to sympathetic stimuli, decreased intravascular pressure or changes in blood rheology, and excessive vasoconstrictive stimuli. Raynaud's phenomenon is categorized into primary and secondary forms. The primary form implies the absence of any disorder or drug treatment that promotes vasospasm.

The secondary causes of Raynaud's phenomenon include connective tissue disorders, arterial occlusive disease, trauma, neurologic disorders, blood dyscrasias, drugs, and toxins. The diagnosis is made by patient history, which, along with physical examination, can indicate possible secondary causes. Diagnostic testing is directed at revealing the underlying causes of Raynaud's phenomenon and includes digital plethysmography, nail-fold capillary microscopy, and selected blood tests such as the erythrocyte sedimentation rate and antinuclear antibody.

Treatment is initiated with patient education emphasizing the importance of dressing warmly and reducing exposure to cold. Pharmacologic therapy is indicated in those patients with debilitating symptoms and/or digital ulcerations despite conservative therapy. Calcium channel antagonists and sympathetic nervous system blockers are often effective in decreasing symptoms of Raynaud's phenomenon. Sympathectomy is not always helpful and is reserved for those patients with persistent digital ischemia refractory to medical therapy.

Other vascular disorders associated with cold exposure include acrocyanosis, pernio, and frostbite. In contrast to Raynaud's phenomenon, these disorders are characterized by some degree of persistent discoloration. Acrocyanosis is an uncommon disorder of peripheral cyanosis that intensifies during cold exposure. Pernio (chilblains), which occurs in acute and chronic forms, is characterized by pruritic burning lesions affecting skin exposed to the cold. Freezing of tissues results in frostbite. Precipitated by increased temperature, erythromelalgia is a disorder that causes pain, redness, and warmth in the feet and hands. In contrast to the ill effects of cold in the three previous disorders, cold temperatures relieve the erythema and burning pain of erythromelalgia.

Raynaud's Phenomenon

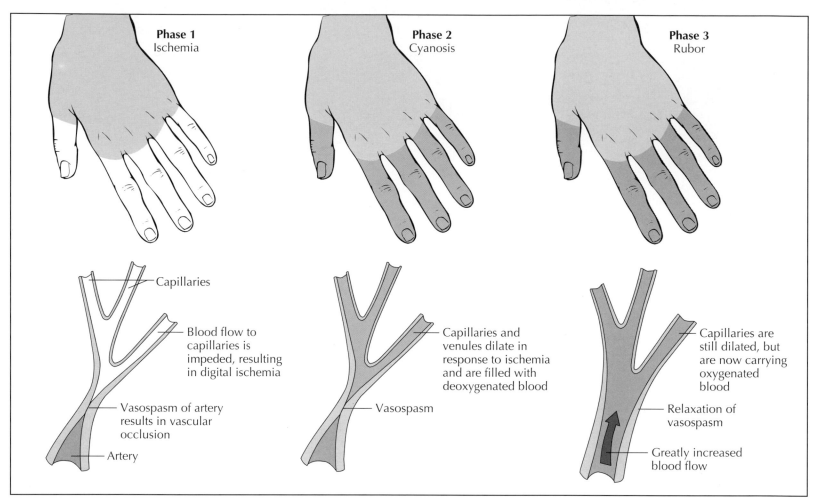

FIGURE 8-1. Raynaud's phenomenon. Raynaud's phenomenon consists of episodic and well-demarcated ischemic color changes that are primarily confined to the fingers and toes. Ischemia (phase 1), which is present in most patients, is secondary to digital vasospasm and results in pallor or blanching. Cyanosis (phase 2) results from the collection of deoxygenated blood in dilated arteri-oles, venules, and capillaries. Cold, numbness, and paresthesia of the digits often accompany phases 1 and 2. Rubor (phase 3) occurs with rewarming, as the digital vasospasm resolves and blood flow into the dilated arterioles and capillaries dramatically increases. Rubor is often accompanied by a throbbing sensation. (*Adapted from* Creager [1].)

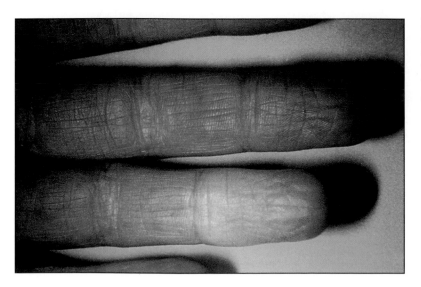

FIGURE 8-2. Raynaud's phenomenon occurring in a single digit. The pallor phase of a vasospastic attack is present in the ring finger of this patient with Raynaud's phenomenon. The ischemic area is characteristically well demarcated. Blanching may affect only one or two fingers early in the course of Raynaud's phenomenon.

CLINICAL CRITERIA OF PRIMARY RAYNAUD'S PHENOMENON

Bilateral episodic attacks of acral pallor or cyanosis

Strong and symmetric peripheral pulses

No digital pitting, ulcerations, or gangrene

No signs or symptoms of systemic disease associated with Raynaud's phenomenon

Symptoms for > 2 y

Normal nailfold capillaries

Negative antinuclear antibody test

Normal erythrocyte sedimentation rate

FIGURE 8-3. Clinical criteria. Raynaud's phenomenon may be primary, *ie*, unassociated with any other disease process, or secondary, *ie*, occurring as a consequence of another disease or drug. Allen and Brown [2] established five minimal criteria for the diagnosis of primary Raynaud's phenomenon after their observation of 150 patients: 1) vasospastic attacks precipitated by cold or emotional stimuli; 2) bilateral involvement of the extremities; 3) absence of gangrene, or gangrene limited to the fingertips; 4) absence of underlying disease to account for the vasospasm; and 5) symptoms for longer than 2 years. These criteria are presented here as modified by LeRoy and Medsger [3] to include the results of laboratory evaluation in addition to history and physical examination. Nailfold capillaries must appear as regularly spaced hairpin loops when examined by microscopy. Antinuclear antibody levels less than a titer of 1:100 for all fluorescence patterns are considered negative. Erythrocyte sedimentation rate less than 20 mm/h is used in these criteria. These criteria permitted classification of 89% of the patients in a retrospective study of 240 patients with Raynaud's phenomenon.

CLINICAL FEATURES OF PRIMARY RAYNAUD'S PHENOMENON

50% of Raynaud's patients have primary Raynaud's phenomenon

Female:male ratio = 4:1

Age of onset: 15–40 y

Vasospastic episodes occur mostly in fingers, less often in toes and tip of nose and earlobes

Spontaneous improvement in 15%; progression in 30%

< 1% lose part of a digit

FIGURE 8-4. Clinical features. Primary Raynaud's phenomenon accounts for 50% of all presentations of Raynaud's phenomenon. It is present in 4.6% to 20% of the population, with a higher prevalence in colder climates. Raynaud's phenomenon occurs more often in females than males, and the average age of onset is 31 years. Vasospastic episodes are usually precipitated by direct or indirect exposure of the extremity to a cool environment and occur most often in the fingers, less often in the toes, and least often in the earlobes and tip of the nose. Primary Raynaud's phenomenon has the most benign prognosis of all the forms of Raynaud's phenomenon. Less than 1% of these patients eventually lose part of a digit to ischemia. Spontaneous improvement occurs in 15%, while progression of symptoms occurs in 30%.

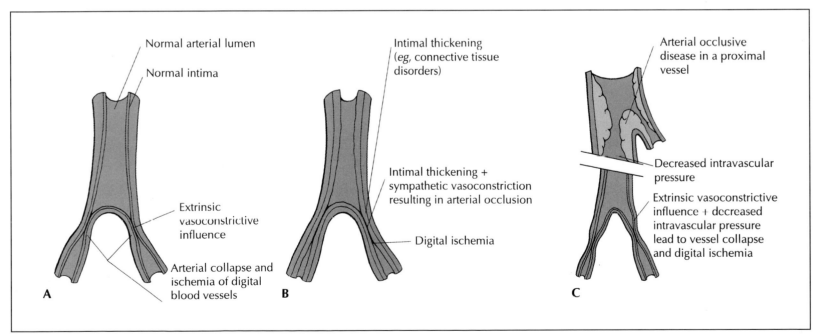

FIGURE 8-5. Pathophysiology. Digital vasospasm results in Raynaud's phenomenon when there is an excessive vasoconstrictor response to stimuli that would normally cause modest smooth muscle contraction, but have instead resulted in obliteration of the vascular lumen (**A**). Sympathetic adrenergic vasoconstriction plays an important role in the phenomenon, since digital cutaneous vessels are not supplied by sympathetic adrenergic vasodilator fibers. An ischemic response to vasoconstrictor stimuli becomes more likely in secondary Raynaud's phenomenon when intimal thickening (*eg*, collagen vascular disease) may result in decreased diameter of the arterial lumen (**B**). Also, when proximal stenosis results in decreased intravascular pressure, the addition of extrinsic vasoconstrictor forces may lead to collapse of the vessel (*eg*, atherosclerosis; **C**).

PATHOPHYSIOLOGY OF RAYNAUD'S PHENOMENON

- Excessive sympathetic efferent activity to digital vessels
- Local vascular fault causes vessels to overreact to normal vasoconstrictor stimuli
- Decreased intravascular pressure allows tissue to collapse when vascular tone increases
- Circulating or local vasoconstrictor substances

FIGURE 8-6. Pathophysiology. A number of mechanisms have been proposed to explain episodic digital vasospasm. Maurice Raynaud suggested that increased sympathetic efferent activity to digital vessels caused the vasospastic attacks [4]. Sir Thomas Lewis subsequently observed that vasospasm could be provoked in fingers that had been exposed to the cold even after nerve blockade or sympathectomy [5]. He concluded that Raynaud's phenomenon occurred because of increased sensitivity of the digital vessels to sympathetic stimuli, *ie*, local vascular abnormalities. Low digital artery pressure may also contribute to the development of Raynaud's phenomenon in the presence of extrinsic vasoconstrictor forces leading to vessel collapse. Both circulating and local vasoconstrictor substances in increased amounts have been suspected to contribute to the development of digital vasospasm.

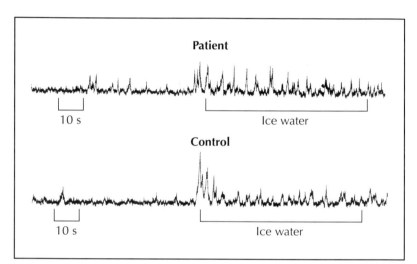

FIGURE 8-7. Role of increased sympathetic activity. Fagius and Blumberg [6] measured skin nerve sympathetic activity from the right median nerve in seven patients with primary Raynaud's phenomenon and in 10 healthy subjects. Sympathetic activity to the right hand was measured both at rest (*left*) and with immersion of the left hand in cold water (*right*). An example of patient and control sympathetic responses is presented. The horizontal lines indicate the immersion time. A clear increase of sympathetic outflow to the right hand was seen in all subjects during immersion of the left hand. Sympathetic efferent activity in response to cold was the same in patients with Raynaud's phenomenon (*top*) and control subjects (*bottom*). These data suggest that increased sympathetic activity does not cause Raynaud's phenomenon. (*Adapted from* Fagius and Blumberg [6].)

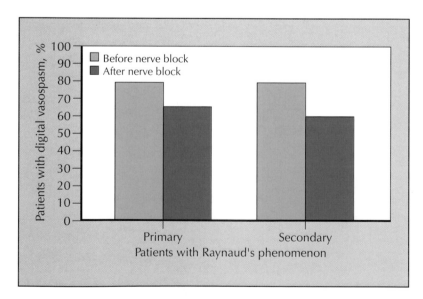

FIGURE 8-8. Local vascular abnormality. A number of investigators have considered the possibility that Raynaud's phenomenon occurs as a result of increased sensitivity of the digital vessels to sympathetic stimuli. To study this possible mechanism, patients with primary Raynaud's phenomenon and control subjects had the temperature of one hand maintained at 36°C and the other at 26°C. When ice was applied to their necks, the magnitude of reflex vasoconstriction was similar in both populations in the warm hand but was exaggerated in the cold hand in the patients with Raynaud's phenomenon. Freedman *et al.* [7] induced vasospastic attacks with environmental and local cooling in patients with primary and secondary Raynaud's phenomenon both before and after digital nerve block. Vasospastic attacks were precipitated in 80% of the subjects with primary Raynaud's phenomenon before digital nerve block and in 66% following digital nerve block. In the subjects with scleroderma and secondary Raynaud's phenomenon, 80% demonstrated vasospastic attacks before digital nerve block and 60% after nerve block. This indicates that the vasospastic attacks of Raynaud's phenomenon can occur without efferent digital nerve activity. (*Adapted from* Freedman *et al.* [7].)

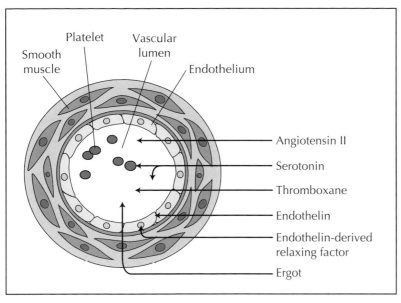

FIGURE 8-9. Vasoactive substances. A number of neurohumoral mediators produced by platelets, leukocytes, and the endothelium have been measured in patients with Raynaud's phenomenon. Serotonin acts directly on the smooth muscle to cause vasoconstric-

tion, and also augments constrictor responses to other neurohumoral mediators. Plasma and platelet serotonin levels are elevated in patients with Raynaud's phenomenon, and they are most elevated in those with secondary Raynaud's phenomenon. The serotonin antagonist, ketanserin, facilitates recovery of digital temperature following vasospasm. Angiotensin II levels are not elevated in patients with Raynaud's phenomenon unless there is coexistent renal artery stenosis or renal parenchymal disease. Urinary excretion of thromboxane B_2 is elevated in patients with Raynaud's phenomenon secondary to scleroderma. However, responses to local cool challenge do not change in either patients or controls after the administration of thromboxane-receptor antagonist and thromboxane synthase inhibitor despite a dramatic reduction of thromboxane levels.

The endothelium produces many potent vasoactive substances. Endothelin-1 levels are elevated in patients with Raynaud's phenomenon, and they increase further in response to a cold stimulus. Free radical activity is known to impair endothelium-dependent vasodilator function. Malondialdehyde levels indicative of free radical activity are elevated in patients with primary and secondary Raynaud's phenomenon. However, agonist-stimulated release of endothelium-derived relaxing factor appears to be similar in patients with Raynaud's phenomenon and control subjects. The administration of exogenous compounds such as ergot derivatives can also result in digital ischemia.

SECONDARY RAYNAUD'S PHENOMENON

SECONDARY RAYNAUD'S PHENOMENON

Connective tissue diseases
Arterial occlusive disease
Thoracic outlet syndrome
Thermal or vibration injury
Blood dyscrasias
Neurologic disorders
Vasoconstrictor medications
Chemotherapeutic agents

FIGURE 8-10. Secondary Raynaud's phenomenon. Connective tissue diseases associated with Raynaud's phenomenon include scleroderma, systemic lupus erythematosus, rheumatoid arthritis, dermatomyositis, polymyositis, Sjögren's syndrome, and necrotizing vasculitis. Arterial occlusive diseases associated with Raynaud's phenomenon include peripheral atherosclerosis, thromboangiitis obliterans, and thromboembolism. Thoracic outlet syndrome results from compression of the neurovascular bundle through the neck and shoulder. This clinical syndrome includes paresthesias, pain, and weakness of the upper extremity as well as Raynaud's phenomenon. Traumatic vasospastic disease includes vibration white finger (caused by exposure to vibrating tools), electric shock injury, percussive injury, and hypothenar hammer syndrome. Blood dyscrasias associated with Raynaud's phenomenon include those causing hyperviscosity such as cold agglutinin disease, cryoglobulinemia, cryofibrinogenemia, and myeloproliferative diseases. Neurologic disorders associated with Raynaud's phenomenon include syringomyelia, poliomyelitis, carpal tunnel syndrome, reflex sympathetic dystrophy, stroke, spinal cord tumors, and intervertebral disk disease. β-Adrenergic antagonists, vasoconstrictor medications such as dopamine and ergot derivatives, and chemotherapeutic agents such as bleomycin and vinblastine are associated with Raynaud's phenomenon.

A. DIGITAL VASCULAR PATHOLOGY IN SCLERODERMA

Thickened intima in small- and
  medium-sized vessels
Thrombosis of medium-sized arteries
Fibrotic, poorly distensible vessels
Elevated tissue pressures

FIGURE 8-11. Digital vascular pathology in scleroderma. Scleroderma is the most common cause of secondary Raynaud's phenomenon. Raynaud's phenomenon occurs in 80% to 90% of patients with scleroderma and may be the presenting symptom in 30%. **A,** Digital vessels are abnormal in diffuse scleroderma and may contribute to the presence of Raynaud's phenomenon. There are fewer cutaneous vessels; thrombosis of medium-sized digital arteries occurs; thickened intima is present in small- and medium-sized vessels; and obstruction of the ulnar artery may occur. The end result is fibrotic, poorly distensible vessels surrounded by an environment with elevated tissue pressures.

Continued on next page

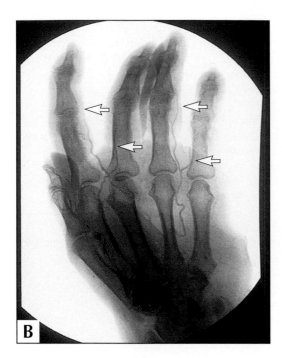

FIGURE 8-11. *(Continued)* **B,** This angiogram demonstrates loss of digital vessels in a patient with scleroderma. Normally, there are both medial and lateral arteries for each digit. In this patient, only a few of the digital arteries are visible, and each of these is occluded (*arrows*).

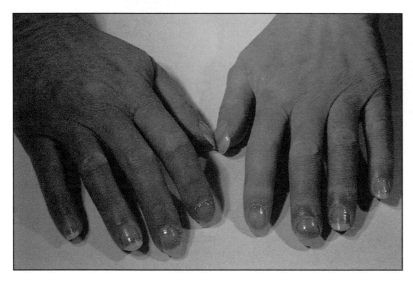

FIGURE 8-12. Raynaud's phenomenon in scleroderma. The hands of a patient with scleroderma are shown during a vasospastic attack induced by environmental cold exposure. Sausage-like swelling is present in the slightly flexed fingers. Well-demarcated areas of cyanosis developed following cold exposure.

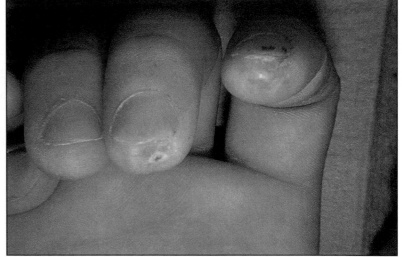

FIGURE 8-13. Scleroderma with digital ulceration. Digital ulceration is present on the first and second fingertips in this patient with scleroderma. Prolonged digital ischemia may lead to ulceration. The manifestations of Raynaud's phenomenon are often more severe in patients with scleroderma compared with patients with primary Raynaud's phenomenon. For example, digital ulceration is more likely to progress to gangrene and amputation in a patient with scleroderma.

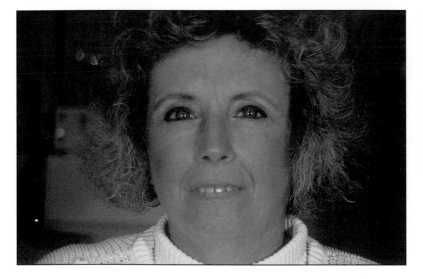

FIGURE 8-14. Proximal scleroderma. The most sensitive and specific indicator of diffuse scleroderma is the presence of proximal scleroderma [8]. Proximal scleroderma involves tightness, thickening, and nonpitting induration of the skin, which occurs proximal to the metacarpophalangeal or metatarsophalangeal joints. It affects the face, neck, and trunk usually in a bilateral, symmetric pattern. In this patient there is tightening of the facial skin with recession of the lips and diminution of mouth size. Sclerodactyly refers to skin involvement and tightening of the fingers, which leads to retraction of the fingers in a flexed position.

OCCLUSIVE ARTERIAL DISEASE

Atherosclerosis
Thromboangiitis obliterans
Thoracic outlet syndrome

FIGURE 8-15. Occlusive arterial disease. Occlusive disease of the small and medium arteries is present in 10% to 20% of all patients presenting to tertiary referral centers with Raynaud's phenomenon. Patients with Raynaud's phenomenon secondary to atherosclerosis are likely to be men with evidence of lower extremity or coronary artery atherosclerosis. Those with thromboangiitis obliterans are likely to be men under 40 years of age who smoke cigarettes. Common clinical presentations in this disorder include Raynaud's phenomenon with digital ulceration, migratory thrombophlebitis, and claudication of the arch of the foot. Thoracic outlet syndrome is encountered frequently in cases of unilateral Raynaud's phenomenon. The clinical presentation includes claudication, weakness, numbness, and paresthesias of the affected arm.

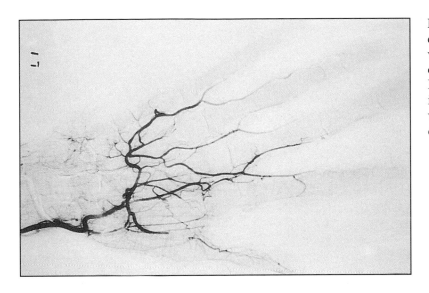

FIGURE 8-16. Digital angiogram of a patient with thromboangiitis obliterans showing multiple digital artery occlusions. Occluded vessels often develop collaterals in a tree root pattern. Biopsy of an acute lesion is required in order to confirm the diagnosis. Polymorphonuclear leukocyte infiltration of all arterial layers, intact internal elastic lamina, and the absence of medial necrosis will be present on arterial biopsy, thereby confirming the diagnosis of thromboangiitis obliterans.

TRAUMATIC VASOSPASTIC DISEASE

Vibration injury
Mechanical percussive injury
Thermal injury

FIGURE 8-17. Traumatic vasospastic disease can result from vibration injury, mechanical percussive injury, and thermal injury. Vibration injury is most common in pneumatic drillers, chain saw operators, and metal grinders and polishers. Raynaud's phenomenon associated with these occupations is known as "vibration white finger." Mechanical percussive injury commonly results from hammering with the palm of the hand, using a walker, and practicing karate. These actions can result in trauma to the ulnar artery at its most vulnerable location (approximately 2 cm distal to the wrist). Examples of thermal injury associated with Raynaud's phenomenon include electric shock injury and frostbite.

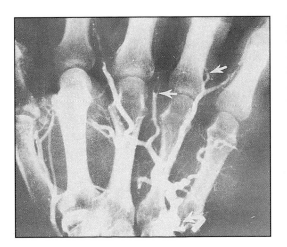

FIGURE 8-18. Hypothenar hammer syndrome. Digital angiogram of a patient with hypothenar hammer syndrome, which results from use of the hypothenar eminence as a hammer. Note aneurysmal dilatation of the ulnar artery (*large arrow*). Angiography in this disorder may also reveal irregularity or thrombosis of the ulnar artery in the region of the hamate bone. Note vasospasm and distal occlusion with the formation of collaterals (*small arrows*). It is postulated that digital artery occlusions in this disorder result from emboli from the site of proximal trauma.

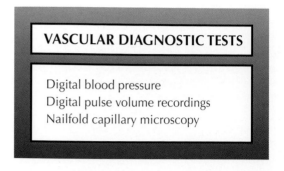

VASCULAR DIAGNOSTIC TESTS

Digital blood pressure
Digital pulse volume recordings
Nailfold capillary microscopy

FIGURE 8-19. Vascular diagnostic tests. Digital blood pressure and pulse volume recordings are obtained using strain gauge plethysmography. Nailfold capillaries are examined using a magnifying glass, microscope, or ophthalmoscope.

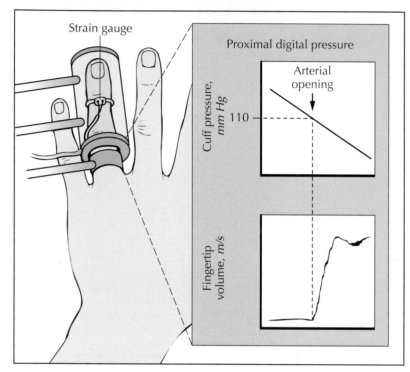

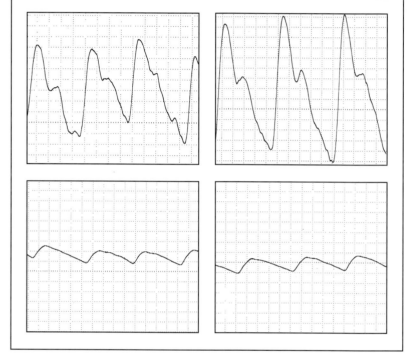

FIGURE 8-20. Digital blood pressure. The finger systolic blood pressure can be measured using plethysmographic techniques. Blood flow into the finger can be detected by measuring changes in fingertip blood volume, or by detecting fingertip pulsation when a sphygmomanometric cuff on the finger is deflated slowly from suprasystolic pressure. In this illustration, finger systolic blood pressure is 110 mm Hg. Fingertip systolic blood pressure falls dramatically when patients with Raynaud's phenomenon are exposed to environmental or local cooling.

FIGURE 8-21. Digital pulse volume recordings. Strain gauge plethysmography or photoplethysmography can be used to measure digital pulse volume waveforms. The amplitude of the digital pulse volume recording normally decreases in a cool environment and increases in a warm environment. In patients with primary Raynaud's phenomenon who are exposed to cool temperatures, the pulse volume recording may flatten if vasospasm occurs. In these patients, however, pulse volume waveforms are restored with rewarming. Digital pulse volume waveforms can be recorded during cooling (*left*; 24°C) and rewarming (*right*; 44°C). In the absence of vascular occlusive disease, the pulse volume increases during warming (*top*). Patients with digital ischemia secondary to vascular occlusion will have diminished pulse volume waveforms during cooling and rewarming (*bottom*).

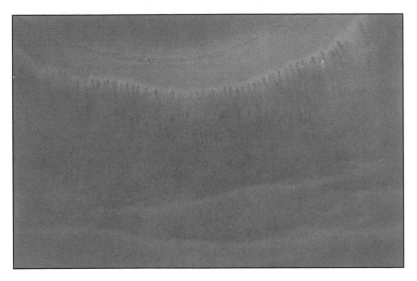

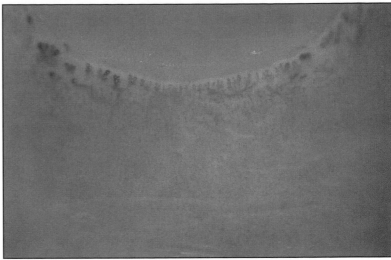

FIGURE 8-22. Nailfold capillary microscopy. is performed using a magnifying glass, ophthalmoscope, or compound microscope (magnification, ×10) to view the clean nailfold covered with immersion oil. Normally, the superficial capillaries are regularly spaced hairpin loops. (*Courtesy of* H. Maricq, MD.)

FIGURE 8-23. Nailfold capillary microscopy. Results of this test are abnormal in patients with connective tissue disorders. Avascular areas and enlarged and deformed capillary loops are present in the nailfold of this patient with scleroderma. Disorganized nailfold capillaries associated with avascular areas and hemorrhage are present in patients with dermatomyositis and polymyositis. (magnification, ×10.) (*Courtesy of* H. Maricq, MD.)

BLOOD TESTS TO DIAGNOSE SECONDARY RAYNAUD'S PHENOMENON

Antinuclear antibody
Rheumatoid factor
Cryoglobulins
Serum protein electrophoresis
Erythrocyte sedimentation rate
Complete blood count

FIGURE 8-24. Blood tests to diagnose secondary Raynaud's phenomenon. Antinuclear antibody levels greater than 1:100 suggest that connective tissue disease may be present. Specific patterns and epitopes of antinuclear antibodies suggest specific connective tissue diseases, *eg*, anticentromere antibody in the CREST syndrome. Features of the CREST syndrome include *c*alcinosis, *R*aynaud's phenomenon, *e*sophageal dysmotility, *s*clerodactyly, and *t*elangectasia. Rheumatoid factor is helpful in determining a secondary cause for Raynaud's phenomenon if it is accompanied by other features of rheumatoid arthritis such as morning joint stiffness, joint swelling, joint pain with motion, subcutaneous nodules, and radiologic and histologic findings of rheumatoid arthritis in the joints. The presence of cryoglobulin precipitation in cold serum is associated with monoclonal and polyclonal gammopathies, which may result in secondary Raynaud's phenomenon. Elevated total protein may suggest the need for serum protein electrophoresis to rule out the presence of myeloma or hyperglobulinemia. Erythrocyte sedimentation rate over 20 mm/h raises the possibility of secondary Raynaud's phenomenon. Both the rheumatoid factor and erythrocyte sedimentation rate tests have much less utility in the elderly.

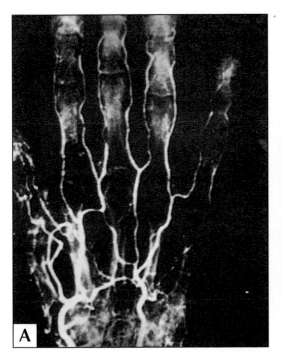
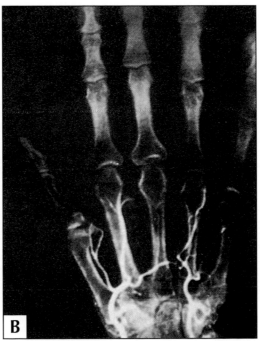

FIGURE 8-25. Angiography. These angiograms are of the palmar arch and digital vessels in a patient with primary Raynaud's phenomenon before (**A**) and after (**B**) cold exposure. Normal digital vessels are present in *A*, and marked digital vasospasm is evident in *B*. Digital artery occlusions can be seen in conjunction with many of the secondary causes of Raynaud's phenomenon (*see* Figs. 18-11, 18-16, and 18-18). Angiography has an extremely limited role in diagnosing Raynaud's phenomenon.

TREATMENT OF RAYNAUD'S PHENOMENON

Avoid cold exposure
Warm clothing
Abstain from nicotine
Behavioral therapy
Treat secondary cause
Pharmacologic therapy
Sympathectomy

FIGURE 8-26. Treatment of Raynaud's phenomenon. Patients should be instructed to avoid unnecessary cold exposure. When dressing for exposure to a cooler environment, they should wear warm and loose clothing. In addition to warm socks and gloves, the head and trunk must be kept warm to avoid reflex vasoconstriction. Nicotine causes vasoconstriction and should be avoided in all forms. Biofeedback training and Pavlovian conditioning have both been used to increase digital temperatures in patients with Raynaud's phenomenon. However, the data on these two forms of behavioral therapy in Raynaud's patients is extremely limited. In patients with secondary Raynaud's phenomenon, the underlying cause should be addressed (*eg*, treat systemic lupus erythematosus, discontinue β-blockers). Pharmacologic intervention is indicated in patients with debilitating symptoms who do not respond to conservative measures. Calcium channel blockers and sympathetic nervous system antagonists are often effective. Sympathectomy has a very limited role in treatment, but could be considered in patients with severe, persistent digital ischemia refractory to medical therapy.

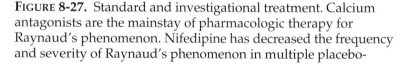

STANDARD AND INVESTIGATIONAL TREATMENT

STANDARD	INVESTIGATIONAL
Calcium channel blockers	Serotonin receptor antagonist
Nifedipine	
Diltiazem	Ketanserin
Nicardipine	Vasodilator prostaglandins and thromboxane synthase inhibitors
Felodipine	
Isradipine	Dazoxiben
Sympathetic nervous system inhibitors	Prostacyclin
Prazosin	Prostaglandin E$_1$
Reserpine	Iloprost
Guanethidine	

FIGURE 8-27. Standard and investigational treatment. Calcium antagonists are the mainstay of pharmacologic therapy for Raynaud's phenomenon. Nifedipine has decreased the frequency and severity of Raynaud's phenomenon in multiple placebo-

controlled trials [9–11]. Diltiazem, felodipine, nicardipine, and isradipine have been studied in fewer trials than nifedipine, but have also shown benefit in the treatment of Raynaud's phenomenon [12–15]. Successful treatment has not been demonstrated with the calcium antagonist verapamil. Although the vasoconstrictor response to cold exposure is mediated by the sympathetic nervous system, sympathetic nervous system inhibitors have had limited success in the long-term treatment of Raynaud's phenomenon. A small placebo-controlled trial of prazosin demonstrated a decreased frequency of Raynaud's phenomenon in patients taking this α-adrenoreceptor antagonist [16]. Reserpine and guanethidine act by depleting norepinephrine from nerve terminals, and both increase fingertip capillary blood flow [17,18]. Both drugs have significant side effect profiles, however, which have limited their use. The serotonin receptor antagonist, ketanserin, was associated with a decreased frequency of vasospastic attacks in one large placebo-controlled trial [19]. Ketanserin is not available in the US. Vasoactive metabolites of arachidonic acid may play a role in digital ischemia. Prostacyclin, prostaglandin E$_1$, and thromboxane synthase inhibitors have all been investigated in the treatment of Raynaud's phenomenon, but no clear beneficial effect has been seen [20–22]. One exception may be the use of iloprost, a prostacyclin analog, in the treatment of severe Raynaud's phenomenon in patients with scleroderma [23].

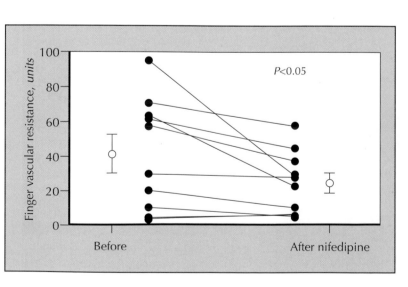

FIGURE 8-28. Treatment with calcium antagonists. Fingertip vascular resistance was measured in 10 patients with Raynaud's phenomenon before and after nifedipine. Fingertip vascular resistance dropped significantly following treatment. The expected corresponding increase in fingertip blood flow following nifedipine was attenuated in this group of patients because of the decrease in mean blood pressure that accompanied nifedipine administration. Objective tests of digital circulation have not uniformly demonstrated improvement with nifedipine. Subjective improvement of Raynaud's phenomenon with nifedipine includes decreased frequency and severity of attacks, decreased functional limitations, and improved healing of digital ulcers. *T-bars* indicate the mean fingertip vascular resistance of the group. (*Adapted from Creager et al.* [9].)

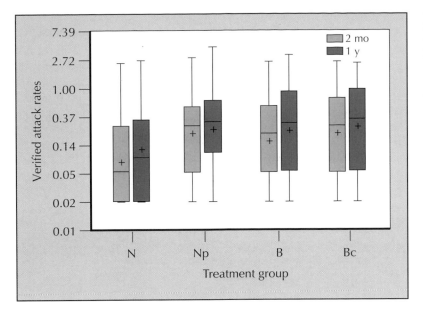

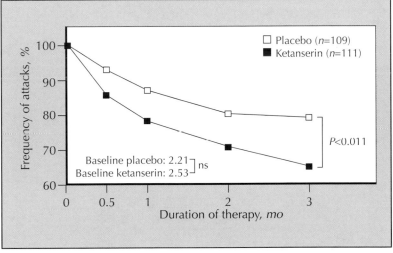

FIGURE 8-29. Effect of nifedipine and temperature biofeedback on Raynaud's phenomenon. Investigators recruited 313 patients with primary Raynaud's phenomenon to evaluate the effectiveness of sustained-release nifedipine and temperature biofeedback for the treatment of primary Raynaud's phenomenon [24]. Measurements were made at 2 months and 1 year. Participants were randomized to one of four treatment groups: sustained-release nifedipine (N), pill placebo (Np), temperature biofeedback (B), or control (electromyographic) feedback (Bc). Patients treated with nifedipine showed a 66% reduction in verified attacks compared with placebo patients (P - .001). Temperature biofeedback did not reduce attack frequency compared with control biofeedback. Comparison of nifedipine with temperature biofeedback treatments favored nifedipine use (P = .08). (Adapted from [24].)

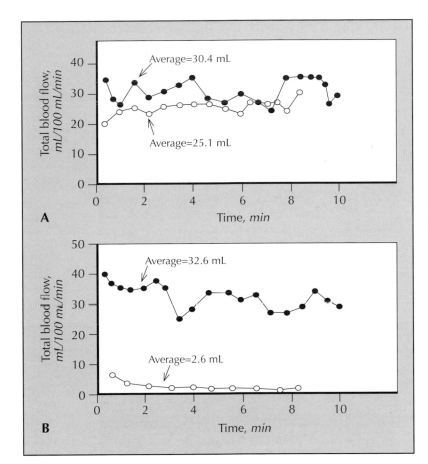

FIGURE 8-31. Effect of ketanserin on Raynaud's phenomenon. A double-blind study of the effects of ketanserin on primary or secondary Raynaud's phenomenon was studied in 222 patients. At 3 months of therapy there was a 34% reduction in the frequency of vasospastic attacks in the treatment group compared with an 18% reduction in the frequency of attacks in the placebo group. Patients with primary and secondary Raynaud's phenomenon responded similarly to treatment. (Adapted from Coffman et al. [19].)

FIGURE 8-30. Treatment with α-adrenoceptor antagonists. The adrenergic antagonist reserpine had once been the mainstay of therapy in patients with Raynaud's phenomenon. These are measurements of total fingertip blood flow via venous occlusion plethysmography from one patient with Raynaud's phenomenon taken before and after treatment with reserpine. A, In the warm room (28° C) there was little difference in total fingertip blood flow before (open circles) and after (closed circles) reserpine. B, In the cold room (20° C), however, there was a significant decrease in fingertip blood flow before reserpine and an increase in fingertip blood flow after reserpine. This suggests that sympathetic activity does contribute to vasoconstriction during cold exposure. Most patients given reserpine report subjective improvement in their Raynaud's phenomenon, as well as side effects attributable to reserpine including nausea, lethargy, depression, nasal congestion, and peptic ulcers. (Adapted from Coffman and Cohen [17].)

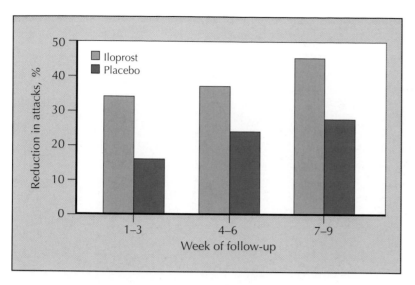

FIGURE 8-32. Effect of iloprost on Raynaud's phenomenon. These data come from a multicenter, placebo-controlled, double-blind trial of intravenous iloprost in 131 patients with Raynaud's phenomenon secondary to systemic sclerosis [23]. Iloprost is a prostacyclin analog with platelet inhibitory as well as vasodilating effects. Either iloprost or placebo was given intravenously for 5 days. The frequency of vasospastic attacks was similar in both treatment groups at baseline. Both groups demonstrated a decrease in attack frequency after treatment, but the magnitude of this decrease was greater in the patients who received iloprost. The attack frequency from baseline for both groups is illustrated. At follow-up week 1 to 3, week 4 to 6, and week 7 to 9 the iloprost treatment group had 34%, 37%, and 45% reductions in the frequency of vasospastic attacks, respectively, compared with 15%, 23%, and 27% reductions in the placebo group. The prolonged effect of iloprost is not due to residual drug levels. (*Adapted from* Wigley *et al.* [22].)

SYMPATHECTOMY IN RAYNAUD'S PHENOMENON

Lumbar
Cervicodorsal
Digital
Radical microarteriolysis

FIGURE 8-33. Sympathectomy. Lumbar sympathectomy is often successful in the treatment of intractable Raynaud's phenomenon involving the lower extremities. However, refractory lower extremity vasospasm is estimated to account for only 2% of all cases of lower extremity vasospasm [23]. Cervical dorsal sympathectomy has been much less successful in the treatment of this disorder. At best it results in improved outcome in only 60% of patients. Relapses are common following upper extremity sympathectomy, making the long-term outcome unclear. This is most likely because there are sympathetic pathways to the brachial plexus that are separate from the cervicothoracic sympathetic trunk [25]. Digital sympathec-tomy is achieved by stripping the adventitia from the common and proximal digital arteries. In small series it has been effective in treating primary Raynaud's phenomenon and Raynaud's phenomenon secondary to trauma [26]. Radical microarteriolysis refers to more extensive adventitiectomy and removal of periarterial scarring of the ulnar artery, palmar arch, and digital arteries. It has been used successfully in a small number of patients to treat severe Raynaud's phenomenon secondary to scleroderma [27].

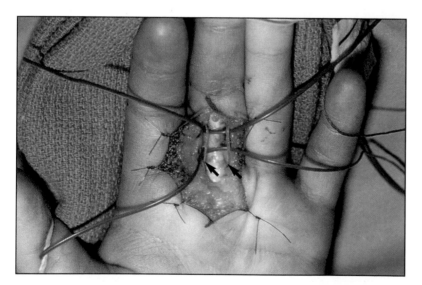

FIGURE 8-34. Treatment with digital sympathectomy. In this patient, digital sympathectomy was used to treat adolescent severe Raynaud's phenomenon refractory to medical therapy. Isolation of the digital vessels and digital nerves of the affected finger or fingers is required for microsurgical digital sympathec-tomy. Operative exposure of the digital arteries (*arrows*) of the finger can be seen here. The small unmyelinated sympathetic nerves in the periarterial adventitia are resected circumferentially for a length of at least 2 cm. Endarterectomy is very rarely used as an adjunctive procedure. (*From* Drake *et al.* [28]; with permission.)

OTHER TEMPERATURE-RELATED DISORDERS

FIGURE 8-35. Other temperature-related vascular disorders. Erythromelalgia, acrocyanosis, pernio, and frostbite are four other vascular disorders associated with discoloration of the extremities in response to cold exposure. Unlike Raynaud's phenomenon, these disorders are not episodic but are characterized by some degree of persistent discoloration.

ERYTHROMELALGIA

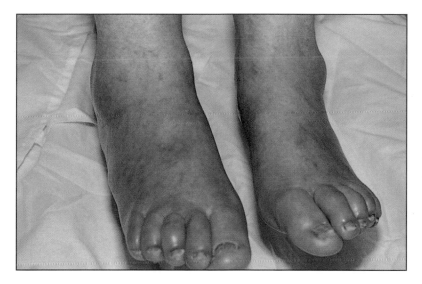

FIGURE 8-36. Erythromelalgia. Erythromelalgia is an uncommon disorder with an incidence of one in 40,000. It is characterized by erythema, intense burning pain, and an increased temperature of the extremities. The hands are less often affected than the feet, especially the soles. Because warmth induces the symptoms and cold relieves them, erythromelalgia is often described as the antithesis of Raynaud's phenomenon. The feet pictured here display the erythema of erythromelalgia. This patient also had intense burning pain in her feet. The mild edema and superficial ulcerations present are complications of continuously soaking her feet in cold water. Aspirin, the mainstay of therapy for this disorder, is not always helpful.

CLASSIFICATIONS OF ERYTHROMELALGIA

PRIMARY ERYTHROMELALGIA

SECONDARY ERYTHROMELALGIA
Myeloproliferative disorders
    Polycythemia vera
    Essential thrombocythemia
Drug-induced
    Nifedipine
    Bromocriptine
    Pergolide
Possible associations
    Spinal cord disease
    Multiple sclerosis
    Diabetic neuropathy

FIGURE 8-37. Classifications of Erythromelalgia. Erythromelalgia is classified as primary, *ie*, unassociated with another disease or treatment, or secondary. Primary erythromelalgia is estimated to account for up to 60% of cases. Polycythemia vera and essential thrombocythemia account for 80% of the cases of secondary erythromelalgia. There are case reports of erythromelalgia occurring in patients with other myeloproliferative disorders. Cutaneous reactions characteristic of erythromelalgia have been reported with nifedipine, bromocriptine, and pergolide treatment. Resolution of erythromelalgia accompanied discontinuation of these therapies. Case reports have suggested associations with several neurologic disorders such as spinal cord disease, multiple sclerosis, and diabetic neuropathy. The prognosis in this disorder is the same as that for the underlying disease.

ACROCYANOSIS

- Symmetric reddish-blue discoloration of hands and feet
- Discoloration exacerbated by cold
- Discoloration extends proximal to wrist and dorsal foot

FIGURE 8-38. Acrocyanosis. Acrocyanosis is an uncommon disorder in which there is symmetric reddish-blue discoloration of the hands and feet that is exacerbated by cold temperatures. The discoloration is persistent rather than episodic, and there is no component of pallor. Cyanosis extends to, and often beyond, the wrist and ankle. The lips, cheeks, chin, and nose are rarely involved. Acrocyanosis is not associated with other disorders. Therapy for these patients is to minimize exposure to cold temperatures. α-Adrenoceptor antagonists may ameliorate the discoloration. The prognosis is very good, with digital loss being extremely uncommon.

PERNIO

Acute
- 12–24 h after cold exposure
- Red to blue edematous lesions
- Itching and burning

Chronic
- Present throughout cold season
- Violet blisters, brown plaques, shallow ulcers
- Itching and burning

FIGURE 8-39. Pernio. Pernio (also known as chilblains) is a cold-induced vascular disorder characterized by inflammatory lesions of the skin. It occurs in both acute and chronic forms. Acute pernio develops within 12 to 24 hours after cold exposure, most frequently involving the areas of skin least protected from the cold. The inflammatory lesions are red to blue in color, edematous, and accompanied by intense burning and itching. Shallow ulcerations with a hemorrhagic base may be present. Varying degrees of cyanosis are often noted. Lesions resolve in 1 to 3 weeks. Chronic pernio follows repeated cold exposure and is characterized by the persistence of lesions with itching and burning. The lesions can appear as brown plaques, violet blisters, yellow blisters, or shallow ulcers. They are typically present throughout the cold season, and may resolve during the warm season.

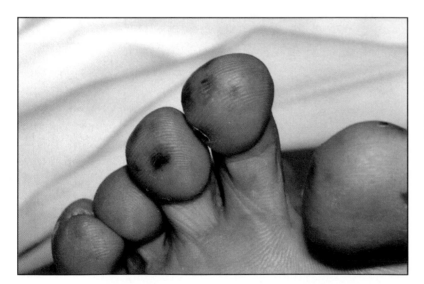

FIGURE 8-40. Chronic pernio. This patient has the characteristic yellow-brown plaques of chronic pernio, as well as a shallow ulcer on the great toe. Treatment of this disorder includes avoiding cold exposure and dressing warmly when cold exposure is unavoidable. Nifedipine has decreased the symptoms of itching and burning in a small number of patients with chronic pernio. Topical steroid creams have not been effective. (*From* Olin and Arrabi [29]; with permission.)

CLASSIFICATION OF FROSTBITE

1st degree	White patches of skin with edema and hyperemia
2nd degree	Blisters
3rd degree	Full skin necrosis, subcutaneous extension
4th degree	Damage to muscle and bone, gangrene

FIGURE 8-41. Frostbite classification. Freezing of the tissues during cold exposure is known as frostbite. Its classification is based on the severity and extent of tissue damage after thawing [30]. First-degree frostbite involves white patches of skin with edema and hyperemia; second-degree involves blisters; third-degree involves full skin necrosis and subcutaneous extension; and fourth-degree involves damage to muscle and bone, and the presence of gangrene. Palpation can assist in differentiating superficial from deep frostbite. The affected area is stony hard or petrified when deeper layers are affected. Initial treatment includes thawing via a warm water bath once the patient is removed from the freezing environment. Refreezing after thawing can accelerate tissue damage. Thereafter, treatment involves débridement of necrotic tissue, whirlpool baths, and antibiotics as indicated.

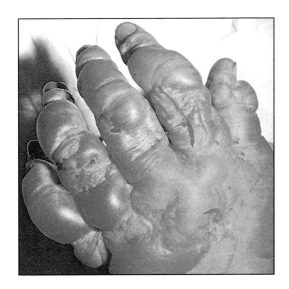

FIGURE 8-42. Blisters and edema are evident in this case of second-degree frostbite. Resorption of blisters usually occurs within 2 weeks, and does not result in tissue loss. Large, fluid-filled blisters extending to the tips of the fingers and toes are common in cases of superficial frostbite (second degree), while small, hemorrhagic blisters are typical of deep frostbite (third and fourth degree). This hand has been thawed by warm water, which has intensified the edema and hyperemia. Before thawing, the frozen parts typically appear white because of intense vasospasm. (*From* Washburn [31]; with permission.)

REFERENCES

1. Creager MA: Raynaud's phenomenon. *Illustrated Med* 1983, 2:84.

2. Allen EV, Brown GE: Raynaud's disease: a critical review of minimal requisites for diagnosis. *Am J Med Sci* 1932, 183:187–200.

3. LeRoy EC, Medsger TA Jr: Raynaud's phenomenon: a proposal for classification. *Clin Exp Rheumatol* 1991, 10:485–488.

4. Raynaud M; Thomas Barlow (translated): *L'Asphyxie locale et de la gangrene symmetrique des extremities.* London: New Sydenham Society; 1862.

5. Lewis T: Experiments relating to the spasmodic arrest of the circulation in the fingers: a variety of Raynaud's disease. *Heart* 1929, 15:7–25.

6. Fagius J, Blumberg H: Sympathetic outflow to the hand in patients with Raynaud's phenomenon. *Cardiovasc Res* 1985, 19:249–253.

7. Freedman RR, Mayes MD, Sabharwal SC: Induction of vasospastic attacks despite digital nerve block in Raynaud's disease and phenomenon. *Circulation* 1989, 80:859–862.

8. Masi AT, Rodnan GP, Medsger TA, *et al.*: Preliminary criteria for the classification of systemic sclerosis (scleroderma). *Arthritis Rheum* 1983, 23:581–590.

9. Creager MA, Pariser KM, Winston EM, *et al.*: Nifedipine induced fingertip vasodilation in patients with Raynaud's phenomenon. *Am Heart J* 1984, 108:370–373.

10. Smith CD, McKendry RVR: Controlled trial of nifedipine in the treatment of Raynaud's phenomenon. *Lancet* 1982, 2:1299–1301.

11. Rodeheffer RJ, Rommer JA, Wigley F, *et al.*: Controlled double blind trial of nifedipine in the treatment of Raynaud's phenomenon. *N Engl J Med* 1983, 308:880–883.

12. Kahan A, Amor B, Menkes CJ: A randomized double blind trial of diltiazem in the treatment of Raynaud's phenomenon. *Ann Rheum Dis* 1985, 44:30–33.

13. Kallenberg CGM, Wouda AA, Meens L, Wessling H: Once daily felodipine in patients with primary Raynaud's phenomenon. *Eur J Clin Pharmacol* 1991, 40:313–315.

14. Leppert J, Jonasson T, Nilsson H, Ringqvist I: The effect of isradipine, a new calcium channel antagonist, in patients with primary Raynaud's phenomenon: a single blind dose response study. *Cardiovasc Drugs Ther* 1989, 3:397–401.

15. French Cooperative Multicenter Group for Raynaud's phenomenon: Controlled multicenter double blind trial of nicardipine in the treatment of primary Raynaud's phenomenon. *Am Heart J* 1991, 122:352–355.

16. Wollersheim H, Thien T: Dose-response study of prazosin in Raynaud's phenomenon: clinical effectiveness versus side effects. *J Clin Pharmacol* 1988, 28:1089–1093.

17. Coffman JD, Cohen AS: Total and capillary fingertip blood flow in Raynaud's phenomenon. *N Engl J Med* 1971, 285:259–265.

18. LeRoy EC, Downey JA, Cannon PJ: Skin capillary blood flow in scleroderma. *J Clin Invest* 1971, 50:930–939.

19. Coffman JD, Clement DL, Creager MA, *et al.*: International study of ketanserin in Raynaud's phenomenon. *Am J Med* 1989, 87:264–268.

20. Clifford PC, Martin MFR, Sheddon EJ, *et al.*: Treatment of vasospastic disease with prostaglandin E1. *BMJ* 1980, 281:1031–1034.

21. Ettinger WH, Wise RA, Schaffhauser D, Wigley FM: Controlled double blind trial of dazoxiben and nifedipine in the treatment of Raynaud's phenomenon. *Am J Med* 1984, 77:451–456.

22. Wigley FM, Wise RA, Seibold JR, *et al.*: Intravenous iloprost infusion in patients with Raynaud's phenomenon secondary to systemic sclerosis. *Ann Intern Med* 1994, 120:199–206.

23. Janoff KA, Phinney ES, Porter JM: Lumbar sympathectomy for lower extremity vasospasm. *Am J Surg* 1985, 150:147–152.

24. Comparison of sustained-release nifedipine and temperature biofeedback for treatment of primary Raynaud phenomenon. Results from a randomized clinical trial with 1-year follow-up. *Arch Intern Med* 2000, 160(8):1101–1108.

25. Baddely RM: The place of upper dorsal sympathectomy in the treatment of primary Raynaud's disease. *Br J Surg* 1965, 52:426–430.

26. Wilgis EFS: Digital sympathectomy for vascular insufficiency. *Hand Clin* 1985, 2:361–367.

27. O'Brien BM, Kumar PAV, Mellow CG, Oliver TV: Radical microarteriolysis in the treatment of vasospastic disorders of the hand, especially scleroderma. *J Hand Surg [Br]* 1992, 17:447–452.

28. Drake DB, Kesler RW, Morgan RF: Digital sympathectomy for refractory Raynaud's phenomenon in an adolescent. *J Rheumatol* 1992, 19:1286–1288.

29. Olin JW, Arrabi W: Vascular diseases related to extremes in environmental temperature. In *Peripheral Vascular Diseases*, edn 1. Edited by Young JR, Graor RA, Olin JW, Bartholemew JR. St. Louis: Mosby–Year Book; 1991:575–586.

30. Purdue GF, Hunt JL: Cold injury: a collective review. *J Burn Care Rehabil* 1986, 7:331–342.

31. Washburn B: Frostbite. *N Engl J Med* 1962, 266:974–989.

9
CHAPTER

KAWASAKI DISEASE

Kathryn A. Taubert and Jane W. Newburger

Kawasaki disease (KD), a leading cause of acquired heart disease in children in the United States, is a generalized vasculitis of unknown etiology. Most affected children are under the age of 2 years, and 85% of cases occur in children under 5 years of age. It is more common in males than in females (1.5:1). Within North America, the reported incidence of KD ranges from 6 to 11 per 100,000 children younger than 5 years of age [1], and while the incidence of KD is higher in children of Asian ancestry, children of all racial backgrounds are affected. KD was first reported by Tomisaku Kawasaki in 1967 in Japan, and was originally referred to as "mucocutaneous lymph node syndrome" [2]. More than 169,000 cases have been reported in Japan through 1998 [3], and KD has been recorded worldwide. Studies from Asia, Europe, and the Americas indicate that KD occurs in both endemic and community-wide epidemic forms [4].

Although the cause of KD remains unknown, its epidemiology and clinical presentation suggest an infectious agent. Speculated etiologic agents include rickettsiae, viruses, bacteria such as group A and other streptococci, propionibacteria, parvovirus, and superantigens—toxins produced by certain staphylococci and streptococci. There has been no documentation of person-to-person transmission (even in day care centers); the rate of cases among siblings is 1%; the recurrence rate is 3%.

Kawasaki disease can cause an arteritis of medium and large vessels, arterial aneurysms, valvulitis, and myocarditis. Coronary artery aneurysms may resolve or persist. These are of particular concern because they can lead to thrombosis, evolve into segmental stenosis, or, in very rare cases, rupture. Studies have shown that approximately 15% to 25% of untreated children develop coronary artery abnormalities. Coronary artery aneurysms are classified as small (< 5 mm in internal diameter), medium (5 to 8 mm in internal diameter), or giant (> 8 mm in internal diameter). While approximately one half of all coronary artery aneurysms regress within 2 years, virtually none of the giant coronary artery aneurysms regresses. Myocardial infarction can occur, typically in patients with giant coronary artery aneurysms. In the current era of diagnosis and treatment, the death rate is approximately 0.3% for all patients with KD.

Because there is no specific diagnostic test for KD, a set of diagnostic criteria have been defined by the American Heart Association [5–7]. Despite the fact that the cause of KD is not currently known, treatment regimens have been developed. In the acute phase of the disease, treatment is directed particularly at reducing inflammation of the coronary arteries and the myocardium and inhibiting platelet activation. This treatment includes aspirin and intravenous gamma globulin.

Long-term follow-up of patients with KD is important. Natural history studies are not currently available, so some type of follow-up of all patients with cardiac involvement should be done. Guidelines for long-term management have been developed [7]. Patients are stratified into five risk levels based on their relative risk for cardiac ischemia. Recommendations for pharmacologic therapy, physical activity, follow-up and diagnostic testing, and invasive testing are included for each risk level.

EPIDEMIOLOGY

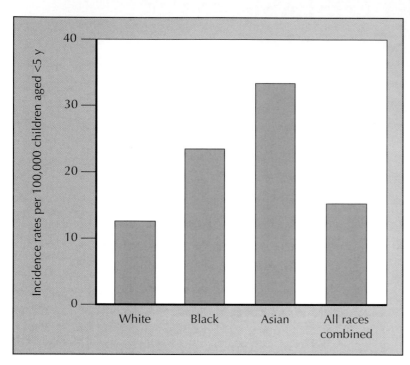

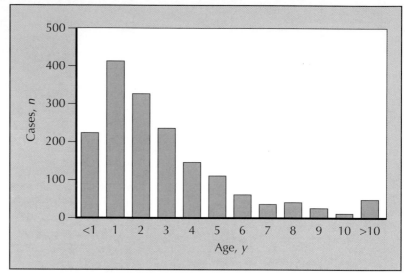

FIGURE 9-2. Peak incidence of Kawasaki disease (KD) by age. KD occurs predominantly in children younger than 5 years of age. For cases of KD reported to the Centers for Disease Control between 1976 and 1984, peak incidence occurred in children between 1 and 2 years of age, and 80% of cases were reported in children less than 5 years of age. (*Adapted from* Rauch [9].)

FIGURE 9-1. Race-specific incidence rates for Kawasaki disease (KD). Rates calculated from 1987–1989 surveillance data in three counties of Washington state indicate that the prevalence of KD is highest among Asians, intermediate in blacks, and lowest in whites (33.3, 23.4, and 12.7 per 100,000 children younger than 5 years of age, respectively). The incidence rates for all races combined is 15.2 per 100,00 children younger than 5 years of age. (*Adapted from* Davis *et al.* [8].)

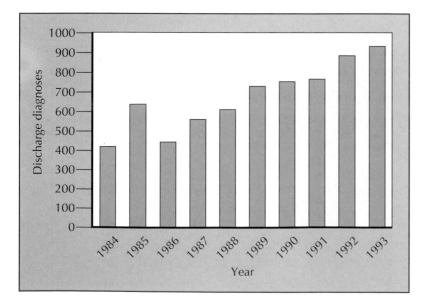

FIGURE 9-3. Discharge diagnoses of Kawasaki disease from a survey of 45 United States children's hospitals. Hospitals were asked to report the number of discharge diagnoses for ICD.9CM diagnostic code 446.1 (Kawasaki disease) for the years 1984 to 1990. (*Adapted from* Taubert *et al.* [10].)

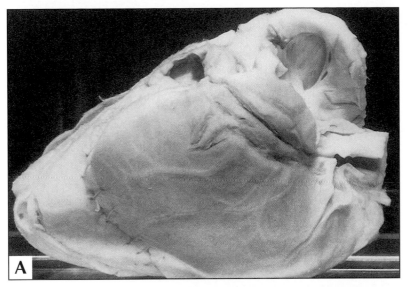

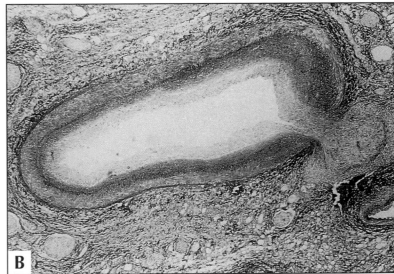

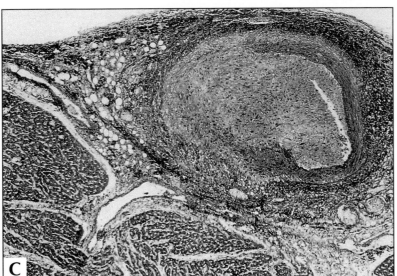

FIGURE 9-4. Possible first case of Kawasaki disease. **A,** The heart of a 7-year-old boy who died in 1870 in London after "scarlatinal dropsy." The heart had been preserved in formalin. Coronary aneurysms can be seen. The child's heart has been recently sectioned and photomicrographed. **B,** Endothelial proliferation. **C,** A thrombus totally occludes a coronary artery. The death of this child is consistent with the sequelae of Kawasaki disease. (*From* Shulman [11]; with permission.)

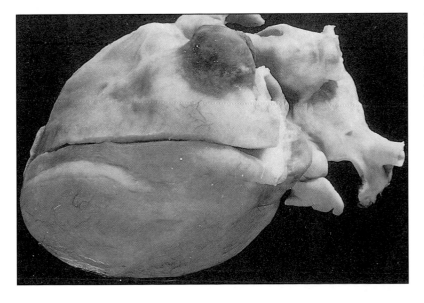

FIGURE 9-5. Aneurysm rupture in Kawasaki disease. Kawasaki disease can lead (rarely) to aneurysm rupture. This photograph shows one such case in a 16-month-old girl, when a saccular aneurysm in the proximal right coronary artery ruptured, leading to cardiac tamponade and death. (*From* Becker [12]; with permission.)

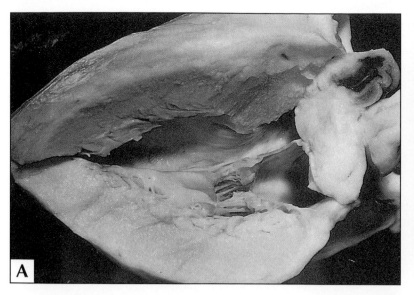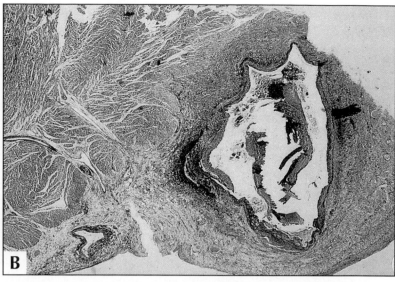

FIGURE 9-6. Two views of fusiform aneurysm. **A,** Dissection of the heart shown in Fig. 9-5 demonstrated a fusiform aneurysm in the left coronary artery. **B,** An elastic tissue stain (× 8) of this aneurysm, demonstrating massive inflammatory infiltration. Autopsy also revealed an arteritis of the principal muscular artery in the hilium of the left ovary. (*From* Becker [12]; with permission.)

DIAGNOSIS AND CLINICAL FEATURES

DIAGNOSTIC CRITERIA OF KAWASAKI DISEASE (PRINCIPAL CLINICAL FINDINGS)

Generally high and spiking fever (often to ≥ 104°F) lasting at least 5 days without other explanation; fever persists in untreated patients for 1–2 weeks or longer

Presence of at least four of the following five principal features

Changes of peripheral extremities: distinctive changes that acutely include redness and swelling, and sometimes induration, of the hands and feet; after 1–3 weeks, desquamation of the fingers and toes; after 1–2 months, Beau's lines (white lines across the fingernails) may appear

Polymorphous exanthem rash: primarily truncal; can take several forms; usually appears within 5 days after the onset of fever

Bilateral conjunctival injection: usually involves the bulbar conjunctivae; is not associated with an exudate; is usually painless

Changes of the lips and oral cavity: including strawberry tongue, redness and cracking of the lips, and erythema of the oropharyngeal mucosa

Cervical lymphadenopathy if at least one lymph node is more than 1.5 cm in diameter: usually presents as unilateral lymphadenopathy, with firm and slightly tender nodes

Exclusion of other diseases with similar findings (*see* Fig. 9-8)

FIGURE 9-7. Diagnostic criteria of Kawasaki disease (KD). Many experts believe that, in the presence of classic features, the diagnosis of KD can be made by experienced observers prior to the fifth day of fever. The first four of the five principal clinical findings are seen in at least 90% of patients. Cervical lymphadenopathy is the least common of the five principal clinical features (observed in 50% to 75% of patients).

Atypical or incomplete cases of KD, in which patients have less than four of the five principal features, have been increasingly reported. Full diagnostic criteria are more often lacking in infants, especially those less than 6 months of age, than in older children. Patients with fever and less than four of the principal clinical features can be diagnosed as having KD when coronary artery disease is detected by two-dimensional echocardiography or coronary angiography. Several studies suggest that coronary arterial involvement is present in almost all infants with atypical KD. (*Adapted from* [5].)

DIFFERENTIAL DIAGNOSIS OF KAWASAKI DISEASE

Measles
Scarlet fever
Epstein-Barr virus
Drug reactions
Stevens-Johnson syndrome
Adenovirus infection
Rocky Mountain spotted fever
Staphylococcal scalded skin
  syndrome
Yersinia pseudotuberculosis
Toxic shock syndrome
Juvenile rheumatoid arthritis
Leptospirosis
Mercury poisoning

FIGURE 9-8. Differential diagnosis of Kawaski disease (KD). These diseases and disorders with similar clinical findings to those of KD should be ruled out. Careful consideration of measles in the differential diagnosis is especially important, particularly in light of outbreaks of measles in some urban areas in the United States. Measles cases misdiagnosed as KD do not allow appropriate measles control measures to be promptly undertaken. Conversely, KD patients diagnosed with measles or other diseases or disorders will fail to receive prompt therapy that may prevent them from having long-term coronary artery disorders.

CARDIAC FINDINGS IN ACUTE KAWASAKI DISEASE

Pericardial effusion, echocardiographically documented in about 30% of patients with acute KD

Myocardial inflammation is common, with signs including

Tachycardia out of proportion to the degree of fever

A gallop rhythm

An electrocardiogram showing decreased R-wave voltage, S–T-segment depression, T-wave flattening or inversion, and prolonged PR and/or QT intervals

Ischemia-induced atrial or ventricular arrhythmias

Congestive heart failure

Coronary artery abnormalities, usually beyond 10 days of onset of illness, including ectasia or aneurysms

FIGURE 9-9. Cardiac findings in acute Kawasaki disease (KD). Cardiovascular manifestations are often prominent in the acute phase of KD; some degree of myocarditis is virtually always present. Coronary artery aneurysms are the leading cause of both short- and long-term morbidity and mortality. These develop in approximately 20% of affected children with untreated KD. The aneurysms usually appear between 10 days and 4 weeks after the onset of symptoms. Certain factors increase the risk of development of coronary artery aneurysms (*see also* Fig. 9-10).

FACTORS ASSOCIATED WITH INCREASED RISK OF DEVELOPING CORONARY ANEURYSMS

Male gender
Age < 1 year
Other signs and symptoms of pancarditis, including arrhythmias
Prolonged period of inflammation, including fever for > 10 days
Recurrence of fever after an afebrile period of at least 24 hours

FIGURE 9-10. Factors associated with increased risk for the development of coronary arterial aneurysms. One should pay particular attention to patients with one or more of the factors listed here.

Figure 9-11. Noncardiac findings in acute Kawasaki disease. Arthritis or arthralgia can occur in the first week of the illness and is usually polyarticular, involving the knees, ankles, and hands. A pauciarticular arthritis commonly appears during the second or third week of illness. Arthritis is more common in older girls. Lumbar puncture shows evidence of aseptic meningitis (presence of white blood cells, predominantly lymphocytes) in approximately one fourth of patients undergoing the procedure. Hydrops of the gallbladder, identified by abdominal ultrasound, is common during the first 2 weeks of the illness. Some other findings are less common. Patients who have giant coronary artery aneurysms are more likely than others to have noncoronary arterial involvement.

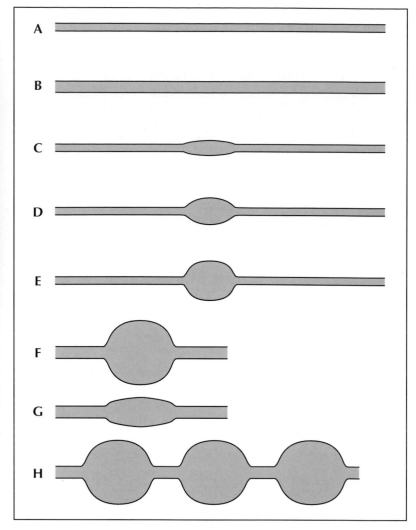

Figure 9-12. Types of coronary artery abnormalities in Kawasaki disease. **A,** A normal coronary artery 2 mm in internal diameter. (Normal coronary artery sizes range from 2 mm in infants and young children to 5 mm in teenagers [13]). **B,** An ectatic artery 3 mm in internal diameter (wider than normal but without aneurysms). **C,** A small aneurysm 4 mm in internal diameter (small aneurysms are < 5 mm in internal diameter). **D,** A medium-sized aneurysm 7 mm in internal diameter (medium aneurysms are 5 to 8 mm in internal diameter). **E,** A giant aneurysm 10 mm in internal diameter (giant aneurysms are > 8 mm in internal diameter). Aneurysms can be saccular (circular-appearing; **F**), fusiform (cigar-shaped; **G**), or segmental (**H**).

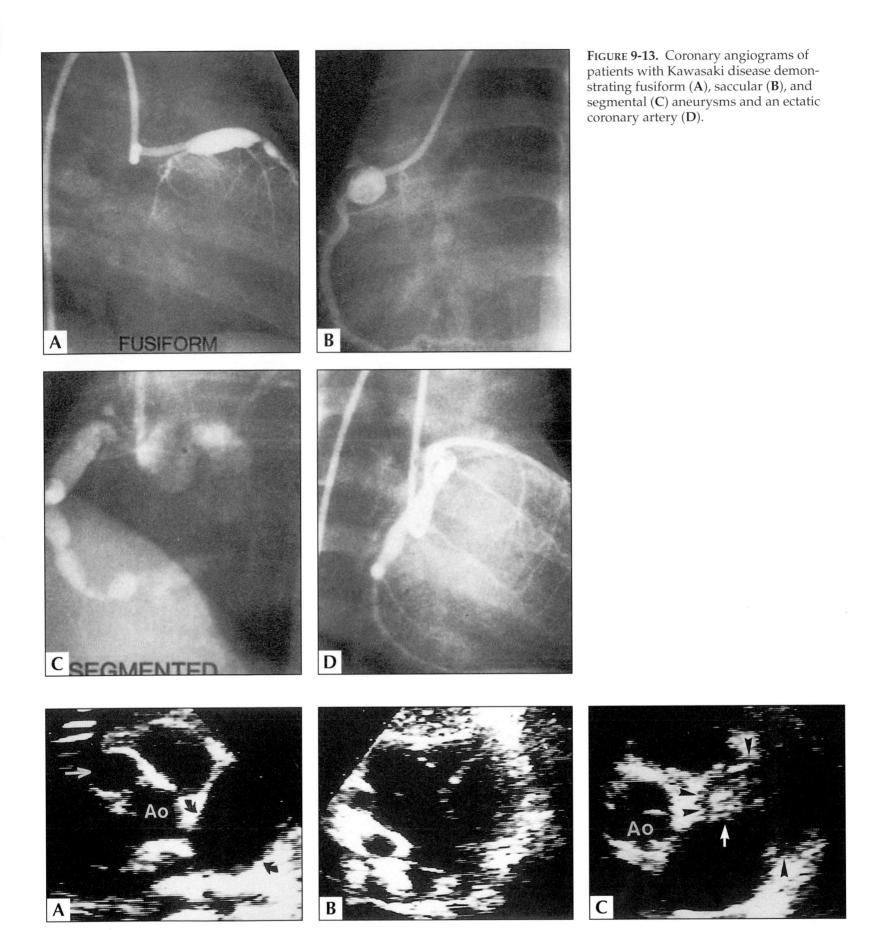

FIGURE 9-13. Coronary angiograms of patients with Kawasaki disease demonstrating fusiform (**A**), saccular (**B**), and segmental (**C**) aneurysms and an ectatic coronary artery (**D**).

FIGURE 9-14. Two-dimensional echocardiograms in a 2-year, 11-month-old boy with acute Kawasaki disease. **A,** Left parasternal short-axis view demonstrating a giant left proximal coronary artery aneurysm (35 × 25 mm, *black arrows*) and an aneurysm in the right coronary artery (*white arrow*). **B,** The subcostal view reveals two giant aneurysms in the right coronary artery. The proximal one is 18 × 18 mm and the distal one is 10 × 10 mm. **C,** A thrombus (*white arrow*) partially occupying the left coronary artery giant aneurysm. The *arrowheads* define the lumen of the aneurysm. Ao—aorta. (*From* Lima *et al.* [14]; with permission.)

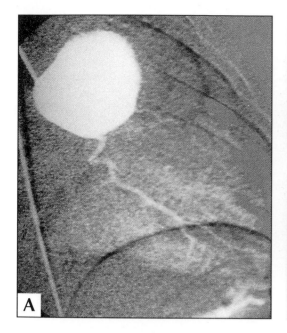

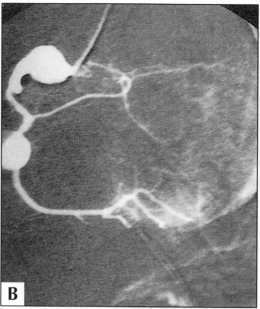

FIGURE 9-15. Coronary arteriograms demonstrating the aneurysms shown in Fig. 9-14. **A,** The giant left proximal coronary artery aneurysm. **B,** The two giant aneurysms in the right coronary artery. Right coronary artery ectasia is seen between the two aneurysms. (*From* Lima *et al.* [14]; with permission.)

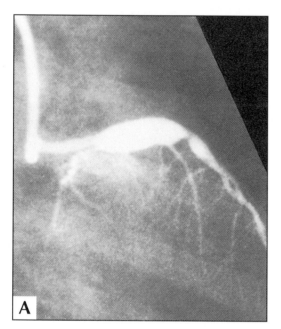

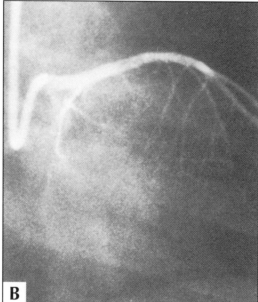

FIGURE 9-16. Left coronary arteriograms from a male infant who contracted Kawasaki disease (KD) at age 6 months. **A,** Arteriogram 1 month after onset of KD. Fusiform aneurysms are observed in the left anterior descending coronary artery. **B,** Arteriogram 16 months later, showing regression of the aneurysm. (*Panel A from* Takahashi *et al.* [15]; with permission.)

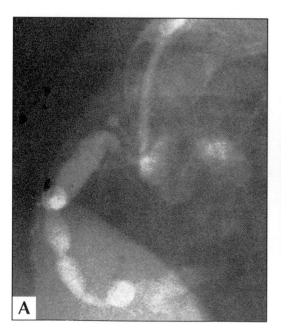

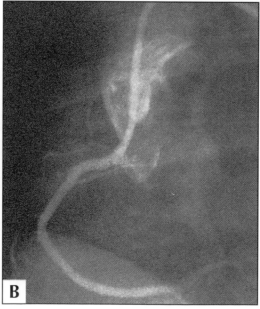

FIGURE 9-17. Right coronary arteriograms from a male infant who contracted Kawasaki disease at age 6 months (same patient as in Fig. 9-16). **A,** Multiple aneurysms can be seen 1 month after onset of the disease. **B,** Regression of the aneurysms 16 months later (17 months after onset of disease).

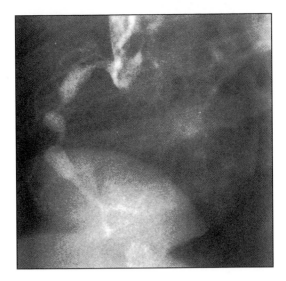

FIGURE 9-18. Right coronary arteriogram from a 17-month-old girl who was diagnosed with Kawasaki disease at age 15 months. Two months after onset of disease, three aneurysms are present, with possible discrete stenoses between aneurysmal segments. (*From* Takahashi *et al.* [15]; with permission.)

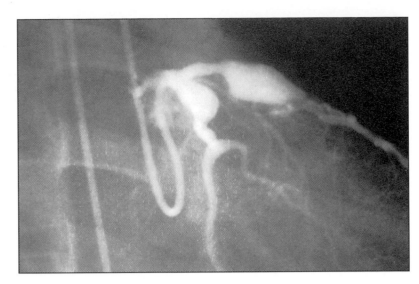

FIGURE 9-19. Giant coronary artery aneurysms. These aneurysms (internal diameter of at least 8 mm) rarely regress. These patients have a worse prognosis than patients without giant aneurysms, and have the greatest risk for development of stenosis, thrombosis, or myocardial infarction. This figure shows aneurysms of the left anterior descending and the left circumflex coronary arteries in a 6-year-old boy who was diagnosed with Kawasaki disease and giant aneurysms 5 years earlier, at age 13 months.

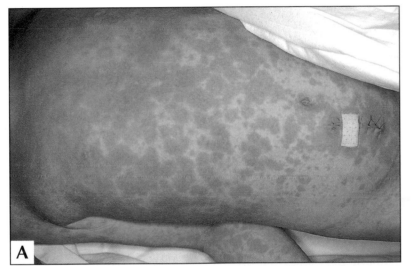

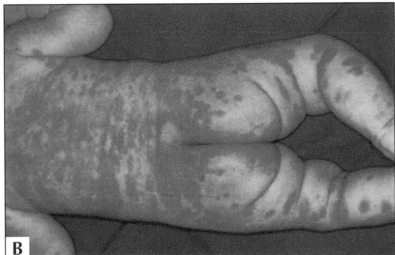

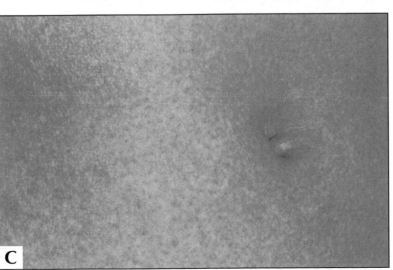

FIGURE 9-20. Examples of rashes seen in patients with Kawasaki disease. The rash is typically polymorphous and appears within 5 days of the onset of fever. Such rashes may take various forms including an urticarial exanthem (**A**), a maculopapular morbilli-form eruption (**B**), a scarlatiniform derma (**C**), or an erythema-multiforme–like (*continued on next page*)

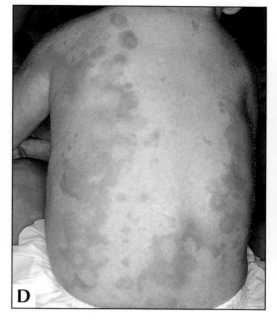

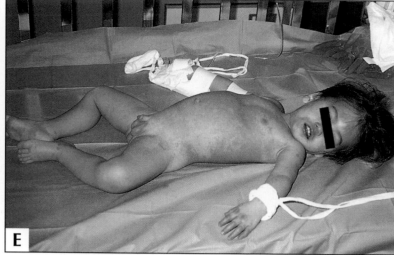

FIGURE 9-20. (*continued*) rash (**D**). Bullous eruptions have not been described. The rash is usually extensive, involving the trunk and extremities with accentuation in the perineal region (**E**). (*Panel B from* [5]; with permission.)

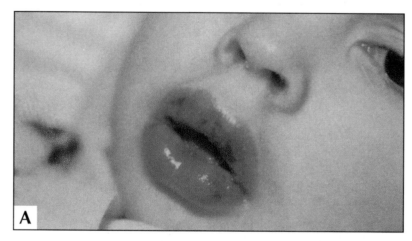

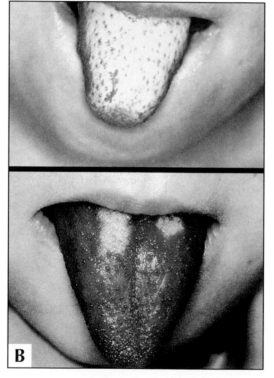

FIGURE 9-21. Mucous membrane changes in Kawasaki disease. These changes involve the conjunctivae, oral cavity and lips (**A** and **B**), and the urethra. Bilateral conjunctival injection usually begins shortly after the onset of fever. It typically involves the bulbar conjunctivae much more than the palpebral or tarsal conjunctivae, is not associated with an exudate, and is usually painless. Changes in the lips and oral cavity include erythema and cracking of the lips, strawberry tongue, and erythema of the oropharyngeal mucosa. No ulcerations are seen. (*From* [5]; with permission.)

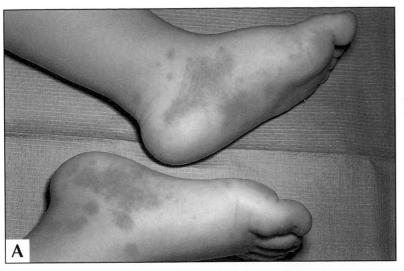
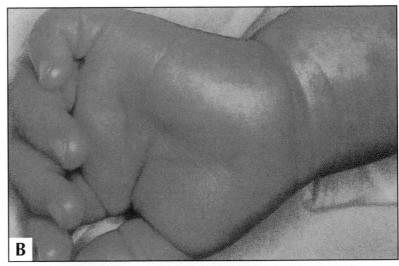
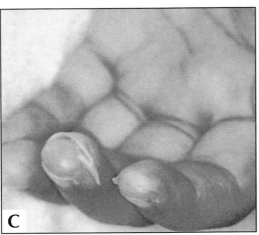
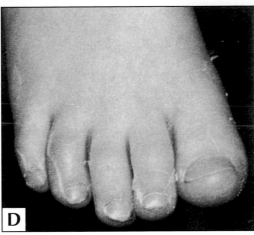
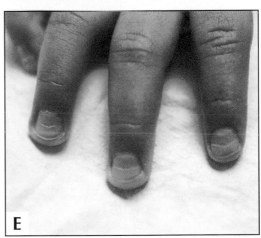

FIGURE 9-22. Changes in the extremities in Kawasaki disease. A and B, Erythema of the palms and soles and/or firm, sometimes painful induration of the hands or feet often occurs in the early phase of the disease. C and D, Desquamation of the fingers and toes usually begins 1 to 3 weeks after onset of fever in the periun-gual region and may extend to the palms and toes. E, Approximately 1 to 2 months after the onset of fever, deep transverse grooves across the nails (Beau's lines) may appear. (*Panels B and C from* [5]; with permission.)

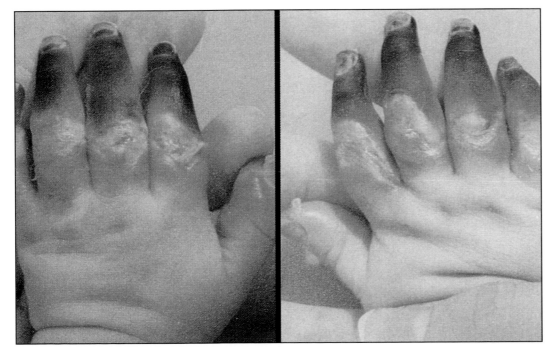

FIGURE 9-23. Peripheral gangrene secondary to arterial involvement in a 2-month-old infant with Kawasaki disease. This is a rare complication of the disease that occurs in young infants (all reported cases have been 7 months of age or younger at onset of disease [16]). Frequently associated findings include giant coronary and peripheral aneurysms.

LABORATORY FINDINGS IN KAWASAKI DISEASE

Neutrophilia with immature forms

Elevated ESR

Positive CRP

Elevated serum α_1-antitrypsin

Anemia

Hypoalbuminemia

Elevated serum IgE

Thrombocytosis

Proteinuria

Sterile pyuria

Elevated serum transaminases

FIGURE 9-24. Laboratory findings in Kawasaki disease (KD). Laboratory findings are nondiagnostic for KD, but may assist in diagnosis. The elevated platelet count usually appears after the first week of illness. The proteinuria is probably secondary to fever. The erythrocyte sedimentation rate (ESR) and C-reactive protein (CRP) are almost invariably elevated.

IMMUNE SYSTEM IRREGULARITIES IN KAWASAKI DISEASE

Activation of monocytes/macrophages

Increased activated T-helper cells

Decreased T-suppressor cells

Increased activated B cells

Cytokine secretion, including:

Interleukin-1β

Interleukin-2

Interleukin-6

Interleukin-10

Tumor necrosis factor-α

Interferon-γ

Circulating soluble selections

Appearance of circulating antibodies
  cytotoxic to vascular endothelial cells

FIGURE 9-25. Immune system irregularities in Kawasaki disease (KD). In response to an unknown triggering process, immunoregulatory abnormalities are observed in KD. It is postulated that the various secreted cytokines target vascular endothelial cells, producing cell-surface antigens. Antibodies produced against these antigens then target the vascular endothelium, resulting in a cascade of events leading to vascular damage.

TARGETS OF THERAPY IN KAWASAKI DISEASE

LIFESTYLE MODIFICATIONS

Implementation of heart-healthy diet, with specific recommendations guided by serum lipid profile

Prevention or cessation of smoking

Physical activity guided by status of coronary arteries and use of antithrombolytic therapy (see Figs. 9-29–9-34 for stratified recommendations)

Maintenance of healthy weight

PHARMACOLOGIC THERAPY

Goals

Decrease overall prevalence and size of coronary artery aneurysms

Prevent coronary artery thrombosis in patients with aneurysms

Treat ischemic heart disease in patients with coronary aneurysms

SURGICAL INTERVENTION

CABG

PTCA

Stents

Cardiac transplantation

FIGURE 9-26. Targets of therapy for Kawasaki disease (KD). Children with KD and their parents should receive lifestyle modification counseling. This is especially important because various follow-up studies in children with coronary aneurysms in the acute phase have indicated that even when these aneurysms regress, there is persisting vascular dysfunction. This may put these children at risk for accelerated atherosclerosis in adulthood. Maintaining a healthy weight is an important factor. Children are considered overweight if their body mass index (BMI) is greater than the 85th percentile for age and sex; they are considered obese if their BMI is greater than the 95th percentile.

Patients will also receive pharmacologic therapy, which should include aspirin and intravenous gamma globulin in the acute phase. They may also receive anticoagulants if giant coronary aneurysms

develop, and other appropriate agents if myocardial ischemia develops. A small number of children will need interventional coronary procedures, coronary artery bypass grafting (CABG), or, rarely, cardiac transplantation [17]. However, CABG may be complex technically because of very small coronary arteries. Technical considerations and choice of graft vessel are discussed in detail by Kitamura *et al.* [18]. Results over the first decade after CABG in childhood are encouraging, but patency later in adulthood is unknown. Therefore, interventional catheterization procedures may postpone further surgery. Percutaneous transluminal coronary angioplasty (PTCA) is not as effective in patients with KD as in adults with atherosclerotic coronary disease because the stenotic lesions in long-term KD are very stiff and are often associated with marked calcifications, especially many years after onset of the illness.

RECOMMENDED THERAPY DURING THE ACUTE STAGE OF KAWASAKI DISEASE

IVGG

2 g/kg as single infusion over 10–12 h

PLUS

Aspirin

80–100 mg/kg/d orally in four equally divided doses until patient is afebrile 48–72 h

THEN

3–5 mg/kg orally once daily up to 6–8 weeks

FIGURE 9-27. Recommended therapy during the acute stage of Kawasaki disease (KD). Initial therapy for KD is currently targeted toward reducing inflammation of the myocardium and coronary artery walls and reducing fever. Intravenous gamma-globulin

(IVGG) given in addition to aspirin has been shown to be superior to aspirin alone in reducing inflammation and preventing the development of coronary artery aneurysms [19–21], especially giant aneurysms [22]. Treatment with high-dose IVGG in the acute phase of KD reduces the prevalence of coronary aneurysms and has become the standard of care. Some patients come to the physician within 10 days of the onset of illness but already have coronary artery ectasia or aneurysms. These patients should receive the above aspirin and IVGG regimen, although current data are lacking on the long-term benefits of such therapy. Aspirin is reduced to a lower dose after the febrile period. This is done for its antithrombotic effect. It should be discontinued 6 to 8 weeks after the onset of illness if no coronary arterial abnormalities are present by echocardiography. Aspirin is continued indefinitely if there are coronary arterial abnormalities. To reduce the very small risk of Reye's syndrome, aspirin therapy should be interrupted temporarily if the patient develops varicella or influenza. Alternate therapy is pyridamole (3–6 mg/kg 2 or 3 times daily) for approximately 2 weeks. Administration of influenza vaccine is recommended in these patients on long-term aspirin therapy.

RETREATMENT STRATEGIES

STANDARD IVGG REGIMEN

Reinfusion of 2 g/kg when fever persists or recrudesces 48 h or more after initial IVGG infusion

Multiple IVGG infusions may be necessary in severe Kawasaki disease

CORTICOSTEROIDS

High-dose pulses of methylprednisolone 30 mg/kg IV over 4 h, once daily for 1–3 d

Note: Patients should undergo continuous cardiac monitoring and blood pressure measurement every 15 min

FIGURE 9-28. Although 80% to 90% of patients respond favorably to initial intravenous gamma-globulin (IVGG) treatment, the remainder have persistent or recrudescent fever. Even when the initial dose fails, most will respond to treatment. Newburger *et al.* [20] demonstrated that peak adjusted serum IgG levels are lower among patients who go on to develop coronary artery abnormalities while they are inversely related to fever duration and laboratory measurements of acute inflammation. This apparent dose-response effect forms the basis for IVGG treatment.

The subgroup of children with acute Kawasaki disease (KD) who are resistant to IVGG therapy have the highest risk for development of coronary artery aneurysms and long-term sequelae of the disease. Corticosteroid therapy for KD was long held in disfavor because a study from Japan in the 1970s showed detrimental effects of the drug. More recently, however, investigators have suggested that steroids may be beneficial in the prevention of coronary artery aneurysm [23–25]. Controlled studies are needed to assess the potential role of steroid administration in KD.

RISK LEVELS USED IN STRATIFICATION

RISK LEVEL	CRITERIA
I	Patients with no coronary artery changes demonstrated by echocardiography at any stage of illness
II	Patients with transient coronary ectasia on echocardiography, which disappears during the acute illness
III	Patients with a small to medium solitary coronary aneurysm demonstrated by echocardiography or angiography
IV	Patients with one or more giant coronary artery aneurysms or multiple small to medium aneurysms, without obstruction on echocardiography, preferably confirmed by coronary angiography
V	Patients with coronary artery obstruction confirmed by angiography

FIGURE 9-29. Clinical experience allows patients with Kawasaki disease to be stratified into risk levels based on their relative risk of myocardial ischemia. The risk level for a patient can change over time when there is a change in coronary artery morphology. A patient could move to a lower risk level (with regression of aneurysms) or to a higher risk level (with development of thrombosis or stenosis).

RECOMMENDATIONS FOR RISK LEVEL I

Pharmacologic therapy: None beyond initial 6–8 weeks

Physical activity: No restrictions beyond initial 6–8 weeks

Follow-up and diagnostic testing: None beyond 1st y unless evidence of cardiac disease suspected

Invasive testing: None recommended

FIGURE 9-30. Recommendations for risk level 1. These patients have no demonstrated coronary artery changes at any stage of their illness. Pharmacologic therapy during the initial 6 to 8 weeks is listed in Figure 9-27. Three recent studies have indicated abnormal convalescent serum lipid profiles in some children after the febrile stage of Kawasaki disease; these abnormalities usually returned to normal by a year after the onset of the disease [26–28]. Counseling of these patients and their parents should adhere to the standard dietary recommendations for children and adolescents [29] and other lifestyle modifications listed in Figure 9-26. The physician may choose to remeasure the lipids a year later. All patients in this risk level should be directed to follow the usual practice of well-child care.

RECOMMENDATIONS FOR RISK LEVEL II

Pharmacologic therapy: None beyond initial 6–8 weeks

Physical activity: No restrictions beyond initial 6–8 weeks

Follow-up and diagnostic testing: None beyond 1st y unless evidence of cardiac disease suspected

Invasive testing: None recommended

FIGURE 9-31. Recommendations for risk level II. These patients demonstrate transient coronary ectasia on echocardiography, which disappears during the acute illness. Pharmacologic therapy during the initial 6 to 8 weeks is listed in Figure 9-27. Because long-term natural history data are not available, some pediatric cardiologists choose to see these patients at 3- to 5-year intervals to monitor their cardiovascular status. For comments on lipid profiles and routine follow-up care, *see* Figures 9-26 and 9-30.

RECOMMENDATIONS FOR RISK LEVEL III

Pharmacologic therapy: Long-term antiplatelet therapy with aspirin at least until aneurysms regress

Physical activity: In 1st decade of life, no restriction beyond initial 6–8 weeks; stress test with myocardial perfusion scan may be useful in 2nd decade as a guide to recommendations for physical activity; competitive contact athletics with endurance training discouraged

Follow-up and diagnostic testing: Annual follow-up with echocardiogram and ECG in 1st decade of life

Invasive testing: Angiography, if patient symptoms, stress testing, perfusion imaging, echocardiogram, or other tests suggest ischemia

FIGURE 9-32. Recommendations for risk level III. These patients demonstrate a small- to medium-sized solitary coronary artery aneurysm on echocardiography. Antithrombotic doses of aspirin are recommended while coronary artery abnormalities are present. For comments on Reye's syndrome, see Figure 9-27. ECG–electrocardiogram

RECOMMENDATIONS FOR RISK LEVEL IV

Pharmacologic therapy: Long-term antiplatelet therapy with aspirin ± warfarin sodium

Physical activity: In 1st decade of life, no restriction beyond initial 6–8 weeks; in 2nd decade, annual stress testing with myocardial perfusion scan guides recommendations; strenuous athletics strongly discouraged; if stress test rules out ischemia, noncontact recreational sports allowed

Follow-up and diagnostic testing: Annual follow-up with echocardiogram ± ECG ± chest radiography ± additional ECG at 6-month intervals; in 1st decade of life, consider pharmacologic stress testing; annual stress testing in patients over age 10 y should include evaluation of myocardial perfusion

Invasive testing: Angiography, if stress testing or echocardiogram suggests stenosis; elective catheterization in the absence of noninvasive evidence of myocardial ischemia may be useful to conclusively rule out subclinical major coronary artery obstructions in certain situations, such as when a patient has atypical chest pain, ability to perform dynamic stress testing is limited by age, or unique activity restrictions or insurability recommendations are needed

FIGURE 9-33. Recommendations for risk level IV. These patients demonstrate one or more giant coronary artery aneurysms, or multiple small to medium aneurysms, without obstruction by echocardiography, preferably confirmed by angiography. If warfarin is used as an adjunct to aspirin therapy (recommended for those with giant aneurysms), an International Normalized Ratio of 2.0 to 2.5 should be maintained. Daily subcutaneous injections of low molecular weight heparin may be an alternative to warfarin in infants and young children in whom blood drawing to measure prothrombin time is difficult. For comments on Reye's syndrome, see Figure 9-27. ECG—electrocardiogram.

RECOMMENDATIONS FOR RISK LEVEL V

Pharmacologic therapy: Long-term antiplatelet therapy with aspirin ± warfarin sodium; β-blockers should be considered to reduce myocardial oxygen consumption

Physical activity: Contact sports, isometrics, and weight training should be avoided; other recommendations for noncompetitive, noncontact dynamic physical activity at low to moderate intensity is guided by outcome of stress testing or myocardial perfusion scan

Follow-up and diagnostic testing: Echocardiogram + ECG at 6-month intervals and annual Holter monitor test; stress testing with evaluation of myocardial perfusion should be performed annually in 2nd decade of life; in younger patients or patients not able to perform dynamic exercise, pharmacologic stress testing with myocardial perfusion can be done

Invasive testing: Cardiac catheterization with selective angiography recommended to aid therapeutic options and identify extent of collateral perfusion; repeat angiography with new-onset or worsening ischemia suggested by noninvasive diagnostic testing or clinical presentation

FIGURE 9-34. Recommendations for risk level V. These patients demonstrate coronary artery obstruction confirmed by angiography. If warfarin is used as an adjunct to aspirin therapy (Fig. 9-33), an International Normalized Ratio of 2.0 to 2.5 should be maintained. For comments on Reye's syndrome, see Figure 9-27. Therapeutic options for patients with severe coronary artery obstruction include coronary artery bypass graft surgery and percutaneous transluminal coronary angioplasty, although data on the use of angioplasty are limited and have not shown consistent improvement. Some patients may experience an acute myocardial infarction, and rapid thrombolytic therapy is indicated. ECG—electrocardiogram.

FATE OF PATIENTS WITH MYOCARDIAL INFARCTION DUE TO KAWASAKI DISEASE

IN A RETROSPECTIVE STUDY OF 195 PATIENTS WITH MI

142/195 had MI within 1 year after KD onset

77/142 had MI within 3 months after KD onset

Mortality rate for first MI was 22% (43 deaths)

Of the 152 survivors of the first MI: 24 had a second MI (16%); mortality was 63% (15 deaths)

Of the nine survivors (from 24 victims) of the second MI: six had a third MI, and only one survived

FIGURE 9-35. Kato *et al.* [30] conducted a nationwide survey in Japan in the mid-1980s. Data were collected on 195 patients with myocardial infarction (MI) due to Kawasaki disease (KD). Seventy-three percent had the MI within 1 year of the diagnosis of KD, with about half of these first-year infarctions occurring within the first 3 months of KD diagnosis. Data from this study and other reports indicate that most patients do not have a history of chest pain prior to the MI. In Kato *et al.*'s study, only three (1.5%) patients had a history of chest pain. (*Adapted from* Kato *et al.* [30].)

REFERENCES

1. Taubert KA, Shulman ST: Kawasaki disease. *Am Fam Physician* 1999, 59:3093—3102.

2. Kawasaki T: Acute febrile mucocutaneous syndrome with lymphoid involvement with specific desquamation of the fingers and toes in children (in Japanese). *Jpn J Allergy* 1967, 16:178–222.

3. Japan Kawasaki Disease Research Committee: The results of the 16th nationwide survey of Kawasaki disease. *Shonika Shinryo* 2002, 65:332–342.

4. Taubert KA: Epidemiology of Kawasaki disease in the United States and worldwide. *Prog Pediatr Cardiol* 1997, 6:181–185.

5. Diagnostic guidelines for Kawasaki disease. *Circulation* 2001, 103(2):335–336.

6. Dajani AS, Taubert KA, Gerber MA, *et al.*: Diagnosis and therapy of Kawasaki disease in children. *Circulation* 1993, 87:1776–1780.

7. Dajani AS, Taubert KA, Takahashi M, *et al.*: Guidelines for long-term management of patients with Kawasaki disease. *Circulation* 1994, 89:918–922.

8. Davis RL, Waller PL, Mueller BA, *et al.*: Kawasaki syndrome in Washington State. Race-specific incidence rates and residential proximity to water. *Arch Pediatr Adolesc Med* 1995, 149(1):66–69.

9. Rauch AM: Kawasaki syndrome: critical review of U.S. epidemiology. In *Kawasaki Disease*. Edited by Shulman ST. New York: Alan R. Liss, Inc; 1987; 33–44.

10. Taubert KA, Rowley AH, Shulman ST: A ten-year (1984–1993) United States hospital survey of Kawasaki disease. In *Kawasaki Disease*. Edited by Kato H. New York: Elsiever Science BV; 1995:34–38.

11. Shulman ST: A commentary on disease mechanism. In *Proceedings of the Fourth International Symposium on Kawasaki Disease*. Edited by Takahashi M, Taubert K. Dallas, TX: American Heart Association; 1993:223–225.

12. Becker AE: Kawasaki disease: reflections on pathological observations. In *Proceedings of the Fourth International Symposium on Kawasaki Disease*. Edited by Takahashi M, Taubert K. Dallas, TX: American Heart Association; 1993:226–230.

13. Arjunan K, Daniels SR, Meyer RA, *et al.*: Coronary artery caliber in normal children and patients with Kawasaki disease but without aneurysms: an echocardiographic and angiocardiographic study. *J Am Coll Cardiol* 1986, 8:1119–1124.

14. Lima M, Kaku S, Macedo A, *et al.*: Echocardiographic diagnosis and surgical treatment of giant coronary arterial aneurysms. In *Proceedings of the Fourth International Symposium on Kawasaki Disease*. Edited by Takahashi M, Taubert K. Dallas, TX: American Heart Association; 1993:404–407.

15. Takahashi M, Schieber RA, Wishner SH, *et al.*: Selective coronary arteriography in infants and children. *Circulation* 1983, 68:1021–1028.

16. Tomita S, Chung K, Mas M, *et al.*: Peripheral gangrene associated with Kawasaki disease. In *Proceedings of the Fourth International Symposium on Kawasaki Disease*. Edited by Takahashi M, Taubert K. Dallas, TX: American Heart Association; 1993:27–31.

17. Checchia PA, Pahl E, Shaddy RE, Shulman ST: Cardiac transplantation for Kawasaki disease. *Pediatrics* 1997, 100(4):695–699.

18. Kitamura S, Kameda Y, Seki T, *et al.*: Long-term outcome of myocardial revascularization in patients with Kawasaki coronary artery disease. A multicenter cooperative study. *J Thorac Cardiovasc Surg* 1994, 107(3):663–673.

19. Newburger JW, Takahashi M, Burns JC, *et al.*: The treatment of Kawasaki syndrome with intravenous gamma-globulin. *N Engl J Med* 1986, 315:341–347.

20. Newburger JW, Takahashi M, Beiser AS, *et al.*: A single infusion of intravenous gamma-globulin compared to four daily doses in the treatment of acute Kawasaki syndrome. *N Engl J Med* 1991, 324:1633–1639.

21. Durongpisitkul K, Gururaj VJ, Park JM, Martin CF: The prevention of coronary artery aneurysm in Kawasaki disease: a meta-analysis on the efficacy of aspirin and immunoglobulin treatment. *Pediatrics* 1995, 96(6):1057–1061.

22. Rowley AH, Duffy CE, Shulman ST: Prevention of giant coronary artery aneurysms in Kawasaki disease by intravenous gamma-globulin therapy. *J Pediatr* 1988, 113:290–294.

23. Newburger JW: Treatment of Kawasaki disease: corticosteroids revisited. *J Pediatr* 1999, 135(4):411–413.

24. Mason WH, Takahashi M: Kawasaki syndrome. *Clin Infect Dis* 1999, 28(2):169–185.

25. Wallace CA, French JW, Kahn SJ, Sherry DD: Initial intravenous gammaglobulin treatment failure in Kawasaki disease. *Pediatrics* 2000, 105(6):E78.

26. Newburger JW, Burns JC, Beiser AS, Loscalzo J: Altered lipid profile after Kawasaki syndrome. *Circulation* 1991, 84:625–631.

27. Inoue O, Sugimura T, Kato H: Long-term lipid profiles in patients with Kawasaki disease. In *Proceedings of the Fourth International Symposium on Kawasaki Disease*. Edited by Takahashi M, Taubert K. Dallas, TX: American Heart Association; 1993:305–309.

28. Salo EPI, Pesonen EJ, Viikari JSA: Serum cholesterol during and after Kawasaki disease. *J Pediatr* 1991, 119:557–561.

29. American Academy of Pediatrics. National Cholesterol Education Program: Report of the Expert Panel on Blood Cholesterol Levels in Children and Adolescents. *Pediatrics* 1992, 89:525–584.

30. Kato H, Ichinose E, Kawasaki T: Myocardial infarction in Kawasaki disease: clinical analyses in 195 cases. *J Pediatr* 1986, 108:923–927.

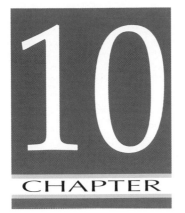

DEEP VEIN THROMBOSIS, PULMONARY EMBOLISM, AND PRIMARY PULMONARY HYPERTENSION

CHAPTER 10

Samuel Z. Goldhaber and Joseph F. Polak

Deep venous thrombosis and pulmonary embolism constitute a cardiovascular illness, venous thromboembolism, and represent an often-unrecognized disease that causes surprisingly frequently disability and loss of life. Overshadowed by acute coronary syndromes, which are more likely to present suddenly with dramatic onset of chest pain, nausea, and diaphoresis, venous thromboembolism is insidious, subtle, and easily overlooked. The consequences of a missed diagnosis of venous thromboembolism can be devastating. The disease, like coronary heart disease, may cause sudden cardiovascular collapse and death due to massive pulmonary embolism. More common, though, is the development of long-term dyspnea on exertion due to chronic pulmonary hypertension, or permanent calf swelling and leg aching due to chronic venous insufficiency.

Progress in understanding the epidemiology and optimization of diagnostic and treatment paradigms for deep venous thrombosis and pulmonary embolism is advancing rapidly. More sophisticated Doppler and ultrasound technology facilitates the rapid identification and exclusion of deep venous thrombosis. The plasma D-dimer enzyme-linked immunosorbent assay has been validated as a reliable blood test to rule out acute pulmonary embolism. Chest CT scanning has overtaken lung scanning as the primary imaging modality for suspected pulmonary embolism. Our ability to utilize an integrated diagnostic strategy has increased the likelihood of early detection of venous thromboembolism.

Treatment of pulmonary embolism has improved because of more rapid and accurate risk stratification, new anticoagulants, novel catheter and mechanical interventions, and a "reinvention" of the open surgical pulmonary embolectomy. Use of clinical assessment, echocardiography to determine right ventricular size and function, and troponin levels to detect microscopic myocardial necrosis permit prognostication of newly diagnosed patients with acute pulmonary embolism. Those at low risk respond well to anticoagulants alone. However, high-risk patients require more aggressive intervention, which can now be initiated more quickly, usually before the clinical condition deteriorates. Thrombolysis can rapidly reverse right ventricular dysfunction, and embolectomy, either in the interventional laboratory or operating room, can be lifesaving for patients who are not candidates for thrombolysis. Chronic thromboembolic pulmonary hypertension, which may occur after unrecognized or inadequately treated pulmonary embolism, can be managed effectively with an entirely different operation (pulmonary thromboendarterectomy).

Primary pulmonary hypertension is an often-devastating illness of uncertain etiology. Fortunately, new therapies are dramatically improving the prognosis of patients with this condition.

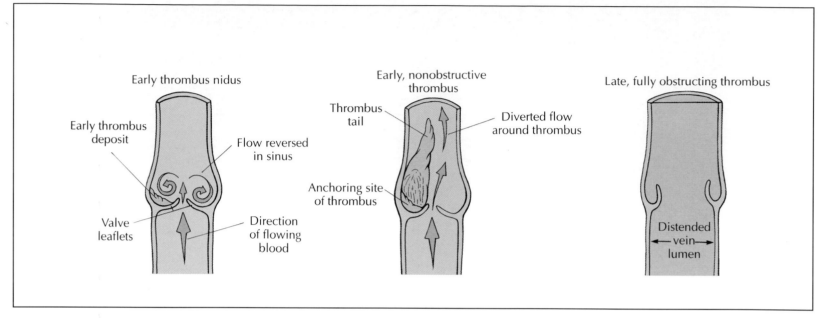

FIGURE 10-1. Different stages of thrombus formation. Early thrombi form in areas of stagnant flow (*left*). This is typically seen at the vein valve sinus where there is stagnation of blood and reversal of blood flow. The inciting events responsible for early thrombus formation are not fully understood and include damage to the endothelial lining of the vein because of trauma, alterations of coagulation factors, and stasis.

Thrombus grows by aggregation of red cells, platelets within a fibrin mesh, and elongation from its anchoring point within the sinus of the vein valve (*middle*). Most thrombi do not evolve beyond this stage.

Thrombus can grow to expand and fully occupy lumen of the vein (*right*). The vein will distend because the volume occupied by the fibrin mesh forming the thrombus is larger than that of the dissolved blood constituents. In obstructing thrombosis, symptoms are likely caused by local distention and activation of pain receptors in the vein wall and surrounding tissues. The finding of vein distention on venous sonography supports the diagnosis of obstructive venous thrombosis. In addition, localized edema or inflammatory changes can activate pain and stretch receptors in the contiguous tissues. Distal to the obstructing thrombus, impairment of venous return causes an increase in hydrostatic pressure, resulting in the extravasation of fluid into the extracellular space.

EPIDEMIOLOGY OF VENOUS THROMBOSIS

250,000–2,000,000 new cases of DVT and/or PE annually in the US

Detection is often difficult and public awareness is low

Case fatality rate for acute PE is surprisingly high; approximately 15% of patients die within 30 days of diagnosis

FIGURE 10-2. Epidemiology of venous thrombosis. Venous thromboembolism, which comprises deep venous thrombosis (DVT) and pulmonary embolism (PE), is the third most common cardiovascular illness after acute coronary syndrome and stroke. The incidence in the US ranges between 250,000 and 2,000,000 cases annually. Precise incidence statistics are not available because detected cases constitute only a small proportion of the total disease burden. Deep venous thrombosis and PE are often occult. Public awareness of venous thromboembolism is low, in contrast to high public recognition of acute myocardial infarction and stroke. It is worthwhile suspecting the possible onset of DVT and PE because the case fatality rate is surprisingly high.

MAJOR RISK FACTORS FOR VENOUS THROMBOSIS

ACQUIRED

Surgery

Trauma

Immobilization

Cancer

Oral contraceptives

Pregnancy

Hormone replacement therapy

Indwelling central venous catheter

Pacemaker

Internal cardiac defibrillator

THROMBOPHILIC

Factor V Leiden mutation

Prothrombin gene mutation

Antiphospholipid antibody syndrome

Hyperhomocystinemia

Deficiencies of antithrombin III, protein C, and protein S

IDIOPATHIC

Long-haul air travel

"None of the above"

FIGURE 10-3. Major risk factors for venous thrombosis. Risk factors for venous thromboembolism can be subdivided into acquired, thrombophilic, and idiopathic factors. Acquired risk factors include situations commonly encountered in hospitalized patients, such as surgery, trauma, and immobilization. Chronic conditions such as cancer also predispose patients to deep venous thrombosis (DVT) and pulmonary embolism (PE). Venous thromboembolism is a women's health issue because oral contraceptives, pregnancy, and postmenopausal hormonal replacement therapy all make DVT and PE more likely. Upper extremity venous thrombosis is becoming more prevalent because of the increased use of indwelling central venous catheters, pacemakers, and internal cardiac defibrillators.

Thrombophilic factors also contribute to the risk of venous thromboembolism [1]. These factors may be genetic and inherited, such as the factor V Leiden or prothrombin gene mutations, or acquired, such as the antiphospholipid antibody syndrome.

Most mysterious and frustrating to patient and clinician are the idiopathic cases of DVT and PE. These may include long-haul air travel or simply thrombophilic risks that have not yet been pinpointed.

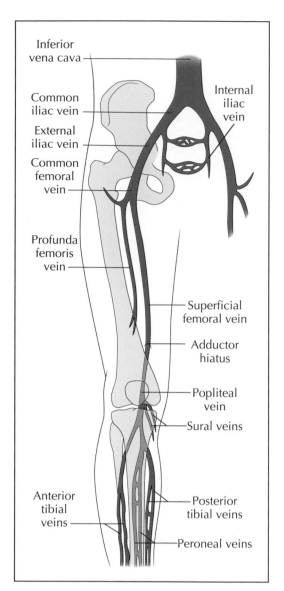

FIGURE 10-4. The major venous channels of the lower extremity. The inferior vena cava, which lies to the right of the aorta, branches into the common iliac veins. On the left, the common iliac vein crosses below the right iliac artery or the aorta. This causes relative compression of the vein and is likely the cause of slower venous blood flow in the left leg as compared with the right lower extremity. The common iliac vein bifurcates into external and internal iliac veins. The internal iliac vein tends to be smaller in diameter and connects with the contralateral internal iliac vein. As the external iliac vein descends through the pelvis, it becomes the common femoral vein at the inguinal ligament.

The common femoral vein then bifurcates into the profunda femoris (deep femoral) and the true (superficial) femoral veins. The profunda femoris (deep femoral) vein is responsible for venous drainage of the proximal two thirds of the thigh. The "superficial femoral vein" accompanies the superficial femoral artery. Despite the name "superficial," this vein is actually a deep leg vein. The superficial femoral vein is responsible for venous drainage of the distal third of the thigh.

As the femoral vein crosses through the adductor hiatus, defined by the adductor muscle in the lower thigh, it becomes the popliteal vein. The popliteal vein has major muscular branches to the gastrocnemius muscle. Approximately 6 cm below the knee joint, the popliteal vein sends off the anterior tibial veins that cross the interosseous membrane and then lie on top of it. Posteriorly, the tibioperoneal trunk branches into the true posterior tibial and peroneal veins. Below the popliteal vein, the deep venous system is almost always duplicated.

DIAGNOSTIC TESTS

PRINCIPAL DIAGNOSTIC TESTS

PULMONARY EMBOLISM

D-dimer ELISA

Lung scan

Chest CT scan

Pulmonary angiogram

DEEP VENOUS THROMBOSIS

Ultrasonography

Doppler

MRI

Duplex ultrasonography

Magnetic resonance venography

Contrast venography

FIGURE 10-5. Principal diagnostic tests for deep venous thrombosis (DVT). Venous ultrasonography with Doppler imaging (duplex) is the most common diagnostic test for DVT. Impedance plethysmography is far less sensitive and is no longer used as a primary diagnostic tool in the US. Magnetic resonance imaging is useful to help differentiate acute, subacute, and chronic clot. It can also help detect extrinsic vascular compression due to fluid or tumor. Contrast venography, which has lost its position as the gold standard for thrombus proximal to the calves, is most useful as a prelude to intervention such as suction thrombectomy, stenting, or catheter-directed thrombolysis.

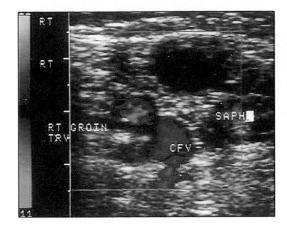

FIGURE 10-6. Ultrasound color Doppler image showing a normal vascular examination with the transducer placed in the right groin. Visualized in cross-section is the common femoral vein (CFV) in *blue*, greater saphenous vein (SAPH) at the junction with the CFV, and the common femoral artery (shown in *red*, adjacent to the CFV, at 10 and 11 o'clock).

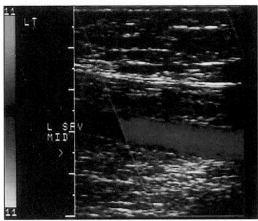

FIGURE 10-7. Ultrasound color Doppler image demonstrating in longitudinal section a normal left mid superficial femoral vein (L SFV MID), which is a deep vein despite its name "superficial."

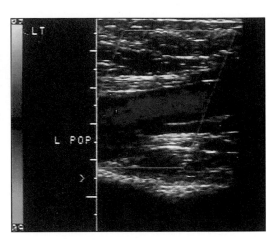

FIGURE 10-8. Ultrasound color Doppler image demonstrating in longitudinal section a normal left popliteal vein (L POP).

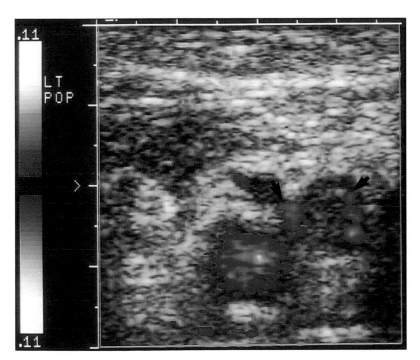

FIGURE 10-9. A rim of *blue color* surrounds a discrete filling defect. This defect is consistent with an acute thrombus. In acute venous thrombosis, blood flow signals are either absent in the affected segment or outline the thrombus within the vein segment.

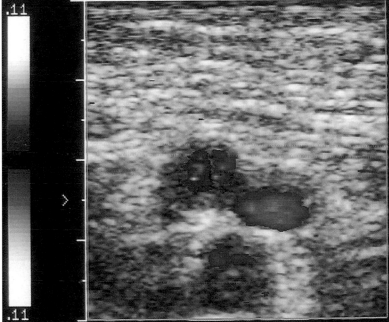

FIGURE 10-10. Blood flow in the central portion of the lumen (*blue area*). The vein wall is thickened. Residual wall thickening following resorption of thrombus is typical of chronic venous thrombosis.

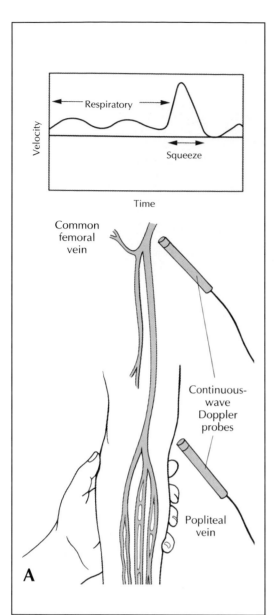

A

FIGURE 10-11. Doppler analysis of blood flow signals providing diagnostic information that complements ultrasound imaging. **A,** Obstructive venous thrombosis can be detected by analyzing flow signals within the veins using either continuous wave or pulsed-wave Doppler. Both types of Doppler use a sound beam to interrogate blood flow velocity within the veins. The motion of erythrocytes within the vein causes frequency shifts in the returning signals. A typical example of the detected waveforms is shown on the *top portion* of the figure. During respiration, there is typically a phasic variation in the velocity waveform detected within the femoral vein ("respiratory phasicity"). This variation is slightly less pronounced at the popliteal vein and difficult to elicit at the calf. During inspiration, there is a relative decrease in blood flow because of the increase in intra-abdominal pressure. During expiration, blood flow velocity is increased. An ancillary maneuver used to exclude the presence of an obstructive process is blood flow augmentation. This is accomplished by externally squeezing the calf. This expels some blood into the popliteal, femoral, and ultimately the iliac veins. A similar effect can be achieved by having the patient dorsiflex and plantarflex the foot. The end result is a marked increase in the velocity signals detected more proximally, within the popliteal and femoral veins (squeeze phase).

The finding of normal respiratory variation and a normal response to flow augmentation excludes the presence of venous obstruction caused either by an intrinsic process, such as venous thrombosis, or an extrinsic process, such as compression by a pelvic tumor.

Continued on next page

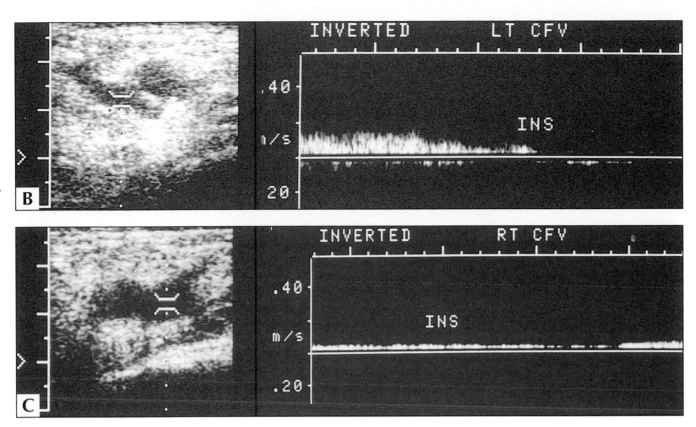

FIGURE 10-11. *(Continued)* **B**, Doppler tracing of a normal response to inspiration (INS) with a decrease in the velocity of blood flow.

C, Doppler tracing showing a decrease in the amplitude of the venous signals and loss of this response to respiratory variation.

This abnormal finding suggests a proximal (iliac vein) obstruction and impaired venous return. In this particular patient, an enlarged lymph node caused extrinsic compression of the iliac vein.

CONTRAST VENOGRAPHY

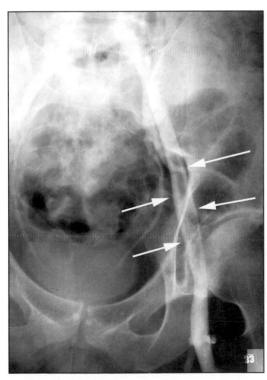

FIGURE 10-12. Left lower extremity contrast venogram showing a filling defect in the external iliac and common femoral veins (*arrows*), diagnostic of pelvic and proximal leg deep vein thrombosis. (*Courtesy of* Richard Baum, MD.)

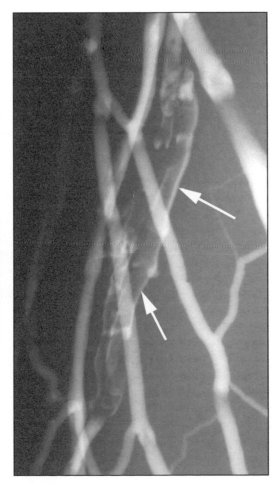

FIGURE 10-13. Left lower extremity contrast venogram showing extensive deep venous thrombosis in the popliteal vein (*arrows*). The image of extensive venous clot on venography resembles long stretches of railroad track. This finding has been called the "tram track" sign. (*Courtesy of* Richard Baum, MD.)

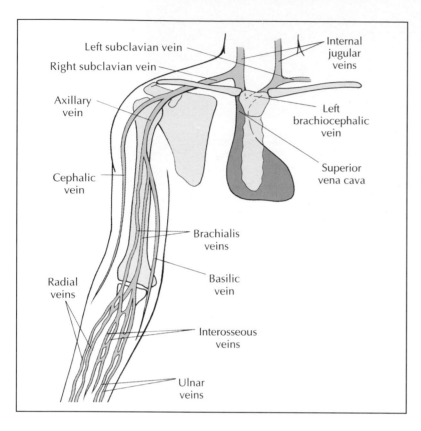

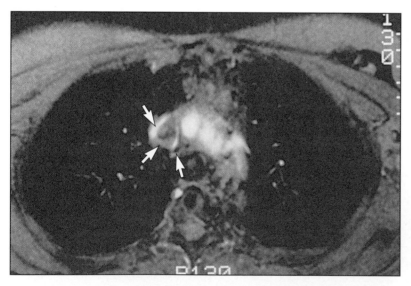

FIGURE 10-14. Venous anatomy of upper extremities. With more frequent use of pacemakers, internal cardiac defibrillators, and chronic indwelling central venous catheters for chemotherapy and hyperalimentation, upper extremity venous thrombosis is becoming more prevalent. The two major superficial veins to the arm are the cephalic and basilic veins. The cephalic vein is situated more laterally and joins the axillary vein at the distal one third of the clavicle. The proximal cephalic vein is often used as the site of insertion of chronic indwelling lines such as Hickman lines, Port-a-Cath catheters, and pacing wires. These can be the source of thrombi that extend into the axillary and subclavian vein. The basilic vein courses medially to become the axillary vein. This is a common location for superficial venous thrombosis, typically at the site of an intravenous line placement. The deep veins of the forearm and the brachial veins are duplicated. Duplications are less common at the level of the axillary vein and are absent at the level of the subclavian vein. The internal jugular veins drain the head and join the subclavian veins. They are often the sites of thrombi associated with central line placements.

The subclavian vein joins the internal jugular vein to become the brachiocephalic vein. On the right side, this venous segment is quite short. On the left, the brachiocephalic vein courses over a large distance behind the sternum. Its length may explain the higher prevalence of left-sided venous thrombi. Both brachiocephalic veins join to form the superior vena cava in the upper mediastinum. The superior vena cava can develop venous thrombi because of the presence of an indwelling catheter. Compression by mediastinal masses may also increase stasis in the superior vena cava and promote de novo thrombosis.

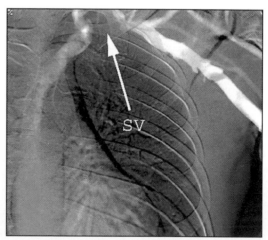

FIGURE 10-16. Left upper extremity contrast venography showing a subclavian vein (SV) thrombosis with large bridging collaterals. (*Courtesy of* Richard Baum, MD.)

FIGURE 10-15. Magnetic resonance venogram showing a typical filling defect in the superior vena cava: an extension of thrombus from the right brachiocephalic vein (*arrows*). The thrombus is located centrally and is surrounded by flow signals, which is typical of an acute venous thrombosis.

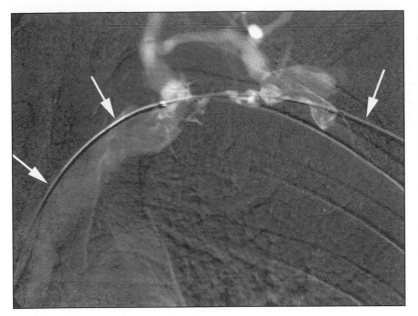

FIGURE 10-17. An infusion wire (*arrows*) placed across the thrombus. (*Courtesy of* Richard Baum, MD.)

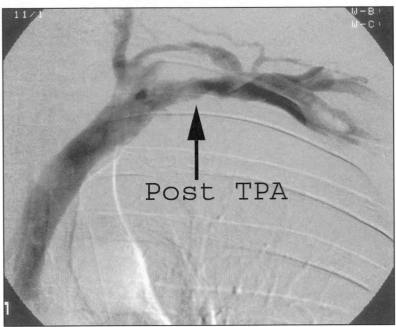

Post TPA

FIGURE 10-18. Catheter-directed administration of a thrombolytic. Flow resumed after therapy (post-TPA [tissue plasminogen activator]). (*Courtesy of* Richard Baum, MD.)

TREATMENT OF DEEP VEIN THROMBOSIS

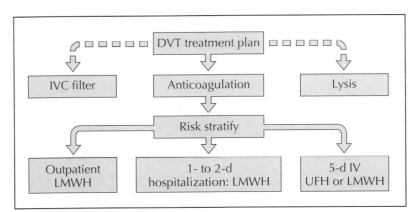

FIGURE 10-19. Anticoagulation. Anticoagulation is the foundation for deep vein thrombosis (DVT) treatment [2]. Patients with intractable hemorrhage or well-documented recurrent pulmonary embolism despite intensive anticoagulation should receive an inferior vena caval (IVC) filter. Patients with iliofemoral DVT or extensive upper extremity DVT may be candidates for catheter-directed thrombolytic therapy. Most patients will simply require anticoagulation with heparin as a "bridge" to oral anticoagulation. Low molecular weight heparin (LMWH) is rapidly replacing unfractionated heparin (UFH) for DVT treatment. In addition, the majority of patients with DVT can be treated as outpatients or with a brief (1- to 2-day) hospitalization. IV—intravenous.

ADVANTAGES OF LOW MOLECULAR WEIGHT HEPARIN VERSUS UNFRACTIONATED HEPARIN

EFFECT	CONSEQUENCE
Much less protein binding	More predictable dose response
Cleared primarily by renal mechanism	Longer plasma half-life
Much less binding to osteoblasts	Less osteopenia
Less binding to PF4	Lower risk of HIT

FIGURE 10-20. Low molecular weight heparin as replacement for unfractionated heparin (UFH) for the treatment of deep vein thrombosis (DVT) [3]. Low molecular weight heparin appears to be more effective than UFH in reducing the size of the venous thrombus and in preventing recurrent DVT [4].

Low molecular weight heparin is suitable for outpatient administration because it can usually be prescribed as a fixed dose with once or twice daily subcutaneous injection. No dose adjustment or blood testing is ordinarily required. The fixed dose is calculated according to the patient's weight. In contrast, continuous intravenous infusion of UFH is cumbersome because the dose necessitates frequent adjustments based on the activated partial thromboplastin time. Low molecular weight heparin also causes less incidence of osteopenia and heparin-induced thrombocytopenia (HIT) when compared with UFH. PF4—platelet factor 4.

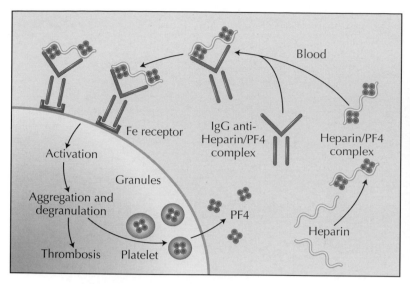

FIGURE 10-21. Pathogenesis of heparin-induced thrombocytopenia. This process involves formation of macromolecular complexes among heparin, platelet factor 4 (PF4), and antibodies generated against heparin/PF4. Platelets release PF4 when they are activated by agonists such as thrombin, collagen, and heparin. The immune complexes comprising heparin, PF4, and antiheparin:PF4 antibodies can interact with platelet receptors and lead to potent platelet activation, aggregation, and thrombin generation [5].

FIGURE 10-22. Diagnosis of heparin-induced thrombocytopenia (HIT). Diagnosis is tricky, because functional laboratory assays lack sensitivity, and quantitative enzyme-linked immunosorbent assays lack specificity. Therefore, clinical observation, analysis, and judgment are of paramount importance. Although the typical onset of HIT occurs 4 to 14 days after heparin exposure, HIT can begin much more rapidly in patients exposed within the previous 100 days [6]. Conversely, HIT can have a delayed onset and can even begin a week or longer after heparin has been discontinued [7]. Such patients may be rehospitalized with venous thromboembolism due to unrecognized HIT, be treated with heparin, and suffer further exacerbation of thrombocytopenia and thrombosis [8]. DVT—deep vein thrombosis.

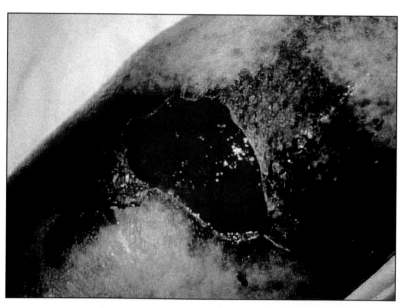

FIGURE 10-23. Gangrene of venules caused by heparin-induced thrombocytopenia.

FIGURE 10-24. Therapy for heparin-induced thrombocytopenia (HIT). Treatment of this illness is challenging because prescribing platelet transfusions or administering warfarin initially worsens the clinical state. Instead, for patients suffering thrombosis due to HIT, treatment is now available with two intravenously administered direct thrombin inhibitors (DTIs): argatroban and hirudin. Argatroban, metabolized by the liver, is especially useful for patients with renal insufficiency [9]. Hirudin, metabolized by the kidney, is especially useful for patients with hepatic failure [10].

FIGURE 10-25. Duration of anticoagulation. The optimal duration of anticoagulation is the most controversial daily management issue in treating patients with deep venous thrombosis (DVT) and pulmonary embolism (PE). Patients with thrombophilic-related or idiopathic venous thromboembolism are at higher risk of recurrence than patients who suffer DVT or PE in the context of surgery or trauma. The current consensus is to treat isolated calf DVT with at least 3 months of anticoagulation, and to treat proximal DVT or PE with at least 6 months of anticoagulation. Ongoing trials, such as PREVENT (Prospective Randomized Evaluation of the Vascular Effects of Norvasc Trial), may eventually provide a definitive answer to the crucial question of optimal duration of therapy.

PULMONARY EMBOLISM

DIAGNOSIS: LUNG SCANNING

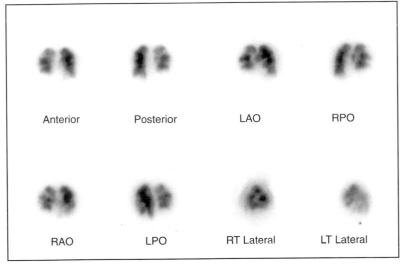

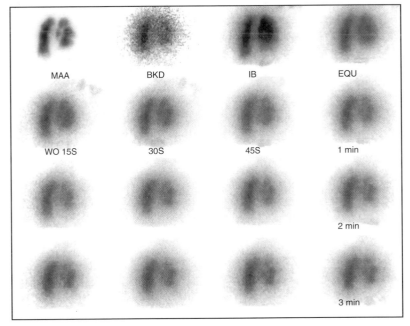

FIGURE 10-26. Perfusion lung scan of a 65-year-old woman who presented after 3 days of unexplained "gasping for breath" with any activity. She underwent a perfusion lung scan with 5.0 mCi of ^{99m}Tc macroaggregated albumin. The eight standard views were obtained: anterior, posterior, left anterior oblique (LAO), right posterior oblique (RPO), right anterior oblique (RAO), left posterior oblique (LPO), and right (RT) and left (LT) lateral. The perfusion scan was abnormal and showed multiple peripheral perfusion defects in both lungs. In the presence of a normal chest radiograph, this perfusion scan shows high probability for acute pulmonary embolism.

FIGURE 10-27. Ventilation lung scan of patient in Figure 10-26. The scan taken in the right posterior oblique (RPO) position demonstrates a "mismatch" between abnormal perfusion and normal ventilation of the right lung. This ventilation-perfusion mismatch indicates a high probability for acute pulmonary embolism.

The *upper left-hand image* is the perfusion scan in the RPO position. All of the other images are ventilation scans in the RPO position. The ventilation is normal. The contrast between the abnormal perfusion scan and the normal ventilation scan is best seen by comparing the perfusion scan in the uppermost left image with the ventilation scan seen in the image to its right.

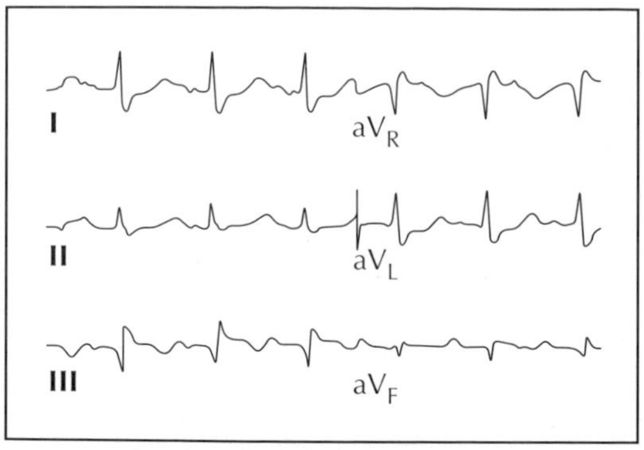

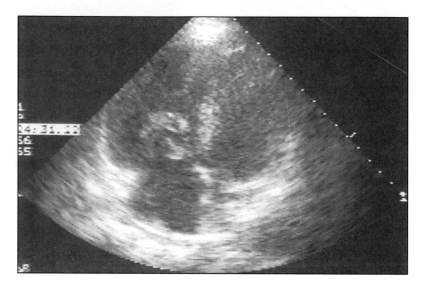

FIGURE 10-28. Electrocardiogram of a 64-year-old woman who was hospitalized with "atypical chest pain." Her electrocardiogram shows sinus tachycardia, incomplete right bundle branch block, and an S1Q3TIII pattern with an S wave in lead I, Q wave in lead III, and inverted T wave in lead III—findings indicative of right ventricular strain. These findings suggest pulmonary hypertension due to massive pulmonary embolism [11].

DIAGNOSIS: ECHOCARDIOGRAPHY

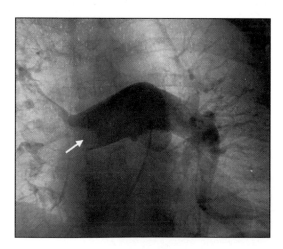

FIGURE 10-29. Echocardiogram of patient in Figure 10-28. In the apical four-chamber view, the right ventricle is abnormally dilated. This is apparent because the right ventricle is larger than the left ventricle, whereas normally the right ventricle should be smaller than (*ie*, no more than 0.6 times the size of) the left ventricle.

A 3 × 4 cm round mass is observed in the right ventricle, just below the tricuspid valve. This mass turned out to be a giant, curled-up venous thrombus, which embolized to the pulmonary arteries and caused massive acute pulmonary embolism.

DIAGNOSIS: PULMONARY ANGIOGRAPHY

FIGURE 10-30. Contrast pulmonary angiogram of patient in Figures 10-28 and 10-29. A massive bilateral saddle embolism is present. The *white arrow* indicates the thrombus in the right main pulmonary artery.

DIAGNOSIS: DIRECT SURGICAL EXTRACTION

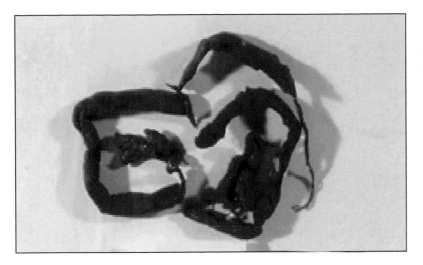

FIGURE 10-31. Acute massive pulmonary embolism. The patient shown in Figures 10-28 to 10-30 was referred for emergency open surgical pulmonary embolectomy. The surgical specimen, demonstrating acute massive pulmonary embolism, is shown here. She had an uncomplicated postoperative course.

DIAGNOSIS: CHEST CT

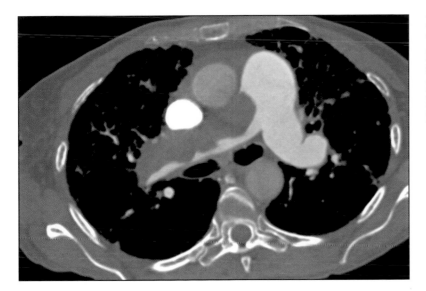

FIGURE 10-32. Computed tomography (CT) scan of a 59-year-old woman with advanced sarcoidosis who underwent evaluation for possible lung transplantation. The CT scan with contrast demonstrated a previously unsuspected large defect filling the right pulmonary artery. The thrombus extends from the right main pulmonary artery into the right upper and right lower lobe pulmonary arteries.

DIAGNOSIS: AUTOPSY

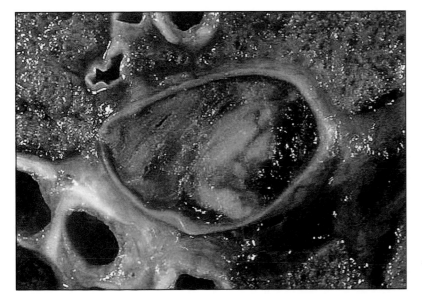

FIGURE 10-33. Thrombus. The patient shown in Figure 10-32 suffered a cardiac arrest and died 3 days later despite maximal resuscitative efforts. At autopsy, the right main pulmonary artery, seen in cross-section, was filled with thrombus of varying ages.

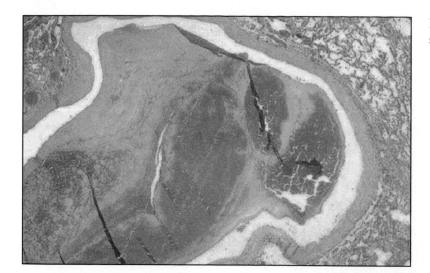

FIGURE 10-34. Microscopy of a right segmental pulmonary artery showing red fibrin clot filling most of the vessel.

MANAGEMENT OF PULMONARY EMBOLISM

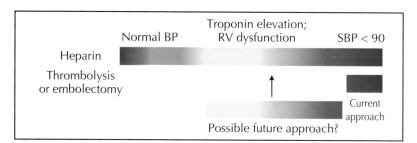

FIGURE 10-35. Acute pulmonary embolism (PE). The majority of patients will recover with anticoagulation alone. However, a surprisingly large minority of patients have adverse prognostic

indicators for a complicated hospital course. A clinical risk scoring system to predict adverse events [12] gives one point each for heart failure, prior deep vein thrombosis (DVT), hypoxemia, or current DVT on ultrasound, and two points each for systemic arterial hypotension and cancer. For those with a total of at least four points, 27% had adverse outcomes. Among those with five points, 57% had adverse outcomes.

Troponin elevation has emerged as an independent prognostic marker of adverse clinical outcome [13] and right ventricular dysfunction [14]. Right ventricular (RV) dysfunction on echocardiogram is an independent risk factor for an adverse outcome such as death or recurrent PE [15]. BP—blood pressure; SBP—systolic blood pressure.

THROMBOLYSIS VERSUS EMBOLECTOMY

WHEN TO CONSIDER THROMBOLYSIS AND/OR EMBOLECTOMY (RISK STRATIFICATION)

Hemodynamic instability
Echocardiogram: right ventricular dysfunction
Elevated troponin
Anatomically extensive clot

FIGURE 10-36. When to consider thrombolysis or embolectomy. One of the most controversial issues within the field of pulmonary embolism management is when to proceed with thrombolysis or embolectomy despite normal systemic arterial pressure [16,17].

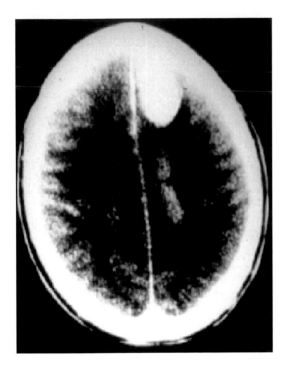

FIGURE 10-37. Computed tomography scan of large front intracranial hemorrhage. The biggest disadvantage of thrombolysis is the potential for intracranial hemorrhage. About half of the intracranial hemorrhages are fatal. Among those who survive this complication, about half have major permanent neurologic deficits. In the International Cooperative Pulmonary Embolism Registry, 3.0% of patients who received thrombolytic therapy developed intracranial bleeding [18]. In a smaller French registry, 4.7% suffered intracranial hemorrhage [19].

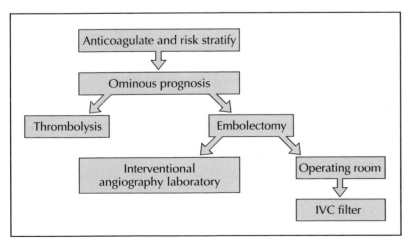

FIGURE 10-38. Risk stratification. The optimal management of acute pulmonary embolism hinges on successful and timely risk stratification. The clinician must initiate prompt and intensive anticoagulation and then use clinical, laboratory, and imaging information to prognosticate whether anticoagulation alone will suffice for a successful outcome. Patients with an ominous prognosis [20] require consideration for thrombolysis [21] or embolectomy. IVC—inferior vena caval.

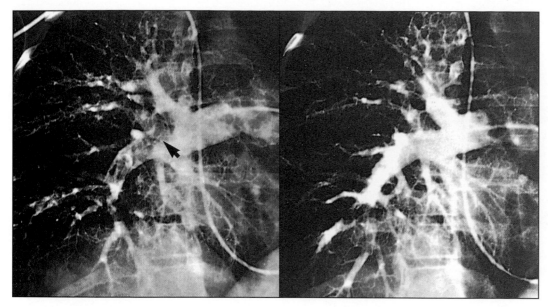

pulmonary artery thromboembolism. Immediately after thrombolysis, a follow-up contrast pulmonary angiogram (*right panel*) shows marked clot lysis.

Thrombolysis can be immediately life-saving by rapidly reversing right heart failure, the usual cause of death from acute PE. In addition, thrombolysis may preserve the normal hemodynamic response to exercise over the long term and may prevent recurrence of venous thromboembolism and the development of chronic pulmonary hypertension [22].

There is a broadly shared consensus that administration of thrombolysis is indicated for patients with massive PE. However, debate rages about the indication for thrombolysis in PE patients with preserved systemic arterial pressure [23]. A large-scale clinical trial to address this controversy is overdue [24].

FIGURE 10-39. Peripheral intravenous administration of thrombolytic therapy (in this case, tissue plasminogen activator administered as a continuous infusion over 2 hours) to lyse pulmonary embolism (PE). In the *left panel*, at baseline, there is a massive right

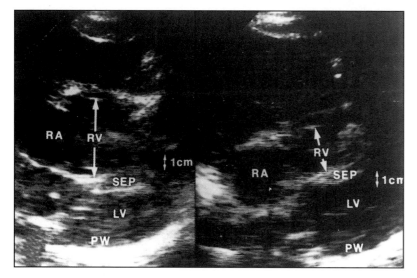

FIGURE 10-40. Successful thrombolysis to reverse right heart failure, including right ventricular hypokinesis, right ventricular dilatation, and tricuspid regurgitation. The *left panel* is a subcostal image in a patient who presented with congestive heart failure and who was diagnosed with acute pulmonary embolism (PE) after this echocardiogram—suspicious for PE rather than left-heart failure—led to further work-up, including contrast pulmonary angiography. The right ventricle (RV) is markedly enlarged, and the diameter of the left ventricle (LV) is reduced. After receiving 2 hours of peripherally administered intravenous tissue plasminogen activator, a remarkable decrease in RV size and corresponding increase in LV size are apparent (*right panel*). PW—posterior wall; RA—right atrium; SEP—interventricular septum.

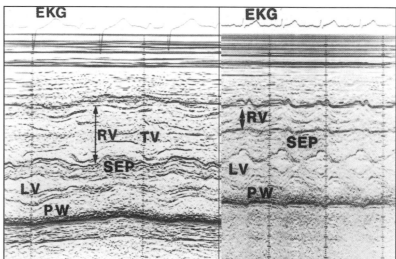

FIGURE 10-41. M-mode echocardiographic recordings of the right ventricle (RV) and left ventricle (LV) from a subcostal transducer position in the patient in Figure 10-39. Before thrombolysis (*left panel*), the RV was markedly enlarged and the LV chamber size was reduced. The interventricular septum (SEP) moved paradoxically. The RV wall motion was markedly hypokinetic. After thrombolysis (*right panel*), the RV became much smaller and the LV became larger. Paradoxical motion of the interventricular septum was no longer present, and right ventricular wall motion normalized. PW—posterior wall; TV—tricuspid valve.

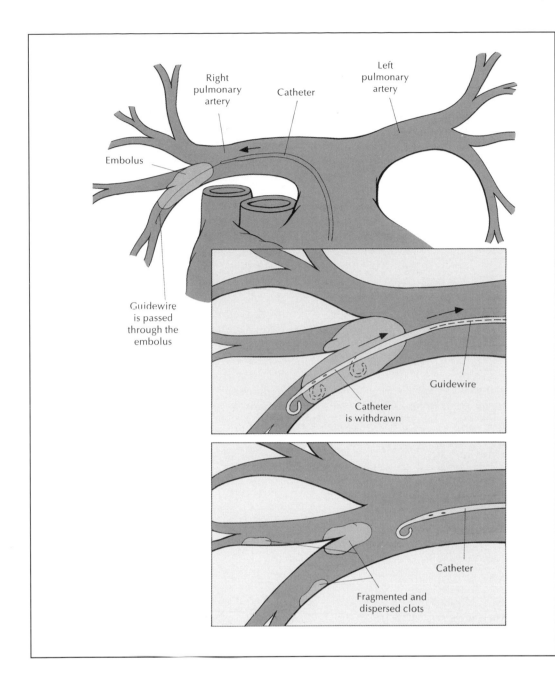

FIGURE 10-42. Catheter embolectomy. Embolectomy can be accomplished with angiographic catheters in the interventional radiology or cardiac catheterization laboratories [25]. A standard angiographic catheter, mounted on a J wire, is advanced to the pulmonary trunk. The thrombus is first pushed forward by advancing the catheter. The guidewire is then passed through the embolus, and the catheter is advanced over the guidewire. The guidewire is withdrawn, thereby allowing the catheter's tip to assume its normal shape (*inset, upper panel*). The catheter is then withdrawn, resulting in fragmentation and dispersion of the thrombus (*inset, lower panel*).

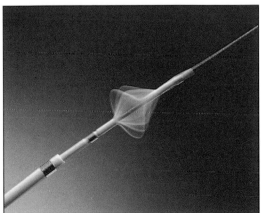

FIGURE 10-43. Mechanical thrombectomy. Special devices have been developed for catheter-based embolectomy. This 5F catheter's distal tip permits high-speed rotation at about 100,000 revolutions per minute. Centrifugal force opens the distal apparatus on the catheter, which forms a helical spiral that pulverizes the thrombus into microscopic particles within a few seconds [26]. Another approach combines mechanical thrombectomy with catheter-directed thrombolytic therapy [27].

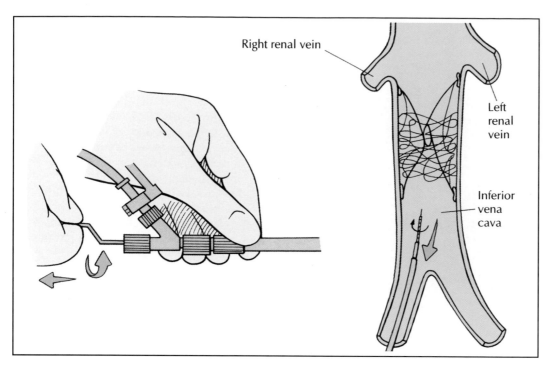

hemorrhage, such as gastrointestinal bleeding that requires multiple blood transfusions or any intracranial bleeding, or recurrent pulmonary embolism despite intensive anticoagulation and laboratory documentation that high-range anticoagulation has been achieved.

Note that the inferior vena caval filter does nothing to halt the thrombotic process. Filters are now being placed more judiciously because a randomized trial [28] and two registries [29,30] have shown that the rate of deep vein thrombosis doubles after filter placement. The filter must serve as a nidus for future thrombus formation.

The Bird's Nest filter (Cook Inc., Bloomington, IN) has low rates of failure, thrombogenicity, and occlusion. The right-angled handle of the wire guide pusher is rotated counterclockwise for 10 to 15 turns to disengage the filter. Then the wire guide pusher is removed, followed by the empty filter catheter. The introducing sheath is temporarily left in place so that a post-procedure cavogram can be obtained.

FIGURE 10-44. Insertion of an inferior vena caval filter. Most inferior vena caval filters are placed percutaneously via the right femoral vein. The two major indications are active major

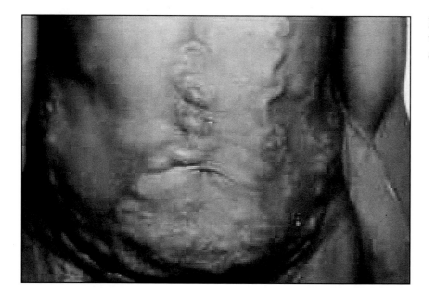

FIGURE 10-45. Abdominal venous collaterals. An occluded inferior vena cava can cause marked bilateral leg swelling (not shown) and massive abdominal wall venous collaterals.

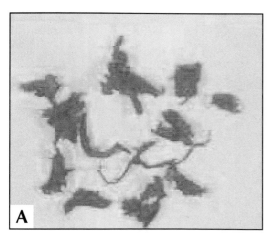

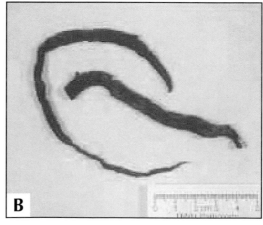

ovale. She underwent emergency surgery that included acute pulmonary embolectomy (**A**), closure of the patent foramen ovale, and removal of the venous thromboembolus that had lodged in the descending thoracic aorta and left subclavian artery (**B**).

Our Venous Thromboembolism Research Group reported on a series of 29 patients who underwent acute pulmonary embolectomy with a contemporary approach that emphasized rapid diagnosis, accurate risk stratification and triage, and improved surgical technique [31]. The 30-day survival rate was 89%. We believe that acute pulmonary embolectomy should no longer be confined to a treatment of last resort reserved for clinically desperate circumstances. Instead, this approach should be used for high-risk patients in whom thrombolysis is contraindicated.

FIGURE 10-46. Paradoxical embolism. This 34-year-old woman presented with marked shortness of breath and left arm discomfort. Computed tomographic scanning indicated both a massive pulmonary embolism as well as a thrombus extending from her left subclavian artery to her descending thoracic aorta. She had suffered a paradoxical embolism with thrombus traveling from her leg veins to both her pulmonary arteries and to her systemic circulation via a patent foramen

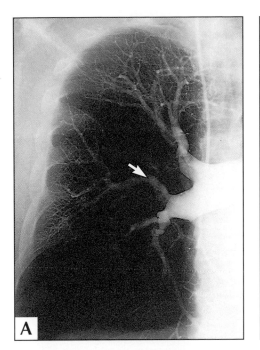

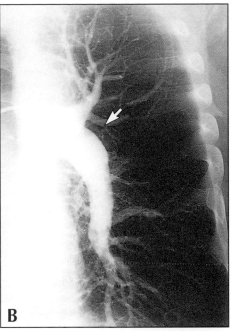

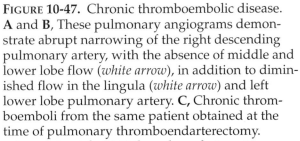

FIGURE 10-47. Chronic thromboembolic disease. **A** and **B**, These pulmonary angiograms demonstrate abrupt narrowing of the right descending pulmonary artery, with the absence of middle and lower lobe flow (*white arrow*), in addition to diminished flow in the lingula (*white arrow*) and left lower lobe pulmonary artery. **C,** Chronic thromboemboli from the same patient obtained at the time of pulmonary thromboendarterectomy.

Approximately 2000 thromboendarterectomy procedures have been performed worldwide, with about 1400 undertaken at the University of California at San Diego Medical Center [32]. The location and extent of the proximal thromboembolic obstruction are the most critical determinants of operability. Occluding thrombi must involve the main, lobar, or proximal segmental arteries. Those that originate more distally are not amenable to surgery [32]. However, such lesions may be managed with balloon pulmonary angioplasty [33].

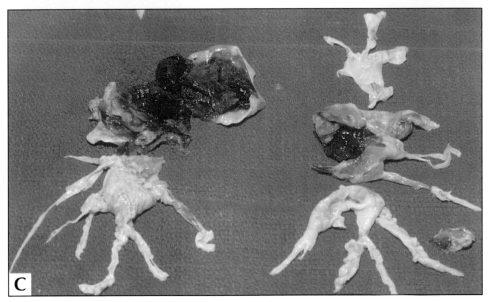

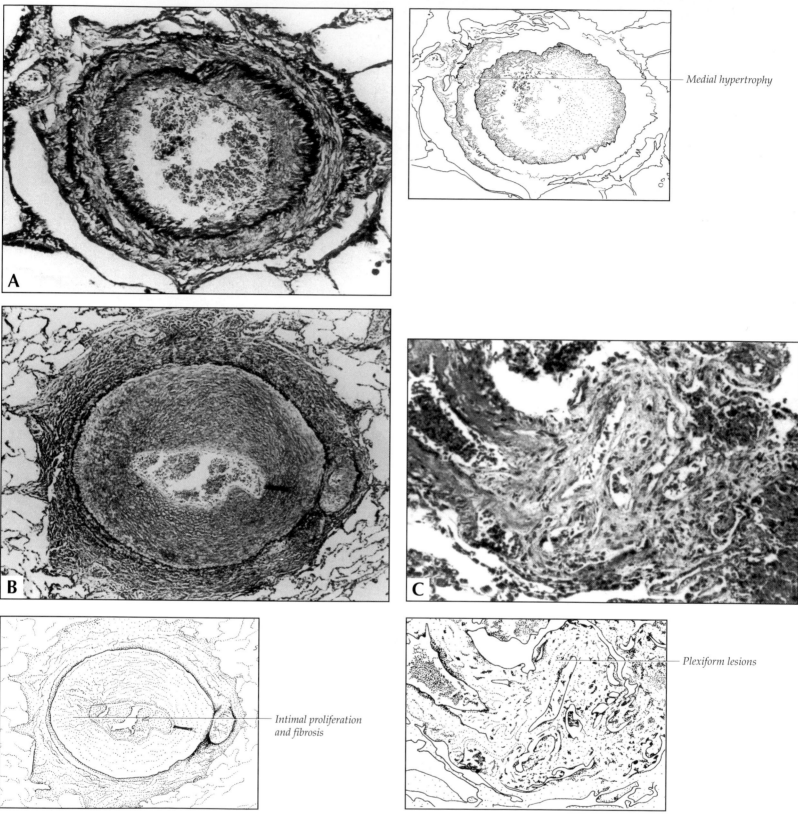

FIGURE 10-48. Primary pulmonary hypertension. Primary pulmonary hypertension is defined clinically as a mean pulmonary arterial pressure of more than 25 mm Hg at rest or 30 mm Hg during exercise, when all known causes of pulmonary hypertension have been excluded [34]. The mean age at diagnosis is during the fourth decade of life. Vascular pathologic features include medial hypertrophy (**A**) and intimal proliferation and thrombosis (**B**). The most common pathologic patterns are plexogenic arteriopathy (**C**) and thrombotic arteriopathy (**D, E**).

Continued on next page

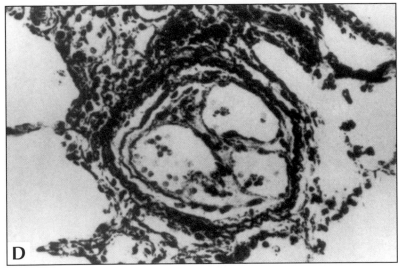

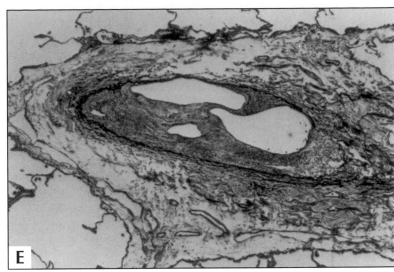

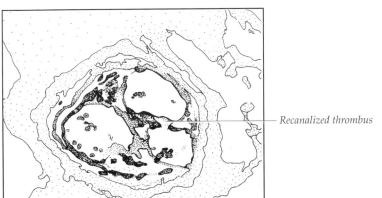

Recanalized thrombus

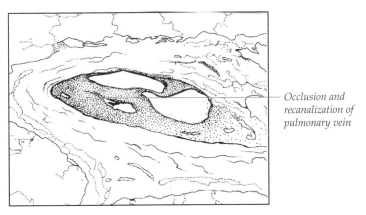

Occlusion and
recanalization of
pulmonary vein

FIGURE 10-48. *(Continued)*

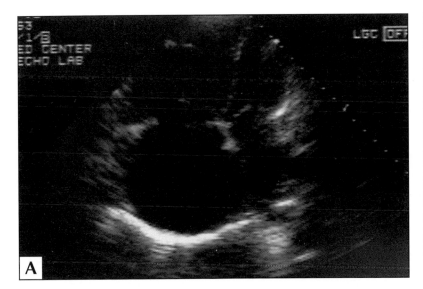

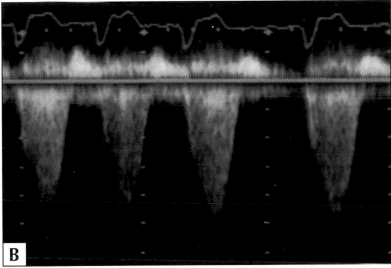

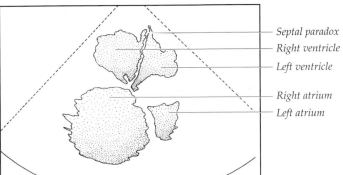

Septal paradox
Right ventricle
Left ventricle

Right atrium
Left atrium

FIGURE 10-49. Echocardiogram in a patient with primary pulmonary hypertension (PPH) demonstrating an enlarged right atrium and right ventricle, and a reduced size of the left ventricle (**A**). **B**, Doppler ultrasound of the tricuspid regurgitant jet is 4.7 m/s, yielding an estimated pulmonary artery systolic pressure of at least 90 mm Hg. Echocardiographic predictors of adverse outcomes in PPH include pericardial effusion, right atrial enlargement, and interventricular septal displacement toward the left ventricle [35].

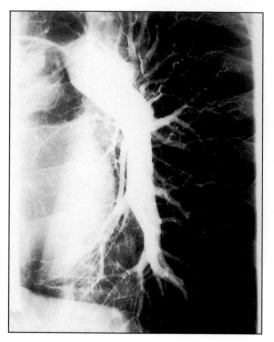

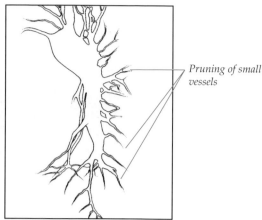

Pruning of small vessels

FIGURE 10-50. Contrast pulmonary angiography in primary pulmonary hypertension (PPH) demonstrating marked "pruning" of small vessels with absent peripheral flow. No segmental or larger vascular abnormalities are noted.

Continuous intravenous infusion of epoprostenol (prostacyclin) is the most effective treatment available for the management of PPH. New therapies include the recently Food and Drug Administration–approved oral antagonist of endothelin receptors, bosentan [36]. Investigational therapies include an aerosolized prostacyclin analogue [37], iloprost, as well as inhaled nitric oxide [38] and combined therapy with aerosolized iloprost plus oral sildenafil [39].

TREATMENT OF PRIMARY PULMONARY HYPERTENSION

Anticoagulation

Round-the-clock oxygen, if necessary

Calcium channel blockers (effective in 10% to 20% of patients)

Continuous intravenous prostacyclin (improves survival and may heal endothelium)

Inhaled prostacyclin or nitric oxide (both investigational)

Oral sildenafil (investigational)

Oral bosentan

FIGURE 10-51. Treatment of primary pulmonary hypertension (PPH). Until recently, the median survival after diagnosis of PPH

was less than 3 years. Since the 1990s, the treatment of this previously rapidly fatal condition has improved to the point where many patients can resume normal or near-normal lives without fear of impending death. Anticoagulation is standard therapy for PPH, and good oxygenation must be maintained, with round-the-clock supplemental oxygen if necessary.

Treatment success is now defined as restoration of normal pulmonary artery pressures. Calcium channel blocking agents may be effective in 10% to 20% of patients. Continuous intravenous prostacyclin, which requires a chronically indwelling central venous catheter, has provided benefit of revolutionary proportions. This therapy may "heal" the endothelium and definitely improves overall survival. Inhaled prostacyclin or nitric oxide are investigational, but the oral agent, bosentan, an analogue of prostacyclin, was recently approved by the Food and Drug Administration. Another investigational agent, sildenafil (used to treat erectile dysfunction), holds promise as oral therapy for PPH.

REFERENCES

1. Joffe HV, Goldhaber SZ: Laboratory thrombophilias and venous thromboembolism. *Vasc Med*, In press.

2. Gelfand EV, Piazza G, Goldhaber SZ: Venous thromboembolism guidebook. *Critical Pathways in Cardiology* 2002, 1:26–43.

3. Hyers TM, Agnelli G, Hull RD, *et al.*: Antithrombotic therapy for venous thromboembolic disease. *Chest* 2001, 119:176S–206S.

4. Breddin HK, Hach-Wunderle V, Nakov R, Kakkar VV: Effects of a low-molecular-weight heparin on thrombus regression and recurrent thromboembolism in patients with deep-vein thrombosis. *N Engl J Med* 2001, 344:626–631.

5 Deitcher SR, Carman TL: Heparin-induced thrombocytopenia: natural history, diagnosis, and management. *Vasc Med* 2001, 6:113–119.

6. Warkentin TE, Kelton JG: Temporal aspects of heparin-induced thrombocytopenia. *N Engl J Med* 2001, 344:1286–1292.

7. Warkentin TE, Kelton JG: Delayed-onset heparin-induced thrombocytopenia and thrombosis. *Ann Intern Med* 2001, 135:502–506.

8. Rice L, Attisha WK, Drexler A, Francis JL: Delayed-onset heparin-induced thrombocytopenia. *Ann Intern Med* 2002, 136:210–215.

9. Lewis BE, Wallis DE, Berkowitz SD, *et al.*: Argatroban anticoagulant therapy in patients with heparin-induced thrombocytopenia. *Circulation* 2001, 103:1838–1843.

10. Greinacher A, Volpel H, Janssens U, *et al.*: Recombinant hirudin (lepirudin) provides safe and effective anticoagulation in patients with heparin-induced thrombocytopenia: a prospective study. *Circulation* 1999, 99:73–80.

11. Daniel KR, Courtney DM, Kline JA: Assessment of cardiac stress from massive pulmonary embolism with 12-lead ECG. *Chest* 2001, 120:474–481.

12. Wicki J, Perrier A, Perneger TV, *et al.*: Predicting adverse outcome in patients with acute pulmonary embolism: a risk score. *Thromb Haemost* 2000, 84:548–552.

13. Meyer T, Binder L, Hruska N, *et al.*: Cardiac troponin I elevation in acute pulmonary embolism is associated with right ventricular dysfunction. *J Am Coll Cardiol* 2000, 36:1632–1636.

14. Giannitsis E, Muller-Bardorff M, Kurowski V, *et al.*: Independent prognostic value of cardiac troponin T in patients with confirmed pulmonary embolism. *Circulation* 2000, 102:211–217.

15. Goldhaber SZ: Echocardiography in the management of pulmonary embolism. *Ann Intern Med* 2002, 136:691–700.

16. Arcasoy SM, Kreit JW: Thrombolytic therapy of pulmonary embolism: a comprehensive review of current evidence. *Chest* 1999, 115:1695–1707.

17. Wood KE: Major pulmonary embolism: review of a pathophysiologic approach to the golden hour of hemodynamically significant pulmonary embolism. *Chest* 2002, 121:877–905.

18. Goldhaber SZ, Visani L, De Rosa M: Acute pulmonary embolism: clinical outcomes in the International Cooperative Pulmonary Embolism Registry (ICOPER). *Lancet* 1999, 353:1386–1389.

19. Hamel E, Pacouret G, Vincentelli D, *et al.*: Thrombolysis or heparin therapy in massive pulmonary embolism with right ventricular dilation: results from a 128-patient monocenter registry. *Chest* 2001, 120:120–125.

20. Feldman JP, Goldhaber SZ: The management of massive pulmonary embolism. In *Thrombosis and Thromboembolism*. Edited by Goldhaber SZ, Ridker PM. New York: Marcel Dekker; 2002:235–245.

21. Goldhaber SZ: Thrombolysis in pulmonary embolism. In *Thrombosis and Thromboembolism*. Edited by Goldhaber SZ, Ridker PM. New York: Marcel Dekker; 2002:247–259.

22. Sharma GV, Folland ED, McIntyre KM, Sasahara AA: Long-term benefit of thrombolytic therapy in patients with pulmonary embolism. *Vasc Med* 2000, 5:91–95.

23. Goldhaber SZ: Thrombolysis in pulmonary embolism: a debatable indication. *Thromb Haemost* 2001, 86:444–451.

24. Goldhaber SZ: Thrombolysis in pulmonary embolism: a large-scale clinical trial is overdue. *Circulation* 2001, 104:2876–2878.

25. Goldhaber SZ: Integration of catheter thrombectomy into our armamentarium to treat acute pulmonary embolism. *Chest* 1998, 114:1237–1238.

26. Fava M, Loyola S, Huete I: Massive pulmonary embolism: treatment with the hydrolyser thrombectomy catheter. *J Vasc Interv Radiol* 2000, 11:1159–1164.

27. De Gregorio MA, Gimeno MJ, Mainar A, *et al.*: Mechanical and enzymatic thrombolysis for massive pulmonary embolism. *J Vasc Interv Radiol* 2002, 13:163–169.

28. Decousus H, Leizorovicz A, Parent F, *et al.*: A clinical trial of vena caval filters in the prevention of pulmonary embolism in patients with proximal deep-vein thrombosis: prevention du Risque d'Embolie Pulmonaire par Interruption Cave Study Group. *N Engl J Med* 1998, 338:409–415.

29. Athanasoulis CA, Kaufman JA, Halpern EF, *et al.*: Inferior vena caval filters: review of a 26-year single-center clinical experience. *Radiology* 2000, 216:54–66.

30. White RH, Zhou H, Kim J, Romano PS: A population-based study of the effectiveness of inferior vena cava filter use among patients with venous thromboembolism. *Arch Intern Med* 2000, 160:2033–2041.

31. Aklog L, Williams CS, Byrne JG, Goldhaber SZ: Acute pulmonary embolectomy: a contemporary approach. *Circulation* 2002, 105:1416–1419.

32. Fedullo PF, Auger WR, Kerr KM, Rubin LJ: Chronic thromboembolic pulmonary hypertension. *N Engl J Med* 2001, 345:1465–1472.

33. Feinstein JA, Goldhaber SZ, Lock JE, *et al.*: Balloon pulmonary angioplasty for treatment of chronic thromboembolic pulmonary hypertension. *Circulation* 2001, 103:10–13.

34. Gaine SP, Rubin LJ: Primary pulmonary hypertension. *Lancet* 1998, 352:719–725.

35. Raymond RJ, Hinderliter AL, Willis PW, *et al.*: Echocardiographic predictors of adverse outcomes in primary pulmonary hypertension. *J Am Coll Cardiol* 2002, 39:1214–1219.

36. Rubin LJ, Badesch DB, Barst RJ, *et al.*: Bosentan therapy for pulmonary arterial hypertension. *N Engl J Med* 2002, 346:896–903.

37. Hoeper MM, Schwarze M, Ehlerding S, *et al.*: Long-term treatment of primary pulmonary hypertension with aerosolized iloprost, a prostacyclin analogue. *N Engl J Med* 2000, 342:1866–1870.

38. Rimensberger PC, Spahr-Schopfer I, Berner M, *et al.*: Inhaled nitric oxide versus aerosolized iloprost in secondary pulmonary hypertension in children with congenital heart disease: vasodilator capacity and cellular mechanisms. *Circulation* 2001, 103:544–548.

39. Ghofrani HA, Wiedemann R, Rose F, *et al.*: Combination therapy with oral sildenafil and inhaled iloprost for severe pulmonary hypertension. *Ann Intern Med* 2002, 136:515–522.

CHRONIC VENOUS INSUFFICIENCY

CHAPTER 11

Andrew W. Bradbury and C. Vaughan Ruckley

The causes of chronic venous insufficiency (CVI) are those diseases that impair function of venous valves or obstruct the venous channels of the limb. Primary valvular insufficiency is believed to result from a congenital or acquired connective tissue disorder in the vein wall. Secondary insufficiency results from direct valve impairment, and follows either venous thrombosis or trauma. Aggravating factors are those that increase the venous backload or interfere with the mechanical function of the muscular pumps of the legs. These include obesity, locomotor disorders, arthropathies, neurologic disorders, pregnancy, cardiac failure, tricuspid incompetence, standing occupations, and senility. Other diseases commonly found in patients with chronic leg ulceration, which may play a role in compounding the diagnosis, impairing healing, or complicating therapy, include arterial insufficiency, rheumatoid disease, hematologic disorders, diabetes, and the vasculitides. Approximately one third of patients with CVI have a history of deep vein thrombosis, in which case it is termed *post-thrombotic syndrome*. Swelling is usually more marked than in nonthrombotic CVI and there is sometimes enough outflow obstruction for the patient to experience venous claudication. More often, however, the crucial finding in the post-thrombotic syndrome is the same as in nonthrombotic CVI, *ie*, valve reflux.

A thorough patient history is essential, with particular attention given to etiologic factors, aggravating factors, and associated diseases. In assessing primary varicose veins, simple physical examination may suffice, but additional investigation is required in patients with CVI, beginning with Doppler measurement of arterial ankle-brachial pressure ratios and color-coded ultrasound imaging of potential sites of reflux. Assessment in the vascular laboratory is classified into tests of function, such as ambulatory venous pressure and the various forms of plethysmography, or imaging, by means of the color-coded duplex scanner. Phlebography is not required unless there is doubt as to the patency of deep veins or if valvular reconstruction is being contemplated.

CEAP CLINICAL CLASSIFICATION

CLASS	CLINICAL SIGNS
0	No visible or palpable signs of venous disease
1	Telangiectasis or reticular veins
2	Varicose veins
3	Edema
4	Skin changes ascribed to venous disease (*eg*, pigmentation, venous eczema, lipodermatosclerosis)
5	Skin changes as defined above with healed ulceration
6	Skin changes as defined above with active ulceration

FIGURE 11-1. CEAP (Clinical signs, *e*tiology, *a*natomy, *p*athophysiology) clinical classification. This is the newest method for classification of chronic venous disease [1]. Patients with chronic venous insufficiency (CVI) are grouped as CEAP 4 to 6. The majority of patients with ulcerated CVI (CEAP 6) are treated conservatively initially by simple physical measures, *ie*, graduated compression therapy, high elevation of the leg at rest, and weight control. Most ulcers can be healed by ambulatory regimens. Surgery should be considered if there are no clear signs of healing after 3 months, because chronic ulcers respond poorly to compression therapy.

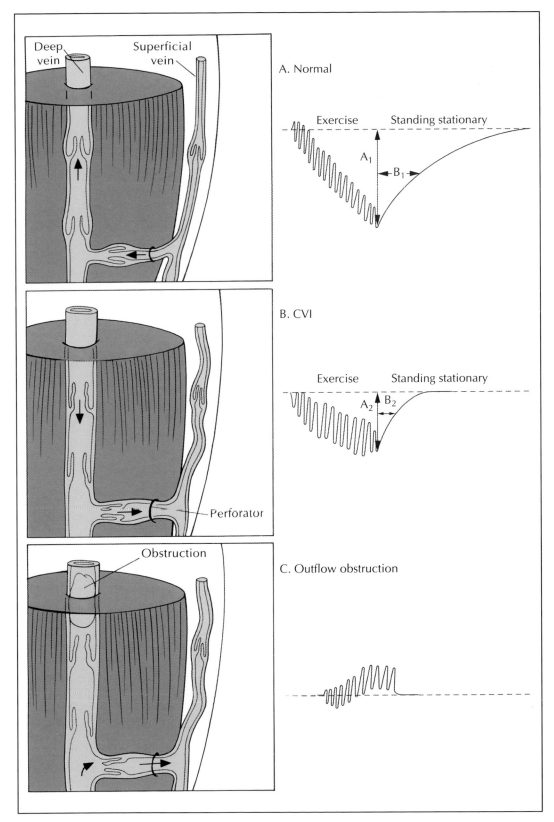

A. Normal

Exercise   Standing stationary

A_1 B_1

B. CVI

Exercise   Standing stationary

A_2 B_2

C. Outflow obstruction

FIGURE 11-2. Pathologic changes in the skin and subcutaneous tissues caused by ambulatory venous hypertension, *ie*, high pressure not only when standing stationary or sitting, which is normal, but also when walking, when the pressure should drop.

A, The normal centripetal direction of venous flow in a perforating vein and the corresponding pressure tracing as obtained following puncture of a foot vein. During exercise the pressure falls (A_1) as a result of the action of the calf muscle pump in the presence of competent valves. Thus, the fall in pressure is a measure of calf pump performance. When standing stationary, the pressure returns to its high baseline level. The slope of the refilling curve and the half refilling time (B_1), the venous valves being competent, reflect venous filling by arterial inflow.

B, In chronic venous insufficiency (CVI), there is outward perforator flow during calf pump contraction and inward flow on relaxation, with little or no fall in pressure (A_2), *ie*, defective pump function. When exercise stops there is an immediate return to high baseline pressure caused by reflux through incompetent superficial or deep valves. Thus, the slope of the curve and the refilling time (B_2) are a measure of the severity of venous insufficiency. **C,** When outflow is obstructed, the pressure does not fall with calf muscle contraction; it may even rise, as is shown in the tracing, which leads to the symptom of venous claudication.

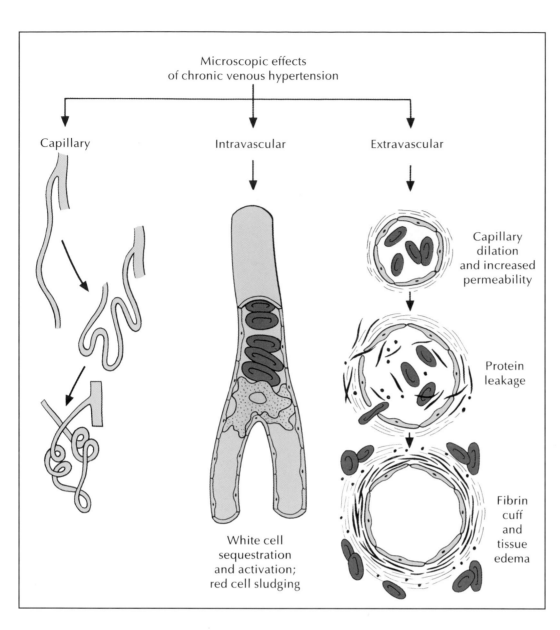

FIGURE 11-3. Microscopic effects of chronic venous hypertension. Sustained hypertension impacts at the venous end of the capillary bed, upsetting the balance between hemodynamic and osmotic pressures (Starling forces). Increased capillary permeability results in the leaking out of proteins, white cells, and red cells, resulting in fibrin pericapillary cuffing, inflammatory infiltration, tissue edema, and pigmentation (hemosiderin) [2]. There is increased capillary tortuosity or "tufting." Sequestration of white cells has been shown to occur in association with chronic venous insufficiency, especially in the dependent limb [3]. Activation of these cells may play an important part in the severe chronic inflammatory change, tissue damage, and scarring that characterize the condition [4]. Observation of these events at the microvascular level has led to a search, with limited success as yet, for pharmacologic agents that may favorably influence chronic venous insufficiency.

CLINICAL PRESENTATION

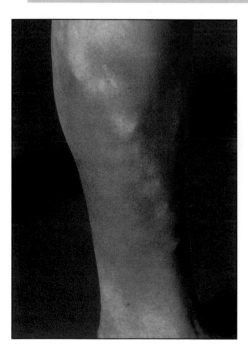

FIGURE 11-4. Pigmentation. As with all of the skin changes involved in chronic venous insufficiency, pigmentation is usually maximal on the postero-medial aspect of the calf, where incompetent perforators connect to the long saphenous vein, specifically the posterior arch vein. When there is short saphenous incompetence, the skin changes are maximal on the posterolateral aspect of the lower calf.

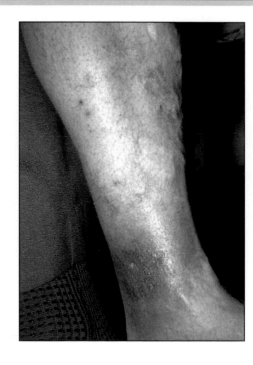

FIGURE 11-5. Lipodermatosclerosis. Acute lipodermatosclerosis should be distinguished from other common causes of acute inflammation in chronic venous insufficiency, such as phlebitis and bacterial cellulitis. Lipodermatosclerosis relates to sites of perforator incompetence. Superficial phlebitis follows the course of a varicose vein. Cellulitis is more diffuse and usually relates to an infected open ulcer or the ingress of infection through a break in the skin of the foot, such as athlete's foot.

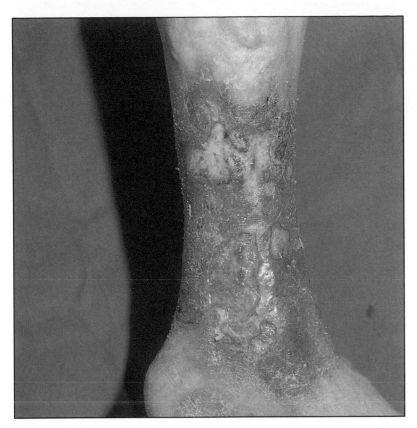

FIGURE 11-6. Ulcers. Ulcers of venous origin are usually single and surrounded, as in this case, by the stigmata of chronic venous insufficiency: pigmentation, subcutaneous edema (induration), and varicose eczema. Because of the numerous medications commonly applied to the skin over the long term of chronic ulcer disease, varicose excema must be differentiated (by careful observation of the distribution and by skin sensitivity tests) from contact dermatitis, to which these patients are especially prone.

ASSESSMENT

PHYSICAL EXAMINATION

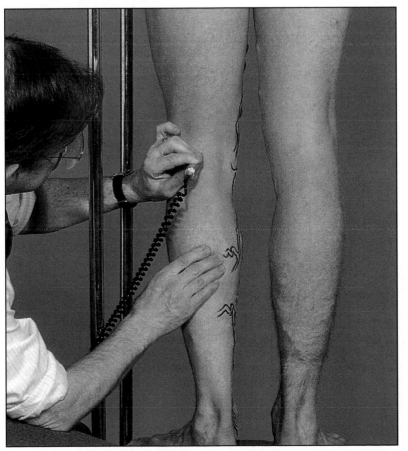

FIGURE 11-7. Physical examination. During the physical examination, aggravating factors including obesity, locomotor problems (especially arthropathies), and skin disorders must be noted. For lower-limb venous assessment the patient is examined while standing on a warm elevated surface, so that the examiner can sit comfortably. The knee is slightly flexed to relax the muscles and deep fascia. The pattern of superficial venous insufficiency is mapped by a combination of inspection, palpation, and percussion. The experienced observer can relate typical patterns of varices to particular sites of incompetence. Some clinicians like to add tourniquet tests in order to ascertain the levels of reflux. Physical examination alone is often insufficient, especially when the limb is obese, swollen, inflamed, or scarred. Continuous-wave hand-held Doppler imaging is an essential office technique both for the identification of reflux sites and for detecting arterial disease by measurement of the ankle-brachial pressure index. It also provides rapid detection of reflux in the groin and behind the knee to aid in planning management. For preoperative assessment, it has been supplanted by color-coded duplex scanning.

TESTS OF THE VENOUS SYSTEM

	TRAINING PERIOD	COST	TYPE
Venous insufficiency			
Doppler	Long	Low	Functional
Duplex	Long	High	Anatomic and functional
Air plethysmography	Short	Medium	Functional
Photoplethysmography	Short	Medium	Functional
Foot volumetry	Short	Medium	Functional
Phlebography	Long	High	Anatomic
Outflow obstruction			
Duplex	Long	High	Anatomic and functional
Air plethysmography	Short	Medium	Functional
Strain-gauge plethysmography	Short	Medium	Functional
Impedance plethysmography	Short	Medium	Functional
Phlebography	Long	High	Anatomic

FIGURE 11-8. Laboratory assessment. Tests of function are based on the response to exercise and the rate of refilling (*see* Fig. 11-2). Such tests enable quantification of the efficacy of the muscle pump, the degree of outflow obstruction, and the severity of valvular insufficiency. The reference standard is direct ambulatory venous pressure measurement, but commonly used noninvasive methods include photoplethysmography, foot volumetry, and air plethysmography.

IMAGING

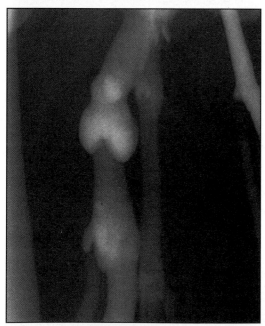

FIGURE 11-9. Phlebography. The phlebogram remains the reference standard for imaging venous disease, although noninvasive imaging is used quite often. For an overall display of the venous pattern of the limbs, phlebography is performed by the ascending route. For assessment of reflux, the descending route is employed. Note the superficial femoral vein, well outlined by contrast injected into the common femoral vein (descending phlebogram), with the patient standing erect. Some leakage of contrast medium through valves into the upper thigh is normal, but reflux down to the knee or beyond is pathologic and may be used as a criterion for valve reconstruction. Duplex scanning has shown that segments of the long saphenous vein fed by thigh perforating veins can be incompetent below a competent sapheno-femoral junction. Similarly, segments of deep vein, such as the popliteal segment, can sometimes be incompetent below competent proximal valves. (*From* Callam and Ruckley [5]; with permission.)

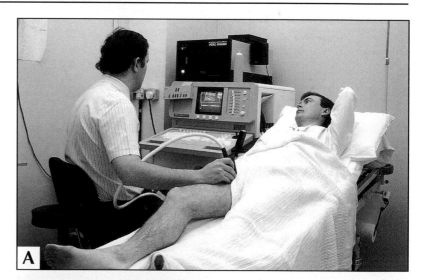

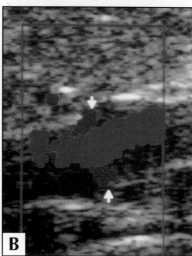

FIGURE 11-10. Color-coded duplex ultrasonography.

A, Because it is noninvasive, color-coded duplex ultrasound scanning represents the major advance in recent years in the investigation of venous disease. The patient is examined standing or lying with foot-down tilt. As well as enabling mapping of the venous system, it provides information on directions and flow velocities. Valve reflux can be directly visualized. However, we still lack a reliable formula for quantifying reflux on duplex scanning. **B,** This duplex scan shows flow through an open valve. The *red areas* indicate reversal of flow in the eddies behind the cusps.

CONSERVATIVE THERAPIES

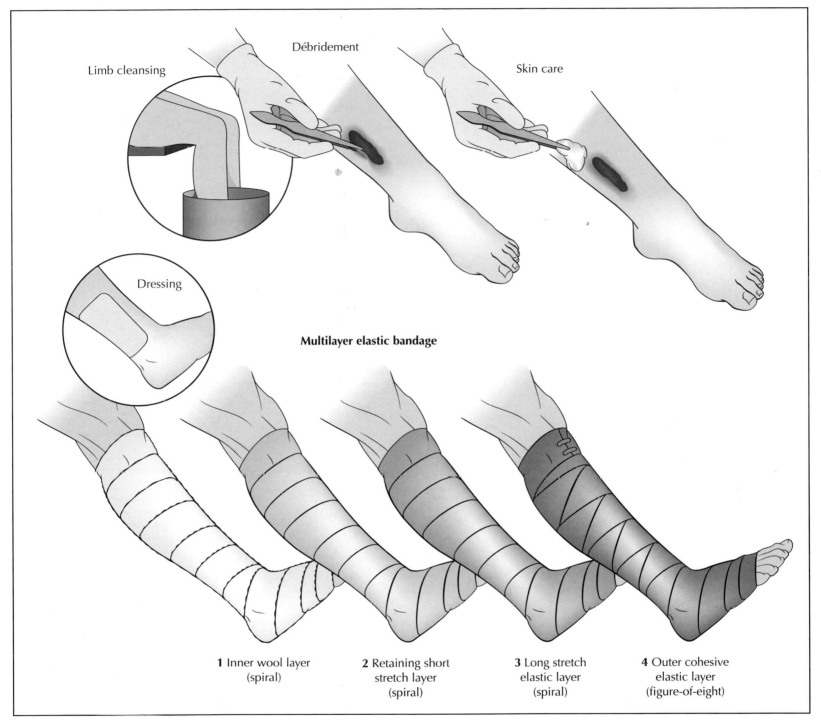

Limb cleansing

Débridement

Skin care

Dressing

Multilayer elastic bandage

1 Inner wool layer (spiral)

2 Retaining short stretch layer (spiral)

3 Long stretch elastic layer (spiral)

4 Outer cohesive elastic layer (figure-of-eight)

FIGURE 11-11. Ulcer care. Because chronic leg ulcers invariably are colonized with bacteria, the technique of ulcer dressing requires cleanliness rather than strict sterility. Ulcer care involves treatment of the whole patient, the limb, and the surrounding skin—as well as the ulcer itself—and is best provided by a trained wound care nurse. A simple regimen applicable to most cases would be as follows. The ulcer and the surrounding skin are washed with plain lukewarm water in a foot bath. Crusts, sloughs, and scaly skin are physically débrided. Dessicated skin is moisturized with arachis oil or 1% ichthammol. Weeping exfoliative eczema is dried with 2% eosin. Itchy eczema is treated sparingly with diluted steroid cream (*eg*, 0.1% hydrocortisone). The ulcer itself is dressed with a hydrocolloid if it needs desloughing or with tulle or a nonadherent dressing once it has entered the clean, healing stage. The most important guiding principle is to avoid agents that may set up skin sensitivity reactions, *eg*, topical antibiotics. Dressings should be bland, but their nature is of minor consequence compared with the crucial importance of dispelling edema and controlling the venous hypertension by physical means. Simple physical measures can effect dramatic improvement in chronic venous insufficiency. These include high elevation of the limb, graduated elastic compression, and weight control.

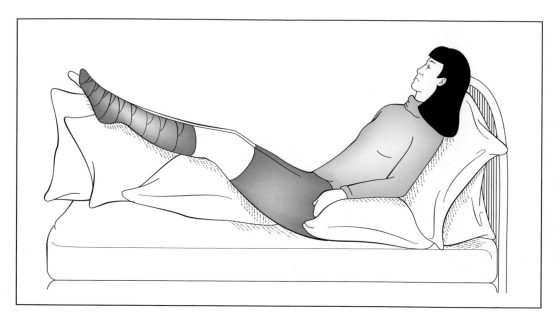

FIGURE 11-12. Elevation. When advised to elevate the legs at rest, few patients will do so properly unless given clear and precise instructions, preferably reinforced by an information sheet and diagram. When sitting, the feet should be higher than the hip, and when lying down, the feet should be higher than the heart. Elevation should be combined with active exercise of calf muscles, consisting of flexion, extension, and rotatory movements at the ankle. The exercises can be reinforced by providing the patient with a latex rubber band, which is held in the hands and looped around the foot so that the patient performs the exercises against elastic resistance.

PHYSIOLOGIC EFFECTS OF COMPRESSION

INCREASE	DECREASE
Local interstitial pressure	Edema
Venous femoral flow velocity	Superficial venous pressure
Plasminogen activator release	Ambulatory venous pressure
Compression of superficial veins	Superficial vein distention
Expelled calf volume on exercise	
Venous refilling time	
Local capillary clearance	
Capillary refilling time	

FIGURE 11-13. Compression therapy. The physiologic effects of compression therapy are beneficial in every type of venous disease ranging from simple primary varicose veins to advanced chronic venous insufficiency. Whether the therapy is bandaging or tailored hosiery, the principles are the same: 1) the pressure exerted must be appropriate to the severity of disease and the build of the patient; 2) the pressure must be maximal at the ankle and in a diminishing gradient as it ascends the leg; 3) the bandage or stocking must be correctly measured and accurately and expertly applied; and 4) in chronic venous insufficiency, unlike extensive post-thrombotic edema or lymphedema, compression should only be applied from the base of the toes to the tibial tuberosity. Severe arterial insufficiency (ankle-brachial pressure index < 0.7) is a contraindication to compression therapy.

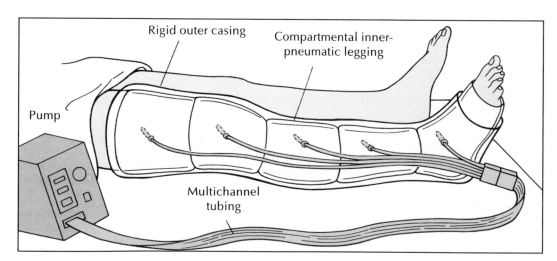

Rigid outer casing
Compartmental inner-pneumatic legging
Pump
Multichannel tubing

FIGURE 11-14. Sequential pneumatic compression. Sequential pneumatic compression may be employed to control edema and hasten ulcer healing. This consists of a plastic sleeve divided into compartments that are inflated in sequence, from distal to proximal, thus enhancing venous return and lymphatic clearance. The patient can use the device at home as required.

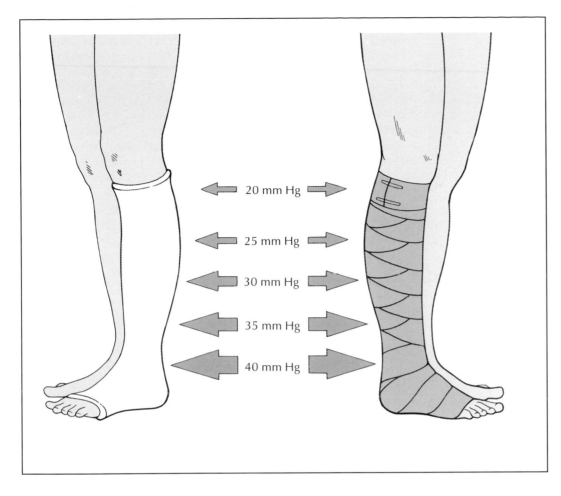

FIGURE 11-15. Compression therapy. To control venous hypertension and heal a venous ulcer, the average patient requires a pressure of approximately 35 to 40 mm Hg at the ankle. A tall, heavily built individual will require higher pressures, and a frail, elderly patient will require lower pressures. The pressures illustrated are not absolute but rather are intended to convey approximate levels and the need for a gradient. Bandaging is the preferred form of compression when there is open ulceration with exudation and when dressings require changing at regular intervals. Effective bandaging requires experience and skill. The bandage characteristics are vitally important, notably elasticity, handling qualities, conformity, and cohesiveness. Long stretch elastic bandaging has been shown to heal ulcers faster than nonstretch bandaging [6], but the latter is safer in patients with arterial compromise. Figure-of-eight application gives better and more sustained compression than a simple spiral. Multilayer elastic bandaging is generally more effective than single-layer bandaging because it results in a more even distribution of pressure and is more likely to stay in place, especially if a cohesive bandage is used as the outer layer [7]. In the late stages of ulcer healing and in the long-term treatment of chronic venous insufficiency, bandaging is replaced by below-knee elastic stockings.

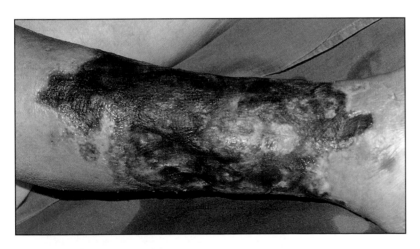

FIGURE 11-16. Risks of compression therapy. Although graduated compression is beneficial for the majority of patients with chronic venous insufficiency, approximately 20% of the population over 60 years of age has some degree of arterial impairment, as demonstrated by Doppler pressure measurements [8]. Compression therapy can be dangerous in these patients, and especially in diabetics [9]. Severe tissue damage can result from the application of tight elastic compression to an ischemic limb. Well-padded short stretch bandaging is the safer option. However, a venous ulcer, if it is to be managed on an ambulatory basis, will not heal without effective compression. Therefore, if the ankle-brachial pressure index is below 0.7, coexisting arterial insufficiency should first be corrected by reconstruction or angioplasty.

OPERATIVE TREATMENT

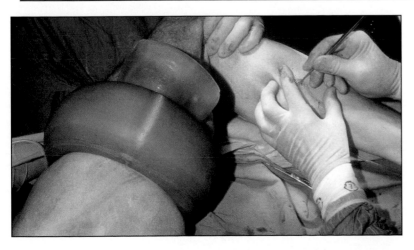

FIGURE 11-17. Operative treatment. Depending on the sites of incompetence, superficial varicose veins are dealt with by conventional techniques including saphenofemoral and saphenopopliteal ligation, stripping of the thigh portion of the long saphenous vein, and multiple avulsions of varices. After saphenofemoral incompetence has been corrected, it is preferred to carry out the remaining venous reconstruction after a sterile pneumatic cuff is inflated to approximately 160 mm Hg, rolled on from the toes to exsanguinate the limb, and then secured in place at thigh level by a latex wedge.

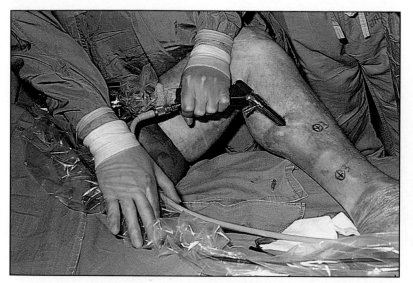

FIGURE 11-18. Subfascial endoscopic perforator surgery (SEPS). Since the advent of SEPS, open calf perforator ligation (Linton's procedure) has become obsolete because of its unacceptable complications, *ie*, wound infection and nonhealing. Subfascial endoscopic perforator surgery consists of placing an operating scope into the posterior compartment of the calf and interrupting perforating veins under direct endoscopic vision. The figure shows the insertion of the endoscope in a patient who had a healed venous ulcer. Note the preoperative markings of perforator sites. Debate continues regarding the use of a tourniquet, one or two ports, use of gas insufflation and preoperative duplex marking, methods for interrupting the perforators, type of operating scope to be used, the need for paratibial fasciotomy, and the utility of repeat SEPS for recurrent disease.

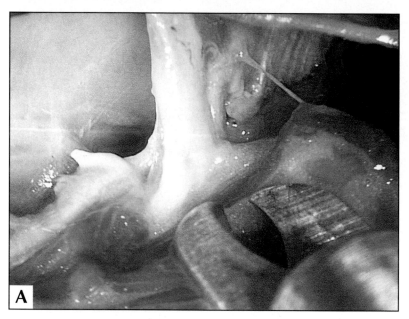

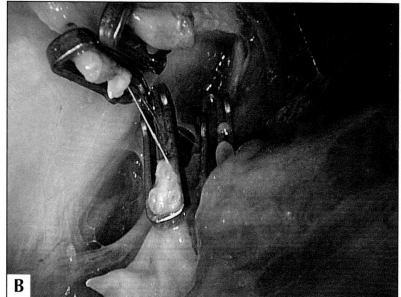

FIGURE 11-19. Subfascial endoscopic perforator surgery (SEPS).. Perforators in the patient in Figure 11-18 before (**A**) and after (**B**) endoscopic clipping and division. Although SEPS can be performed in patients with open ulceration with little or no additional morbidity over conventional saphenous surgery, its role remains highly controversial. There is no evidence that open calf perforator ligation confers added clinical or hemodynamic benefit to saphenous surgery, or that either procedure was better than the best medical therapy. The same is true of SEPS. In patients without deep venous disease, there is considerable evidence to show that eradication of superficial (saphenous) reflux will lead most incompetent medial calf perforators to regain competence [10]. Therefore, SEPS may be limited to patients with deep reflux in whom incompetent perforators remain despite saphenous surgery, especially when such perforators lie close to or beneath the ulcer.

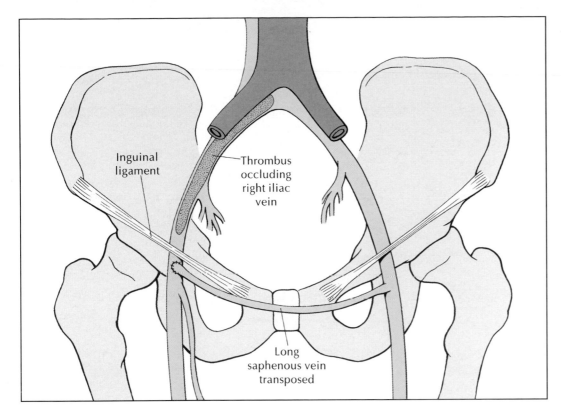

FIGURE 11-20. Obstruction. Deep venous obstruction is a significant contributor to venous hypertension in only about 10% of patients with chronic venous insufficiency. However, this figure may be artificially low because of the inability, until the recent advent of endovenous catheterization with pressure measurement and intravascular ultrasound, to identify venous obstruction both anatomically and hemodynamically. Patients with obstruction in addition to reflux tend to have the most severe symptoms (venous claudication), gain the least benefit from high-grade compression, and suffer the worst long-term prognosis in terms of ulcer recurrence. In patients whose symptoms, signs, and investigations indicate a functionally significant proximal (aorto-iliac) venous obstruction, a Palma crossover femorofemoral venous bypass using contralateral long saphenous vein may be indicated. Some authors advocate the simultaneous construction of an arteriovenous fistula, which is closed a few weeks later. In the future, there is likely to be an increasing role for endovenous therapy including balloon angioplasty, stent placement, and, in certain cases, thrombolysis.

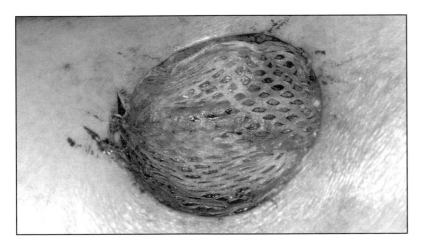

FIGURE 11-21. Ulcer. An excised ulcer that has been covered with a mesh graft. The majority of ulcers (< 10 cm^2) can be healed within 3 months by an ambulatory regimen of dressings and graduated compression therapy. Larger ulcers and those proving intractable to ambulatory care should be skin-grafted. Recurrence is likely unless the underlying vascular abnormality is also corrected.

There is controversy over the role of split skin grafting (SSG) in patients with venous ulceration. While SSG can increase the rate of epithelial coverage, many skin grafts that initially "take" quickly fail upon discharge from the hospital. It is debatable, therefore, whether this rapid but often transient re-epithelialization actually equates with true and durable healing. Split skin grafting carries significant morbidity, and usually requires a prolonged hospital stay. Pinch grafts can be performed on an outpatient basis. While this technique cannot be used to cover large ulcers, some suggest that the creation of islands of re-epithelialization encourages the ulcer healing process through the release of growth factors and the donation of fresh epithelial cells and fibroblasts. Artificial skin substitutes have been developed and proposed for use in chronic wounds including venous ulcers. However, these products can be difficult to use, are extremely expensive, and may not provide any benefit over the patient's own skin.

REFERENCES

1. Beebe HG, Bergan JJ, Bergqvist D, *et al.*: Classification and grading of chronic venous disease in the lower limbs: a consensus statement. *Phlebology* 1995, 10:42–45.

2. Browse NL, Gray L, Jarrett PE, Morland M: Blood and vein-wall fibrinolytic activity in health and vascular disease. *Br Med J* 1977, 1:478–481.

3. Thomas PR, Nash GB, Dormandy JA: White cell accumulation in dependent legs of patients with venous hypertension: a possible mechanism for trophic changes in the skin. *Br Med J (Clin Res Ed)* 1988, 296:1693–1695.

4. Coleridge Smith PD, Thomas P, Scurr JH, Dormandy JA: Causes of venous ulceration: a new hypothesis. *Br Med J (Clin Red Ed)* 1988, 296:1726–1727.

5. Callam MJ, Ruckley CV: Chronic venous insufficiency and leg ulcer. In *Surgical Management of Vascular Disease*. Edited by Bell PRF, Jamieson CW, Ruckley CV. London: Saunders; 1992:1267–1303.

6. Callam MJ, Harper DR, Dale JJ, *et al.*: Lothian and Forth Valley Leg Ulcer Healing Trial. Part 1: elastic versus nonelastic bandaging in the treatment of chronic leg ulceration. *Phlebology* 1992, 7:136–141.

7. Blair SD, Wright DD, Backhouse CM, *et al.*: Sustained compression and healing of chronic venous ulcers. *BMJ* 1988, 297:1159–1161.

8. Callam MJ, Harper DR, Dale JJ, *et al.*: Arterial disease in chronic leg ulceration: an underestimated hazard. *BMJ* 1987, 294:929–930.

9. Callam MJ, Ruckley CV, Dale JJ, Harper DR: Hazards of compression treatment of the leg: an estimate from Scottish surgeons. *Br Med J (Clin Res Ed)* 1987, 295:1382.

10. Stuart WP, Adam DJ, Allan PL, *et al.*: Saphenous surgery does not correct perforator incompetence in the presence of deep venous reflux. *J Vasc Surg* 1998, 28(5):834–838.

CHAPTER

LYMPHATIC DISEASE

Stanley Rockson

Lymphedema can be defined as a clinical presentation characterized by an excessive regional interstitial accumulation of protein-rich fluid. This common clinical disorder most typically arises when regional microcirculatory imbalances are created by a loss of lymphatic transport capacity. Whenever the lymphatic circulation is damaged, diseased, or malformed, a spectrum of derangements can result.

Under normal circumstances, circulatory equilibrium is established through the balance of arteriovenous hydrostatic and oncotic pressures. Limited quantities of protein-rich interstitial fluid are returned to the central circulation by the lymphatic system. Disruption of this equilibrium can occur as a result of changes in intra- or extracellular protein concentration or altered arteriovenous hemodynamics. Any imbalance of the lymphatic load and the lymphatic transport capacity, whether congenital or acquired, can lead to lymphedema, the clinical expression of this imbalance.

The simplest classification of lymphedema requires a differentiation between secondary and primary causes [1,2]. The secondary lymphedemas, often iatrogenic or post-infectious, arise after acquired destruction of the lymphatic structures, including nodes, lymphatic channels, or both. The primary lymphedemas, which reflect heritable defects in lymphatic development and function, are often classified according to the age of the patient when the edema first occurs [3].

The classification of primary lymphedema may be based clinically on the age of onset, with anatomic and functional classifications confirmed by diagnostic lymphangiography or lymphoscintigraphy. Congenital lymphedema, apparent at birth or recognizable within the first 2 years of life, represents about 15% of cases. Aplasia, the absence of lymphatic trunks, and hypoplasia, the presence of a reduced number or caliber of lymphatic channels, are the most common lymphangiographic findings. Lymphedema praecox is first detected most commonly at puberty, but may also appear as late as the patient's third decade of life. This form, which comprises 75% of the primary cases, is typified by a hypoplastic lymphangiographic pattern. In lymphedema tarda, which typically first appears in affected patients after age 35 years, the lymphatic vasculature can be either hypo- or hyperplastic. In the latter circumstance, primary lymphatic valvular incompetence is usually accompanied by an increased number of lymphatic channels with varicosities of the major collecting vessels.

Generalized developmental insufficiency of the lymphatic circulation is not compatible with post-embryonic survival [4]. In life, these disorders commonly disrupt the regional lymphatic drainage of the extremities, either upper or lower, or both. Visceral lymphatic abnormalities can also occur, either in isolation or as an accompaniment to the superficial extremity edema. In addition to the effect upon bodily structure and function, the presence and severity of lymphedema has a substantial impact on the quality of life and the perception of well being in the affected patients [5]. A variety of medical and surgical therapies have been attempted in the management of lymphedema, but have often led to mixed or disappointing functional and cosmetic results. Comprehension of the mechanisms of lymphatic dysfunction in disease may lead to effective utilization of an existing treatment modality and, ultimately, the delineation of improved therapeutics for lymphedema.

ANATOMY AND PHYSIOLOGY OF THE LYMPHATIC CIRCULATION

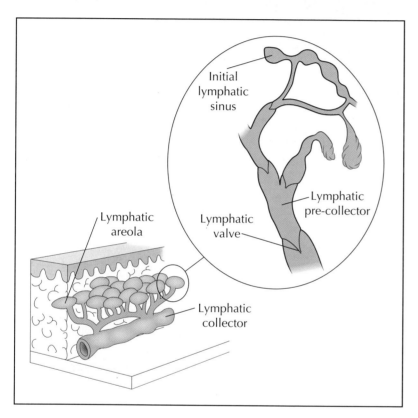

FIGURE 12-1. Lymphatic microcirculation. The lymphatic vasculature consists of initial lymphatics, the lymphatic pre-collectors, which coalesce into the lymphatic ducts that drain into the lymph nodes. In the skin, the initial lymphatics are found in the papillae as blind-ended sinuses lined by a single layer of lymphatic endothelial cells. The lymphatic system consists of a superficial (epifascial) system that collects lymph from the skin and subcutaneous tissue and a deeper system that drains subfascial structures such as bone, muscle, and deep blood vessels. In the extremities, the two drainage systems merge within the pelvis or axilla, respectively. These parallel systems function in an interdependent fashion, such that the deep lymphatic system in all likelihood participates in lymph transport from the skin during lymphatic obstruction [6]. It has been estimated that deep lymphatic transport accounts for only 7.7% of the lymph flow through the superficial system [7].

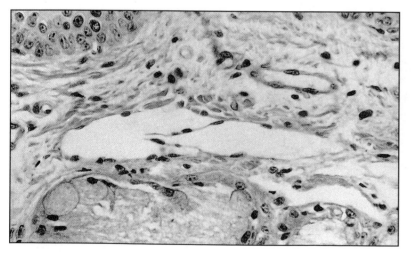

FIGURE 12-2. Photomicrograph of an oblique section of a lymphatic capillary demonstrating the valvular structure. Valves are more numerous here than in veins and consist of folds of intimal endothelial cells. The wall structure of a lymphatic vessel incorporates intimal and adventitial layers. The smooth muscle content of the media increases in prominence as the lymphatic vessel ascends. In skeletal muscle, lymphatics are usually paired with arterioles, so that arterial pulsation and muscle contraction contribute to the periodic expansion and compression of initial lymphatics to enhance fluid uptake. Intrinsic lymphatic contractility increases in response to tissue edema, temperature change, mechanical stimulation, exercise, and hydrostatic pressure.

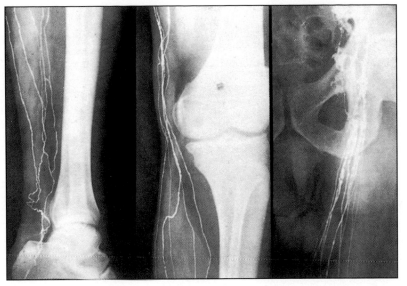

FIGURE 12-3. Normal lymphangiograms demonstrating three to five lymphatic trunks at the mid-calf and tibial plateau regions. A total of five to 15 major lymph trunks are present in each thigh, with each trunk measuring 1 to 1.5 mm in diameter. Contrast lymphography is performed through the direct injection of iodine-based, lipid-soluble agents into subcutaneous lymphatics, following the subcutaneous injection of dye to facilitate their identification and cannulation [8]. Historically, the method has been useful for the direct visualization of lymphatic anatomy and has had some utility prior to reconstructive lymphatic surgery. More recently, however, lymphangiography has been largely supplanted by the ready availability of radioisotope lymphoscintigraphy. In addition to the greater ease of application of nuclear imaging, contrast lymphography may, in fact, induce exacerbation of lymphatic malfunction through accumulation and pooling of the oil-based contrast media within the lymphatic structures.

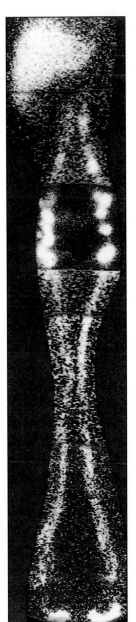

FIGURE 12-4. Normal lymphoscintigram demonstrating uniform columns of isotope with concentration in the femoral, iliac, and para-aortic lymph nodes as well as in the liver. Radionuclide lymphoscintigraphy is the most common clinically utilized imaging modality for lymphatic function. It is a reliable and reproducible method for the diagnostic confirmation of lymphedema. A radio-labeled macromolecular tracer, such as ^{99}Tc-labeled sulfur colloid, is administered parenterally into the subdermal interdigital region of the affected limb. The lymphatic transport of the macromolecule can be imaged quantitatively with a gamma camera. Visualization of major lymphatic trunks and lymph nodes is feasible. Typical abnormalities observed in lymphedema include absent or delayed transport of tracer, absent or delayed visualization of lymph nodes, crossover filling with retrograde backflow, and dermal backflow.

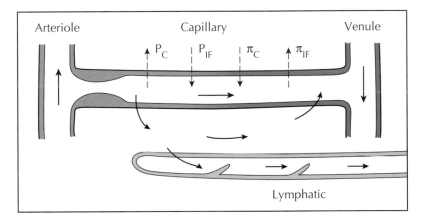

FIGURE 12-5. Schematic representation of the dynamics of interstitial fluid exchange. Based on the Starling hypothesis [9], movement of fluid across the capillary wall is determined by the intravascular hydrostatic pressure (P_C), the capillary osmotic pressure of the plasma (π_C), the interstitial hydrostatic pressure (P_{IF}), and the osmotic pressure (π_{IF}) of the surrounding interstitial fluid [10]. Albumin is primarily responsible for intravascular and interstitial oncotic pressures. The effect of hydrostatic pressure driving fluid out of the capillary is represented by $P_C - P_{IF}$. The osmotic pressure, which acts to retain fluid in the capillary, is represented by $\pi_C - \pi_{IF}$. Under normal conditions a net outflow of fluid across the capillary wall results from a pressure gradient estimated to be 0.3 mm Hg. This excess fluid, which approximates 0.003 mL/min/100 g of tissue in the moving limb, is removed by the lymphatics [11]. A relative increase in the intravascular hydrostatic pressure or a decrease in oncotic pressure favors an increased filtration of fluid across the capillary membrane. Elevated intravascular hydrostatic pressures may also occur as a result of elevated venous outflow pressures due to obstruction or insufficiency. The inability of the lymphatic network to collect and to drain interstitial fluid and protein results in edema. A rise in the interstitial hydrostatic pressure occurs until a new intra- and extravascular equilibrium is established.

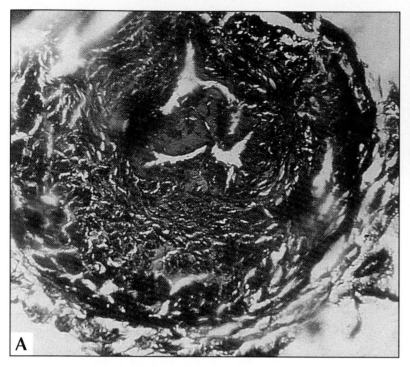

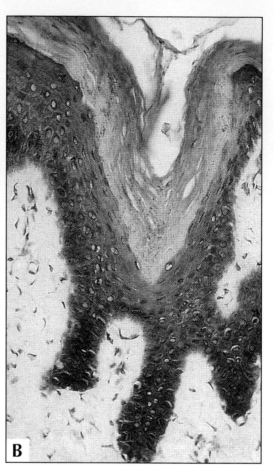

FIGURE 12-6. Chronic changes in tissue architecture accompanying chronic lymphedema. **A**, With chronic lymph stasis, obliterative changes in the conduit lymphatic vessels eventually render the process irreversible. **B**, Lymph stasis ultimately leads to hyperkeratosis and hypercellularity of the dermal and subdermal structures.

PRIMARY LYMPHEDEMA

PRIMARY LYMPHEDEMA

Congenital lymphedema
   Autosomal dominant, familial (Milroy's disease,
    lymphedema-distichiasis syndrome)
   Autosomal recessive, syndrome-associated
   Sporadic
Lymphedema praecox
   Familial (Meige's disease)
   Sporadic
Lymphedema tarda

FIGURE 12-7. Primary lymphedema. Classification of primary lymphedemas is often made according to the age of the patient when the edema first appears. Congenital lymphedema is apparent at birth or becomes recognized within the first 2 years of life. Lymphedema praecox is most commonly first detected at the time of puberty, but its appearance may be delayed until the patient's third decade of life. Lymphedema tarda typically becomes manifest after age 35 years.

In congenital lymphedema, the swelling can involve only a single lower extremity, but edema of multiple limbs, the genitalia, or the facial structures can be seen. Bilateral leg swelling and involvement of the entire lower extremity is more likely in congenital cases than in other forms of primary lymphedema. Lymphedema tarda is relatively uncommon, accounting for no more than 10% of the cases of primary lymphedema.

Although congenital lymphedema clusters in families with an autosomal dominant pattern of transmission, the isolated instances of lymphedema are much more common [12]. A strong association has been described between various heritable chromosomal abnormalities and the detection of intrauterine and congenital lymphatic pathology. Most recently, the heritable defect of Milroy's disease has been associated with missense mutations in the gene that encodes the vascular endothelial growth factor (VEGF)-3 receptor [13]. The disease-associated alleles prevent downstream gene activation, thereby impairing the process of lymphangiogenesis. Similar progress is underway with lymphedema-distichiasis [14].

SECONDARY LYMPHEDEMA

Post-surgical (lymph node dissection, after vascular surgery)
Parasitic (filariasis)
Post-infectious
Post-traumatic
Neoplastic (intrinsic and extrinsic obstruction)
Lymphedema complicating chronic venous insufficiency

FIGURE 12-8. Secondary lymphedema. This condition develops after disruption or obstruction of lymphatic pathways by other disease processes, or as an iatrogenic consequence of surgery or radiotherapy. Secondary lymphedema is much more common than the primary form. Edema of the arm after axillary lymph node dissection is probably the most common cause of lymphedema in the Western world [15]. Edema of the leg is also comparatively common following pelvic or genital cancer surgeries, particularly when there has been inguinal or pelvic lymph node dissection and/or irradiation. Pelvic irradiation correlates with an increase in the frequency of leg lymphedema seen after cancer surgery.

Recurrent pyogenic infections can also cause secondary lymphedema. Although β-hemolytic Streptococcus is the most frequently isolated bacterium in these infections, *Staphylococcus aureus* and gram-negative aerobes have also been implicated. The infectious process causes an obliteration of the lymphatic vessels and fibrosis of the afferent lymph nodes. Obliteration of lymphatics due to repeated bouts of cellulitis may exacerbate the chronic edema observed in the post-thrombotic limb and may precipitate a combined disorder. Worldwide, the incidence of all other forms of secondary lymphedema is overshadowed by filariasis, a nematode infection that accounts for over 90 million cases of secondary lymphedema.

DIFFERENTIAL DIAGNOSIS OF LYMPHEDEMA

Chronic venous insufficiency and post-phlebitic syndrome
Myxedema
Lipedema
Malignant lymphedema

FIGURE 12-9. Differential diagnosis of lymphedema. Several features of lymphedema serve to distinguish the physical presentation from other causes of chronic edema of the extremities. Among these are the unique changes of dermal and subdermal fibrosis (peau d'orange) and the characteristic Stemmer's sign, in which the skin and soft tissue changes produce an inability to tent the skin of the interdigital webs. When present in the lower extremities, lymphedema often produces preferential swelling of the dorsum of the foot, as well as characteristic squaring-off of the digits. Both of these features serve to distinguish lymphedema from other local and systemic causes of edema.

Chronic venous insufficiency and post-phlebitic syndrome are the disorders that are perhaps most readily confused with lymphedema of the legs. Distinguishing clinical features include aching discomfort in the lower extremities during sitting or standing, and chronic pruritus, particularly overlying the incompetent communicating veins. Physical findings include characteristic cutaneous deposits of hemosiderin, dusky discoloration, and venous engorgement with dependency of the extremity, cutaneous varicosities, and, if advanced, characteristic ulceration of the skin. Myxedema occurs in thyroid disease when abnormal deposits of mucinous substances accumulate in the skin. Hyaluronic acid-rich protein deposition in the dermis produces edema that, in turn, disrupts structural integrity and reduces the elasticity of the skin. In thyrotoxicosis, this process is focal, in the pretibial region; in hypothyroidism, the myxedema is more generalized. Concomitant physical findings such as roughening of the skin over the palms, soles, elbows, and knees; brittle, uneven nails; dull, thinning hair; yellow-orange discoloration of the skin; and reduced sweat production may help to distinguish this presentation from lymphedema. Lipedema affects women almost exclusively. It almost certainly has a hormonal basis, since it arises in men only when they have concomitant feminizing disturbances. In lipedema, the edema accompanies the abnormal accumulation of fatty substances in the subcutaneous regions. Although the mechanisms of this disease are still incompletely understood, it is clear that there is excess elaboration of subcutaneous adipocytes along with characteristic structural alterations in the small vascular structures within the skin. In lipedema, the characteristic distribution, with sparing of the feet, suggests the correct diagnosis. The absence of a Stemmer's sign is an additional clue that diminishes the likelihood of lymphedema. Malignant lymphedema can cause the appearance or worsening of lymphedema. This typically occurs because of spread of tumor cells through the lymphatics, leading to obstruction of lymph flow. Extrinsic obstruction of the lymphatics by tumor can also occur. In conditions caused directly by tumor spread or compression, there is a tendency for rapid development and relentless progression. In addition, pain, generally absent in benign lymphedema, may be a feature.

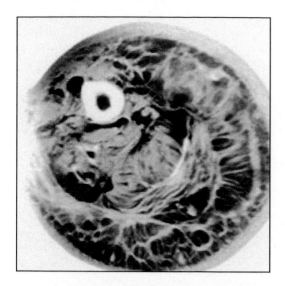

FIGURE 12-10. Fibrosis in lymphedema. Chronic lymphedema of an extremity inexorably leads to thickening of the skin and fibrosis of cutaneous and subcutaneous structures, as illustrated in this cross-sectional magnetic resonance image.

PHYSICAL FINDINGS AND DIAGNOSIS

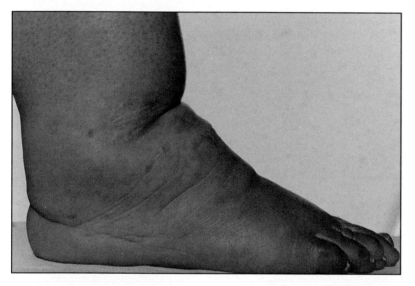

FIGURE 12-11. The diagnosis of lymphedema can be made by simple observation because of the pathognomonic shape of the limb due to the distribution of edema. This photograph of a lymphedematous ankle and foot in profile demonstrates typical findings. These include concentric calf edema with a loss of normal contour, sparing at the level of the ankle joint, and significant hindfoot edema relative to the forefoot, yielding a "buffalo hump" profile. The toes are usually tensely edematous with a sausage shape.

The fluid distribution in the lymphedematous limb differs from that in chronic venous insufficiency or systemic causes of dependent edema. In the latter instances, fluid accumulation is greatest in the ankle area and is least over the toes.

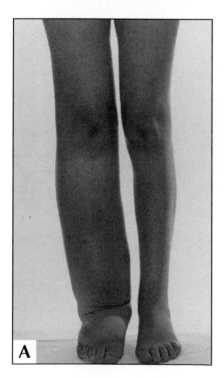
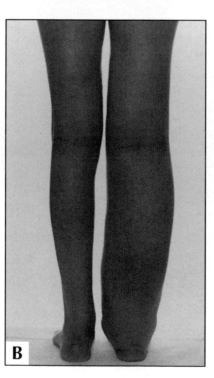

FIGURE 12-12. The cosmetic deformity produced by limb swelling is usually the reason patients seek medical care. **A,** Anterior view. **B,** Posterior view. As the process becomes more severe, the level of the edema advances to involve the more proximal portions of the extremity and may not diminish at night with simple elevation. Increased fluid retention in the limb contributes to a sense of limb heaviness. Early fatigue of the limb is common.

Lymphangitis frequently complicates lymphedema; when present, this may produce an acutely painful limb marked by a diffuse, superficial burning sensation. The skin changes associated with lymphedema help to classify its severity. In mild lymphedema the skin retains its normal texture but may appear flushed or pink because of cutaneous vasodilatation and increased cutaneous blood flow. In moderate lymphedema there is thickening of the skin due to chronic edema, and "peau d'orange" is observed. In advanced stages of lymphedema skin changes are characterized by thickening and coarseness. Lichenification of the toes develops and intermittent bacterial infection occurs at sites of skin fissures, minor trauma, or breakdown induced by interdigital fungal infection.

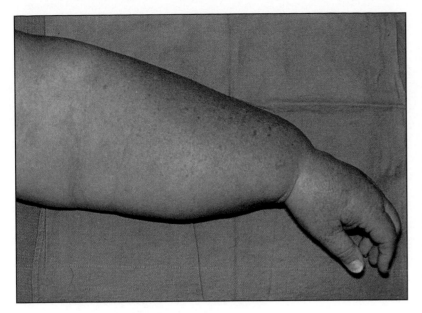

FIGURE 12-13. Lymphedema of the arm is commonly a complication of mastectomy or adjuvant radiation therapy. The distribution of edema in the arm is similar to that in lower-extremity lymphedema, with tense edema throughout the hand and fingers. Although post-mastectomy lymphedema is precipitated by iatrogenic trauma to the lymphatic vessels and nodes, it is not uncommon to encounter a mixed pathogenesis of edema, with concomitant venous obstruction. In cancer patients with iatrogenic forms of edema, the pathobiology of the disease distinctly favors the likelihood of venous obstruction [16,17]. In addition to venous injury arising from surgical intervention, radiation damage, chemotherapy, or local invasion of the tumor, there is also the predisposition to hypercoagulability that often accompanies the underlying malignancy. Furthermore, venous stenosis can be mediated by post-surgical scarring, tumor compression, or radiation-induced fibrosis. Noninvasive venous studies are important in the initial evaluation of the edematous limb to eliminate venous insufficiency or occlusion as an etiology of edema. In the lower extremities, plethysmography or duplex imaging is performed to rule out venous obstruction. Duplex assessment of the superficial and deep systems and spectral scan modes are then obtained to document evidence of valvular insufficiency.

DIAGNOSTIC EVALUATION OF THE EDEMATOUS EXTREMITY

Degree of lymphedema
  Measurement of limb circumference
  Limb volume displacement
Venous noninvasive imaging
  Plethysmography
  Duplex ultrasonography
Lymphatic imaging
  Lymphoscintigraphy
  Multiple frequency bioelectrical impedance analysis
  CT
  MRI

FIGURE 12-14. Diagnostic evaluation of the edematous extremity. In the patient with suspected lymphedema, there are three goals of diagnostic studies: to establish the diagnosis, to assess lymphatic function, and to document objectively the degree or

severity of lymphedema. In cases of moderate to severe lymphedema the diagnosis can be made by clinical examination alone. In patients with mild or early-onset lymphedema, correlative studies may be required to differentiate it from other disorders. When the physical examination alone does not conclusively support the diagnosis of lymphedema, additional objective evidence may be necessary to confirm the presence of impaired lymphatic function. Available tests include isotopic lymphoscintigraphy, lymphatic capillaroscopy, bioelectrical impedance analysis [18], magnetic resonance (MR) imaging, axial tomography [19], and ultrasonography. Although less commonly employed in the clinical assessment of lymphedema, MR and computed tomography (CT) imaging have potential applicability. The characteristic absence of muscle involvement in lymphedema provides a distinguishing feature that can be resolved in radiographic imaging. In addition, the honeycomb distribution of edema within the epifascial plane, along with thickening of the skin, is characteristic. The anatomic delineation of lymphatic and nodal architecture derived from MR imaging can complement the functional assessment provided by lymphoscintigraphy.

The two standard methods for assessing the degree of lymphedema are measurement of limb circumference at specific anatomic sites and measurement of limb volume by water displacement. The degree of lymphedema is represented by a ratio of the abnormal to the normal limb caliber [(abnormal - normal)/normal].

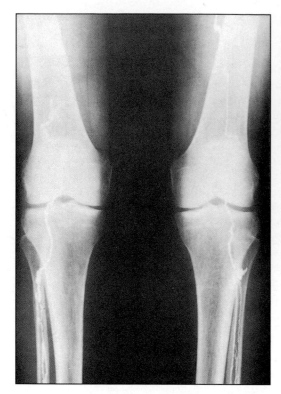

FIGURE 12-15. Lymphoscintigram demonstrating bilateral primary lymphedema in a hypoplastic pattern, marked by a reduced number of trunks. Eighty percent to 90% of patients studied with lymphangiography demonstrate a hypoplastic pattern. A review of lymphangiograms confirmed that patients with hypoplastic patterns averaged 2.1 major lymphatic trunks at the proximal thigh level as opposed to 12 trunks found in normal controls [20]. Hypoplasia may be primary (consequent to lymphatic dysgenesis) or secondary (as a result of recurrent lymphangitis causing fibrosis and obliteration of channels).

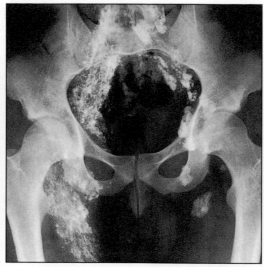

FIGURE 12-16. Pelvic lymphangiogram in a patient with lymphedema involving the entire right lower extremity. Note multiple opacified femoral lymph nodes and pelvic trunks consistent with lymphatic hyperplasia. A delayed contrast transit time on the right compared with the left supports the clinical diagnosis of lymphedema. Ten percent of patients with primary lymphedema have hyperplastic lymphangiographic patterns. Lymphatic hyperplasia is associated with an average of 18.5 trunks at the thigh level that have a varicosed appearance. Hyperplasia can be a bilateral lymphangiographic finding associated with obstruction to lymphatic outflow at the cisterna chyli or thoracic duct.

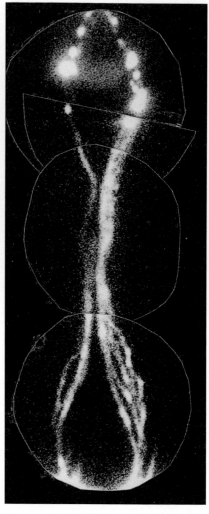

FIGURE 12-17. Bilateral lower extremity lymphoscintigraphy confirmed a hyperplastic pattern of the left leg and a delayed disappearance of radioactivity in this patient with lymphedema. In a comparison of lymphangiography and lymphoscintigraphy, Stewart *et al.* [21] demonstrated that the findings of each technique were closely correlated. Lymphoscintigraphic transit time and radioactive disappearance curves may be useful in the functional evaluation of lymphedema. 99mTc–labeled antimony trisulfide colloid is the commonly used isotope.

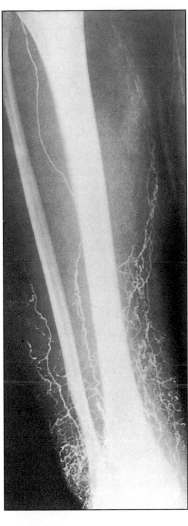

FIGURE 12-18. Lymphoangiogram in a patient with chronic venous insufficiency complicated by severe limb swelling and recurrent infected ulcers. This study demonstrates multiple fine collateral channels below a reduced number of more proximal lymphatic trunks. It suggests that the refractory edema is partly a consequence of secondary lymphedema, most likely caused by destruction of lymphatics due to recurrent infection.

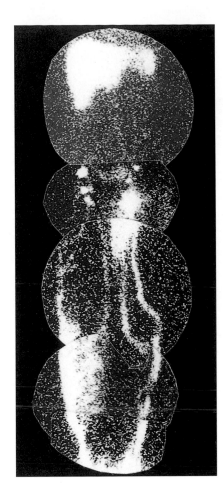

FIGURE 12-19. Bilateral lower extremity and abdominal lymphoscintigraphy in a patient with traumatic soft tissue injury to the right leg complicated by lymphedema. The diffuse pattern of activity in the injured region indicates dermal backflow, a reflection of radionuclide reflux into fine dermal collateral vessels at the level of lymphatic trunk disruption. This study also identifies lymphatic congestion in the left iliofemoral region where prior pelvic surgery had been performed. Normal opacification of the liver is noted. Dermal backflow is diagnostic of secondary lymphedema [21–23].

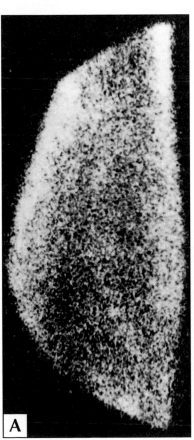
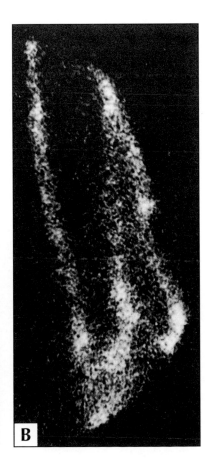

FIGURE 12-20. Modified radical mastectomy may be complicated by secondary lymphedema, particularly when adjuvant therapy for breast cancer includes radiation therapy. **A** and **B,** These simultaneous forearm lymphoscintigraphic studies in a postmastectomy patient with left arm lymphedema document loss of the normal forearm lymphatic trunk anatomy (*B*). Truncal disruption has resulted in extensive dermal backflow (*A*).

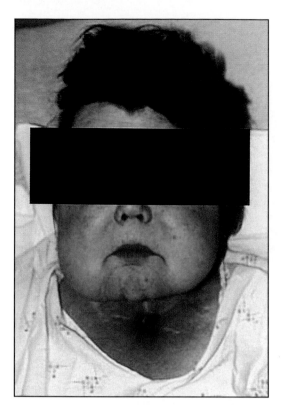

FIGURE 12-21. Facial lymphedema. Lymphedema of the head, neck and facial structures, while uncommon, can follow radical surgery, usually in the setting of neoplasia. If there is involvement of the airway, this can pose a medical emergency.

TREATMENT OF LYMPHEDEMA

TREATMENT OF LYMPHEDEMA

Nonsurgical
   Proper skin care with topical emollients
   Manual lymphatic therapy
   Multilayer, short stretch bandaging
   Exercise
   Well-fitted compressive garments
   Intermittent multi-compartmental compression pump therapy
Surgical
   Lymphaticovenous anastomosis
   Excisional procedures
   Liposuction

FIGURE 12-22. Treatment of lymphedema. The treatment of chronic lymphedema is best achieved through the application of multiple, interrelated treatment strategies. The goals of therapy are to reduce limb size, preserve and improve the quality of the skin and subcutaneous tissue, and prevent infection [24].

Decongestive lymphatic therapy is comprised of several component modalities, including skin care, manual lymphatic massage, multilayer bandaging, compressive garments, and exercise. Intermittent biocompression can be adjunctively accomplished with mechanical pumps designed for this purpose. Surgical therapies are reserved for the minority of patients who continue to experience unacceptable dysfunction despite maximal utilization of conservative therapies.

Fungicidal agents should be liberally applied interdigitally. Bacterial infections should be treated aggressively, often requiring intravenous therapy followed by prolonged oral antibiotics. Patients with recurring infections may require lifelong prophylactic antibiotics.

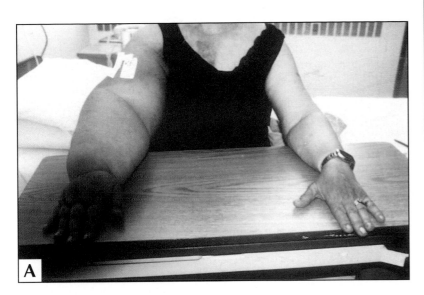

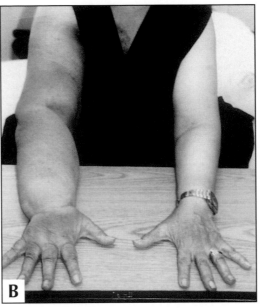

FIGURE 12-23. Decongestive lymphatic therapy in post-mastectomy lymphedema of the upper extremity. **A,** Before physiotherapy. **B,** Follow-up photograph taken after 7 consecutive daily sessions of manual lymphatic massage and multilayer bandaging.

Such approaches have been shown to provide substantial, durable relief of extremity swelling and dysfunction when coupled with chronic maintenance techniques and diligent use of fitted, compressive garments [25].

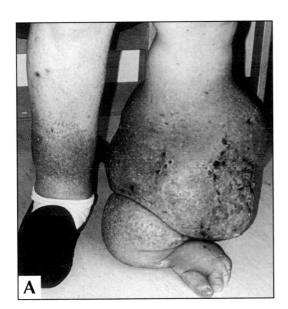

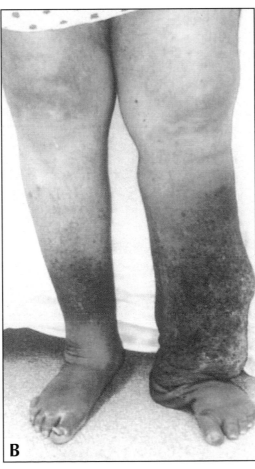

FIGURE 12-24. Decongestive lymphatic therapy in advanced lymphedema. A patient's lymphedematous left leg before (**A**) and after (**B**) successful physiotherapy. These photographs illustrate the benefits to be derived from protracted, intensive application of the standard techniques of massage and multilayer bandaging.

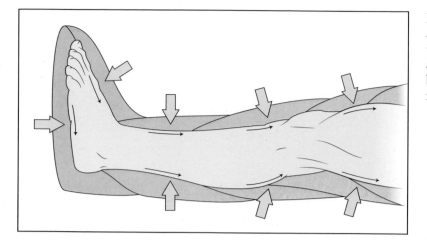

FIGURE 12-25. Intermittent mechanical compression. Although not a substitute for the other components of decongestive lymphatic therapy, intermittent mechanical compression can be used as an adjunct to other modalities. It is recommended that this form of biocompression be applied at relatively low prevailing pressures for not more than 30 to 60 minutes at a time.

SURGICAL TREATMENT

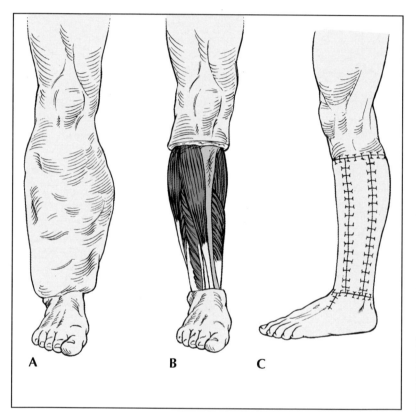

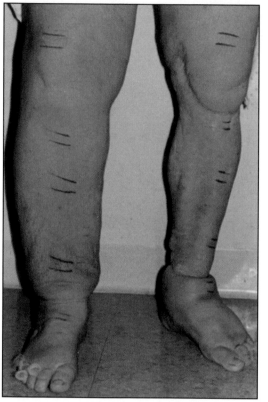

FIGURE 12-26. Excisional procedures. Charles [26] worked in an area endemic for tropical elephantiasis (**A**) and developed an operation that consisted of removing both skin and subcutaneous tissue (**B**) followed immediately by split-thickness skin graft coverage of exposed fascia (**C**). The Charles procedure is an *excisional* procedure, which is meant to improve symptoms by surgical reduction of limb size, and has primary application in cases of lymphatic obliteration. Shown are the pre-, intra-, and postoperative details of this procedure. At present, the Charles procedure is restricted to those patients with severe skin changes that prevent the use of vascularized skin flaps or subcutaneous lipectomy.

FIGURE 12-27. Excisional procedures. Although good clinical results have been achieved in some patients with the Charles procedure, the outcome of surgery is not always satisfactory due to excessive keloid formation and verrucous overgrowth. This technique has been largely abandoned. Lymphaticovenous anastomosis is still performed in some patients, and there has been substantial recent enthusiasm for liposuction, in properly selected individuals, when adipose overgrowth in the subdermis substantially contributes to the excess volume of chronically lymphedematous extremities [27].

REFERENCES

1. Szuba A, Rockson S: Lymphedema: anatomy, physiology and pathogenesis. *Vasc Med* 1997, 2: 321–326.

2. Rockson SG: Lymphedema. *Am J Med* 2001, 110:288295.

3. Rockson SG: Primary lymphedema. In *Current Therapy in Vascular Surgery*, edn 4. Edited by Ernst CB, Stanley JC. Philadelphia: Mosby; 2000: 915–918.

4. Dumont DJ, Jussila L, Taipale J, *et al.*: Cardiovascular failure in mouse embryos deficient in VEGF receptor-3. *Science* 1998, 282:946–949.

5. Velanovich V, Szymanski W: Quality of life of breast cancer patients with lymphedema. *Am J Surg* 1999, 177(3):184–187.

6. Brautigam P, Foldi E, Schaiper I, *et al.*: Analysis of lymphatic drainage in various forms of leg edema using two compartment lymphoscintigraphy. *Lymphology* 1998, 31:43–55.

7. Mostbeck A, Partsch H: Isotope lymphography—possibilities and limits in evaluation of lymph transport [in German]. *Wien Med Wochenschr* 1999, 149:87–91.

8. Kinmonth JB, Taylor GW, Tracy GD, Marsh JD: Primary lymphoedema. Clinical and lymphangiographic studies of a series of 107 patients in which the lower limbs were affected. *Br J Surg* 1957, 45:1–10.

9. Starling EH: On the absorption of fluids from the connective tissue spaces. *J Physiol* 1896, 19:312.

10. Landis EM, Pappenheimer JR: Exchange of substances through capillary walls. In *Handbook of Physiology*, Section 2, Circulation, vol II. Edited by Hamilton WF, Dow P. Washington, DC: American Physiological Society; 1963:961–1034.

11. Guyton AC, Grangher HJ, Taylor AE: Interstitial fluid pressure. *Physiol Rev* 1971, 51:527–563.

12. Wolfe JHN, Kinmonth JB: The prognosis of primary lymphedema of the lower limbs. *Arch Surg* 1981, 116:1157–1160.

13. Karkkainen MJ, Ferrell RE, Lawrence EC, *et al.*: Missense mutations interfere with VEGF-3 signalling in primary lymphoedema. *Nat Genet* 2000, 25:153–159.

14. Mangion J, Rahman N, Mansour S, *et al.*: A gene for lymphedema-distichiasis maps to 16q24.3. *Am J Hum Genet* 1999, 65:427–432.

15. Segerstrom K, Bjerle P, Graffman S, Nystrom A: Factors that influence the incidence of brachial oedema after treatment of breast cancer. *Scand J Plast Reconstr Surg Hand Surg* 1992, 26(2):223–227.

16. Svensson WE, Mortimer PS, Tohno E, Cosgrove DO: Colour Doppler demonstrates venous flow abnormalities in breast cancer patients with chronic arm swelling. *Eur J Cancer* 1994, 30A:657–660.

17. Rockson SG: Precipitating factors in lymphedema: myths and realities. *Cancer* 1998, 83: 2814–2816.

18. Ward LC, Bunce IH, Cornish BH, *et al.*: Multi-frequency bioelectrical impedance augments the diagnosis and management of lymphoedema in post-mastectomy patients. *Eur J Clin Invest* 1992, 22:751–754.

19. Vaughan BF: CT of swollen legs. *Clin Radiol* 1990, 41:24–30.

20. O'Donnell TF, Edwards JM, Kinmonth JB: Lymphography in congenital mixed vascular deformities of the lower extremities. *J Cardiovasc Surg* 1976, 17:535–540.

21. Stewart G, Gaunt JI, Croft DN, Browse NL: Isotope lymphography: a new method of investigating the role of the lymphatics in chronic limb oedema. *Br J Surg* 1985, 72:906–909.

22. Ter SE, Alavi A, Kim CK, Merli G: Lymphoscintigraphy: a reliable test for the diagnosis of lymphedema. *Clin Nucl Med* 1993, 18:646–654.

23. Gloviczki P, Calcagno D, Schirger A, *et al.*: Noninvasive evaluation of the swollen extremity: experiences with 190 lymphoscintiographic examinations. *J Vasc Surg* 1989, 9:683–690.

24. Rockson SG, Miller LT, Senie R, *et al.*: American Cancer Society Lymphedema Workshop. Workgroup III: Diagnosis and management of lymphedema. *Cancer* 1998, 83:2882–2885.

25. Szuba A, Cooke JP, Yousuf S, Rockson SG: Decongestive lymphatic therapy for patients with cancer-related or primary lymphedema. *Am J Med* 2000, 109:296–300.

26. Charles RI I: *A System of Treatment*, vol 3. Edited by Latham A, English TC. London: J & A Churchill Ltd; 1912:504.

27. Brorson H, Svensson H: Liposuction combined with controlled compression therapy reduces arm lymphedema more effectively than controlled compression therapy alone. *Plast Reconstr Surg* 1998, 102:1058–1067.

13
CHAPTER

NEOPLASTIC AND NON-NEOPLASTIC VASCULAR TUMORS

Alexander J. F. Lazar and Scott R. Granter

Vascular neoplasms are a heterogeneous group of disorders that are derived from blood vessels or their cellular components: endothelial lining cells, smooth muscle cells, and pericytes. Since vessels are present throughout the body, vascular tumors may be seen in nearly any organ at any age. This diverse group encompasses congenital malformations such as the vascular ectasia or port-wine stain of Sturge-Weber syndrome and non-neoplastic inflammatory vascular proliferations such as bacillary angiomatosis. The spectrum of vascular neoplasms ranges from benign hemangiomas to intermediate-grade hemangioendotheliomas to highly malignant angiosarcomas. In addition, neoplasms of uncertain histogenesis, such as Kaposi's sarcoma and hemangioblastoma, fall under this rubric.

Because of the heterogeneous nature of these neoplasms, classification schemes are complex. Integration of clinical context and histologic features allows a definitive diagnosis in most cases. A definitive diagnosis is essential for proper treatment and prognostication. This chapter will serve as an overview for the clinical and pathologic spectrum of vascular tumors and tumor-like conditions.

BENIGN VASCULAR TUMORS

CLASSIFICATION OF BENIGN VASCULAR TUMORS AND TUMOR-LIKE CONDITIONS

Hemangioma
  Capillary hemangioma
    Cherry (senile) hemangioma
    Pyogenic granuloma (lobular capillary hemangioma)
    Tufted angioma
    Verrucous hemangioma
  Hobnail ("targetoid hemosiderotic") hemangioma
  Spindle cell hemangioma
  Cavernous hemangioma
  Venous hemangioma
  Arteriovenous hemangioma
  Soft tissue hemangioma
Glomus tumor
Angioleiomyoma
Reactive or acquired vascular proliferations
  Granulation tissue
  Bacillary angiomatosis
  Intravascular endothelial hyperplasia (Masson's tumor)
  Angiokeratoma
  Glomeruloid hemangioma

Vascular ectasia or malformation
  Nevus flammeus
  Port-wine stain
  Arteriovenous malformation
  Telangiectasia
  Arterial spider
Uncertain etiology
  Angiolymphoid hyperplasia with eosinophilia (epithelioid hemangioma)
  Hemangioblastoma

FIGURE 13-1. Classification of benign vascular tumors and tumor-like conditions. Hemangiomas are vascular proliferations whose components recapitulate normal vascular components and are thus classified according to the type of vessel composing the tumor. The importance of recognizing and subtyping reactive and acquired vascular proliferations is twofold. First, the distinction of a benign process from a malignant one is required to prevent overtreatment. Second, recognition of each entity is important since some may have important clinical implications. For example, bacillary angiomatosis, which is an infectious disease, must be distinguished from pyogenic granuloma, in order that antibiotic treatment be instituted in the former. In addition, certain types of vascular tumors are associated with disease syndromes (*see* Fig. 13-19).

CAPILLARY HEMANGIOMA: CLINICAL SUMMARY

Age:	Usually present in early childhood
Gender:	Females affected more commonly
Location:	Skin and subcutaneous tissue of head and neck most common location
Clinical:	Red, purple, or blue depending on proximity to skin surface; blanches with pressure; spontaneous involution and resolution in most cases arising during childhood

FIGURE 13-2. Clinical summary of capillary hemangioma, including age, sex, location, and clinical presentation.

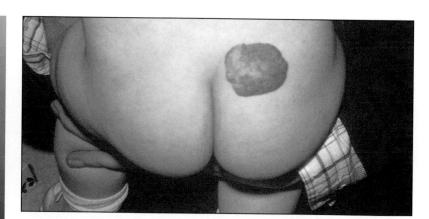

FIGURE 13-3. A typical example of a capillary hemangioma of infancy. The characteristic bright red color is due to the superficial position of the neoplastic blood vessels in the dermis and results in the alternate appellation, strawberry nevus. Lesions typically appear in the first few months of infancy as flat red patches and rapidly enlarge to develop a raised surface. Capillary hemangiomas tend toward regression during childhood. Treatment is often avoided because spontaneous regression tends to give better cosmetic results. (*Courtesy of* Stephen Gellis, MD, Boston Children's Hospital, Boston, MA.)

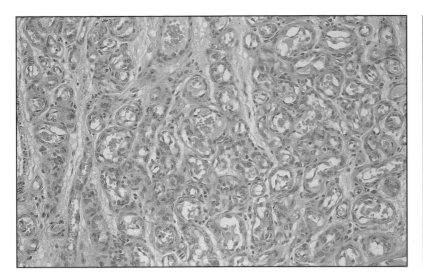

FIGURE 13-4. Capillary hemangioma. The dermis is expanded and nearly replaced by uniform small-caliber vessels lined by flattened endothelium. Despite the increased cellularity commonly present in capillary hemangiomas in children, the lack of necrosis, nuclear pleomorphism, and atypical mitotic figures are consistent with the benign nature of this tumor.

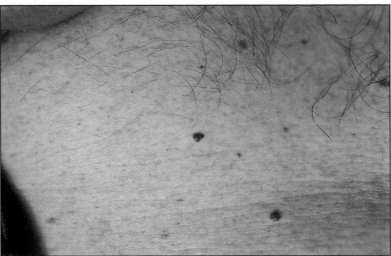

FIGURE 13-5. Cherry (senile) hemangioma. This extremely common capillary hemangioma is seen in young adults and increases in number and size with age. Two lesions on the chest of a middle-aged man are shown here. Characteristically, these lesions are single or multiple bright red, dome-shaped papules occurring on the trunk, proximal extremity, or head and neck. They are harmless and are only of cosmetic concern in some patients. They may be removed surgically or with electrocoagulation. (*Courtesy of* Rick Mitchell, MD, PhD, Brigham and Women's Hospital, Boston, MA.)

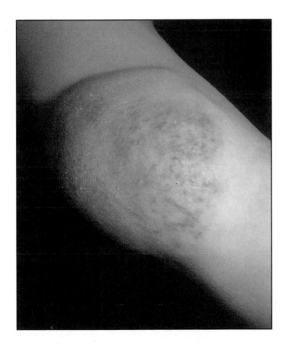

FIGURE 13-6. Cavernous hemangioma. Cavernous hemangiomas are paler than capillary hemangiomas because they occur deeper in the skin and subcutaneous tissue, even extending into the deep soft tissue. In some cases, however, a component of the vascular lesion extends to the cutaneous surface, giving a focal bright red color. Cavernous hemangiomas tend not to regress and may require surgical intervention if the vascular pressures are destructive to adjacent structures. Cavernous hemangiomas, like their capillary counterparts, tend to present in the head and neck area of children, predominantly girls. They may also involve visceral organs as well as deep soft tissue [1]. (*Courtesy of* Stephen Gellis, MD, Boston Children's Hospital, Boston, MA.)

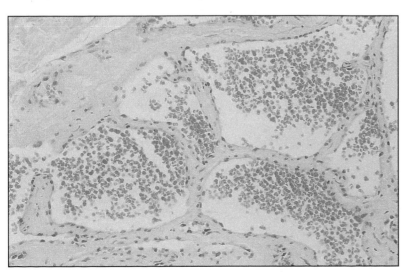

FIGURE 13-7. Cavernous hemangiomas. This photomicrograph shows the characteristic large, dilated, thin-walled vascular channels lined by flattened endothelial cells. These large dilated vascular channels give this lesion its name. Unlike capillary hemangiomas, cavernous hemangiomas show little or no tendency toward involution.

GLOMUS TUMOR: CLINICAL SUMMARY

Age:	2nd to 4th decade
Gender:	Male-to-female ratio roughly equal
Location:	Subcutaneous tissue of extremities, especially sub-ungual region; rarely stomach, cervix, vagina, nose
Clinical:	Small, red to blue, firm nodule; paroxysmal, burning elicited by trauma or temperature change

FIGURE 13-8. Clinical summary of glomus tumor, including age, sex, location, and clinical presentation [2].

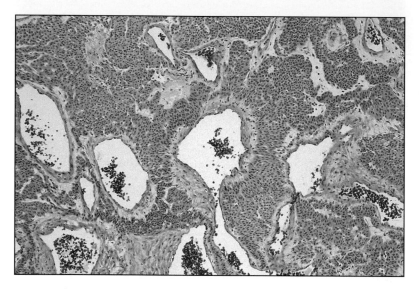

FIGURE 13-9. Glomus tumor. The glomus tumor is thought to be derived from modified smooth muscle cells of the glomus body, a specialized arteriovenous anastomosis that plays a role in thermoregulation. This photomicrograph shows a typical glomus tumor from the finger of a young adult. In the mid-dermis is an ectatic vascular space surrounded by uniform glomus cells. Complete removal is curative and provides welcome prompt symptomatic relief to the patient.

LOBULAR CAPILLARY HEMANGIOMA (PYOGENIC GRANULOMA): CLINICAL SUMMARY

Age:	All age groups
Gender:	Both sexes, with particular predilection for gingival lesions during pregnancy (pregnancy epulis)
Location:	Face, hands, oral and nasal mucous membranes
Clinical:	Friable red papules or polyps; tend to ulcerate and bleed; may recur locally after removal and rarely as multiple satellite lesions

FIGURE 13-10. Clinical summary of lobular capillary hemangioma (pyogenic granuloma), including age, sex, location, and clinical presentation [3].

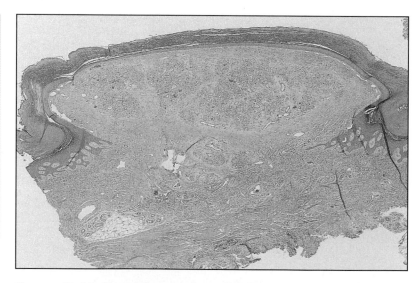

FIGURE 13-11. Pyogenic granuloma. These are mushroom-shaped lesions with a thin attenuated surface epithelium and a thickened (acanthotic) collar. The central vascular proliferation has a lobular array as in the capillary hemangiomas. Many cases have superficial ulceration with hemorrhage and inflammation resembling granulation tissue. Despite the often conspicuous presence of inflammation and granulation tissue, this benign lesion is believed to be neoplastic rather than reactive [1].

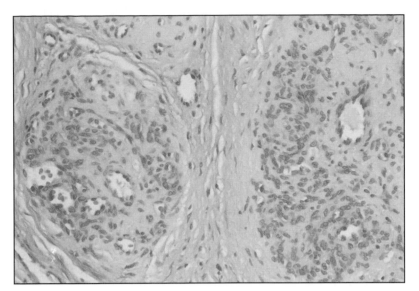

FIGURE 13-12. Pyogenic granuloma. Two discrete lobules are depicted with central patent vessels surrounded by clusters of small, incompletely canalized vessels. This architecture may be obscured by acute or chronic inflammation. The pyogenic granuloma that occurs during pregnancy, "pregnancy epulis," is histologically indistinguishable.

BACILLARY ANGIOMATOSIS: CLINICAL SUMMARY	
Epidemiology:	Primarily seen in AIDS patients, but has also been reported in immunocompetent patients
Location:	Skin, most common; also bone, spleen, liver, lymph nodes, and brain
Clinical:	Polypoid, red nodules in skin; peliosis in liver and spleen; resolves with erythromycin therapy

FIGURE 13-13. Clinical summary of bacillary angiomatosis, including epidemiology, location, and clinical presentation [4]. The incidence of this condition has fallen dramatically in populations where HIV-antiretroviral therapy is available.

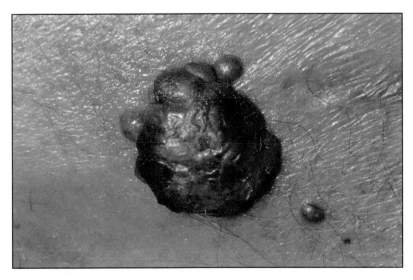

FIGURE 13-14. Bacillary angiomatosis (BA). These tumors are characterized by a reactive vascular proliferation secondary to infection by *Rochalimaea* species. Skin lesions, either solitary or multiple, are the most common manifestation. This red, dome-shaped nodule in an HIV-infected patient is typical. The lesions may be superficial or may involve subcutaneous and soft tissue. Some lesions are friable and prone to ulceration and bleeding with even minor trauma. Cutaneous BA may closely resemble Kaposi's sarcoma and pyogenic granuloma on clinical examination. While cutaneous BA is the most common presentation, other sites can also be affected. (*Courtesy of* Richard A. Johnson, MD, New England Deaconess Hospital, Boston, MA.)

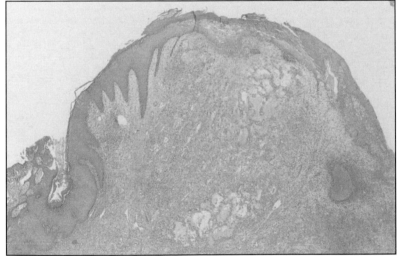

FIGURE 13-15. Bacillary angiomatosis (BA). This low-power micrographic view demonstrates the striking resemblance of BA to pyogenic granuloma (*see* Fig. 13-11). A thickened acanthotic collar that is so characteristic of pyogenic granuloma is present in this case. Both lesions also show a predilection for surface ulceration and bleeding after even mild trauma. The lesion is dome-shaped and is markedly edematous, forming clear spaces of fluid in some areas.

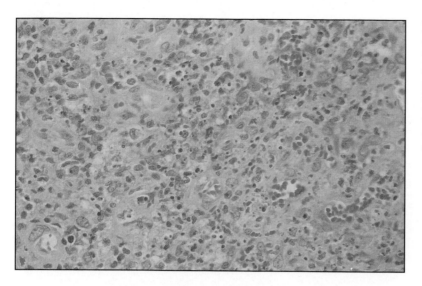

FIGURE 13-16. Bacillary angiomatosis (BA). This high-power view of the same case depicted in Fig. 13-15 demonstrates the salient histologic features. There is a proliferation of small capillary-sized vessels lined by plump histiocytoid endothelial cells, which may be so atypical as to warrant a consideration of angiosarcoma. However, helpful differentiating features are the prominent neutrophilic infiltrate and associated nuclear debris (karyorrhexis) that is the hallmark of BA. In addition, organisms are identified with silver stains or electron microscopy.

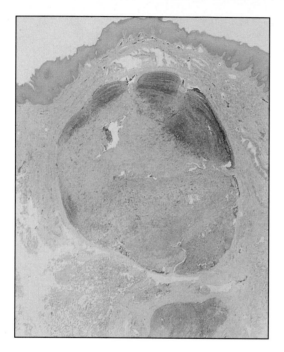

FIGURE 13-17. Intravascular papillary endothelial hyperplasia. This benign lesion, also known as Masson's tumor, is most likely a form of intravascular organization of thrombus rather than a true neoplasm. The lesions tend to occur in the hands, feet, or the head and neck region as a slowly enlarging red-blue papule or nodule. This low-power view shows a subcutaneous mass associated with thrombus.

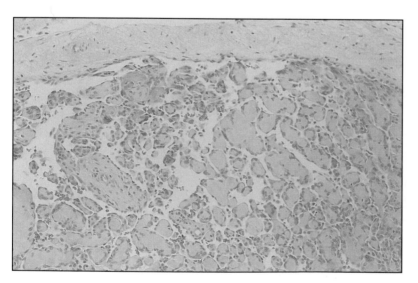

FIGURE 13-18. Intravascular papillary endothelial hyperplasia. Higher magnification demonstrates numerous delicate and bulbous papillary projections and anastomosing vascular channels that can simulate angiosarcoma. The Masson's tumor can be distinguished from angiosarcoma or nodular Kaposi's sarcoma by its intravascular location, infrequent mitoses and lack of necrosis, significant nuclear pleomorphism, or destructive invasion. The border of this proliferation has a sharp line of demarcation between the papillary projections and the surrounding connective tissue. The circumscribed nature of the specimen is also a very helpful feature in the distinction from malignant vascular tumors, especially angiosarcoma.

SYNDROMES ASSOCIATED WITH VASCULAR PROLIFERATIONS

Hereditary hemorrhagic telangiectasia (Osler-Weber-Rendu) syndrome	Autosomal dominant syndrome characterized by aggregates of small ectatic vessels (telangiectasias) involving skin and mucous membranes of the aerodigestive and urinary tracts that are prone to bleeding; may also involve the brain, liver, and spleen
Fabry's disease	While not a syndrome, this lyosomal storage disease caused by an absence of α-galactosidase A leading to accumulation of ceramide trihexoside is now treatable. The reactive angiokeratomas seen in this condition have a clinical appearance quite similar to cherry (senile) angiomas and can regress with treatment
Kasabach-Merrit syndrome	Large, giant cavernous hemangioma with thrombocytopenia and local consumption coagulopathy
Klippel-Trenaunay syndrome	Nevus flammeus involving one or more extremities; associated with soft tissue and bony hypertrophy as well as venous varicosities
Maffucci's syndrome	Multiple enchondromas associated with hemangiomas of the skin and subcutaneous tissues; patients are susceptible to developing chondrosarcomas and other types of sarcomas
Parke-Weber syndrome	Nevus flammeus of one or more extremities associated with soft tissue or bony hypertrophy and arteriovenous malformation
POEMS syndrome	Syndrome of polyneuropathy, organomegaly, endocrinopathy, M-protein, and skin changes combined with multicentric Castleman's disease. Glomeruloid hemangiomas, reactive ectatic vascular spaces filled with capillary aggregations reminiscent of renal glomeruli, can be seen
Sturge-Weber syndrome	Nevus flammeus in the distribution of the ophthalmic branch of the trigeminal nerve, sometimes with ipsilateral meningeal angioma resulting in secondary retardation, seizures, and hemiplegia
von Hippel-Lindau disease	Autosomal dominant syndrome characterized by hemangioblastomas of the cerebellum and retina in association with renal cysts and renal cell carcinoma, pancreatic cysts, cystadenoma of the epididymis, pheochromocytoma, and hemangiomas of the liver

FIGURE 13-19. Syndromes associated with vascular proliferations.

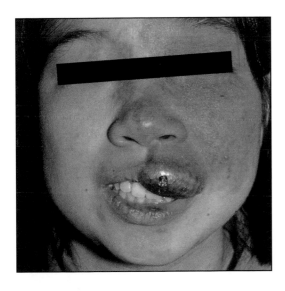

FIGURE 13-20. Sturge-Weber syndrome. This young woman with Sturge-Weber syndrome has a vascular malformation (nevus flammeus) involving skin in the distribution of the ophthalmic division of the trigeminal nerve. Involvement of oral mucosa can be seen. This patient also has associated glaucoma and hypertrophy of the maxilla. Patients with Sturge-Weber syndrome also suffer from seizures and neurologic deficits due to leptomeningeal vascular malformations. There are other syndromes associated with vascular proliferations as well (*see* Fig. 13-19). (*Courtesy of* John B. Mulliken, MD, Boston Children's Hospital, Boston, MA.)

FIGURE 13-21. Clinical summary of angiolymphoid hyperplasia, including age, sex, location, and clinical presentation [5]. This lesion is also designated epithelioid hemangioma.

ANGIOLYMPHOID HYPERPLASIA: CLINICAL SUMMARY

Age:	Usually in the 2nd to 4th decades
Gender:	More prevalent in women
Location:	Head and neck is the most common site, often around the ear
Clinical:	Single or multiple pruritic red papules; may have regional adenopathy and peripheral eosinophilia; lesions usually persist if untreated or incompletely excised

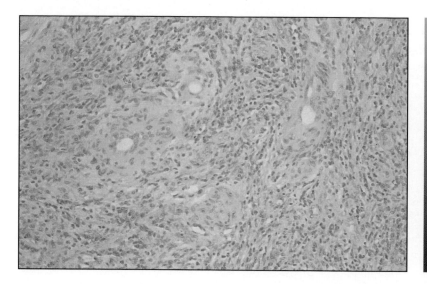

HEMANGIOBLASTOMA: CLINICAL SUMMARY

Age:	Most common in adulthood
Location:	Cerebellum is the most common location; less common in the brainstem and spinal cord; tumors of the retina are seen in the von Hippel-Lindau syndrome
Clinical:	Often presents with ataxia; benign; may be sporadic or associated with the von Hippel-Lindau syndrome, which is an autosomal-dominant disorder; other manifestations include renal cysts and renal cell carcinoma, pancreatic cysts, cystadenoma of the epididymis, pheochromocytoma, and hemangiomas of the liver

FIGURE 13-22. Angiolymphoid hyperplasia with eosinophilia. It is not clear whether this disease represents a reactive process or a benign neoplasm. The salient histologic features are dermal replacement by a proliferation of small vessels surrounded by a dense inflammatory infiltrate. Abundant eosinophils and lymphocytes are characteristic of this lesion. This lesion is also designated epithelioid hemangioma [4].

FIGURE 13-23. Clinical summary of hemangioblastoma, including age, location, and clinical presentation.

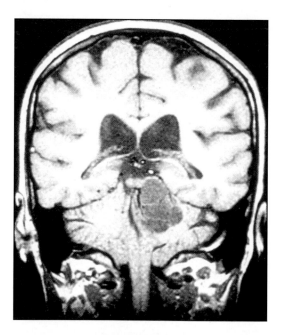

FIGURE 13-24. Hemangioblastoma. This magnetic resonance image of the brain is from a patient with von Hippel-Lindau disease (VHL). A mass is located in the cerebellum, which is by far the most common location for hemangioblastomas; it can also arise in the retina. This patient developed a pheochromocytoma in addition to the hemangioblastoma. Von Hippel-Lindau disease is also associated with renal cell carcinoma, islet cell tumor of the pancreas, pheochromocytoma, and cysts in a variety of internal organs. The *VHL* gene responsible for this syndrome acts as a tumor suppressor gene. Patients with VHL disease carry a germline inactivation of one *VHL* allele inherited in an autosomal dominant fashion. Tumors arise when the remaining allele is inactivated in a cell. The precise function of the protein encoded by *VHL* is not known, but it appears to be involved in the regulation of the cellular response to hypoxia. This function is intriguing in light of the high vascularity of the hemangioblastomas and other VHL disease-associated neoplasms [6].

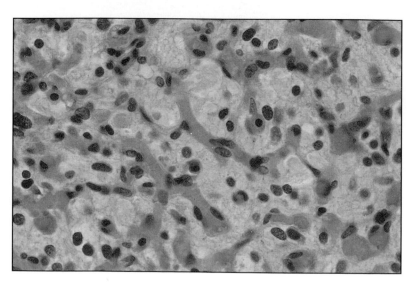

FIGURE 13-25. Hemangioblastoma. Microscopic examination demonstrates the two cell populations that are seen in hemangioblastomas: blood vessels and interstitial cells. Current research indicates that the interstitial cells are neoplastic, while the blood vessels are reactive and may arise in response to factors secreted by the interstitial cells. The origin of these interstitial cells is not known. The large round to polygonal interstitial cells have abundant foamy cytoplasm that contains fat. Some of these tumors produce erythropoietin or a similar factor that may lead to polycythemia [6].

CLINICAL FORMS OF KAPOSI'S SARCOMA

European-endemic (or classic)	Most commonly seen in elderly Mediterranean, Eastern European, and Ashkenazi Jewish males. The disease is characterized by chronic skin involvement, usually limited to dermal involvement, with patients usually dying of an unrelated disease
African-endemic (non–HIV-associated)	Affects young children with predominantly lymph node involvement. The disease runs an aggressive, usually deadly course. A second clinical group of young adults is seen in sub-Saharan Central Africa. This group usually has limb involvement and may develop locally aggressive disease with lesions extending into soft tissue and bone or generalized disease. It is this latter form of the disease that some authorities consider to be a true neoplasm with recurrent and locally aggressive potential, thus falling into the intermediate or borderline group of vascular tumors
Transplantation- (or immumosuppression-) associated	Transplant allograft recipients on immunosuppressive therapy may develop a cutaneous and lymph node–based disease. The lesions may regress with withdrawal of immunosuppressive therapy
Epidemic (AIDS-associated)	Generalized mucocutaneous, lymph node, and visceral involvement in AIDS patients, especially homosexual or bisexual men

FIGURE 13-26. Four clinical forms of Kaposi's sarcoma are recognized: European-endemic, African-endemic, transplantation-associated, and epidemic [7]. All four clinical variants are now known to be associated with human herpes virus VIII (HHV8) infection. The association of this disease with HHV8 infection and immunocompromised patients would seem to indicate that it is a reactive process.

However, some researchers believe that a truly neoplastic or sarcomatous tumor may arise in this condition, perhaps in a manner analogous to cervical cancer arising in human papillomavirus-infected cells. Certain clinical subsets of this lesion can behave in a very aggressive manner. Though some researchers believe that Kaposi's sarcoma originates in the endothelium, the pathogenesis is controversial [7].

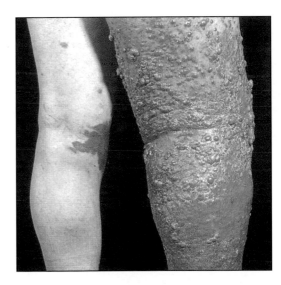

FIGURE 13-27. Endemic Kaposi's sarcoma (KS). This elderly patient with endemic KS has diffuse involvement of one leg with multiple nodules that coalesce in areas. Despite this striking involvement, KS typically will remain limited to the limbs without causing death of the patient. (*Courtesy of* Richard A. Johnson, MD, New England Deaconess Hospital, Boston, MA.)

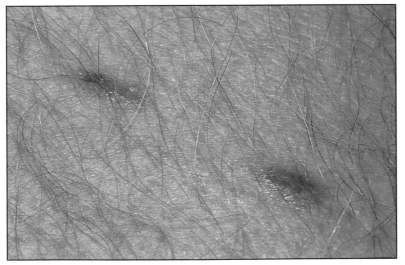

FIGURE 13-28. Epidemic Kaposi's sarcoma (KS). The spectrum of lesions seen in AIDS-associated KS progresses from small red-pink macules to plaques and finally to nodules and masses. These slightly elevated red-purple papules on the upper chest of a young HIV-infected man represent early KS lesions. (*Courtesy of* Richard A. Johnson, MD, New England Deaconess Hospital, Boston, MA.)

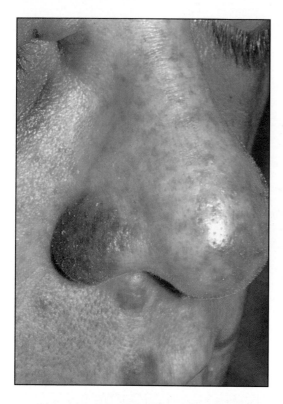

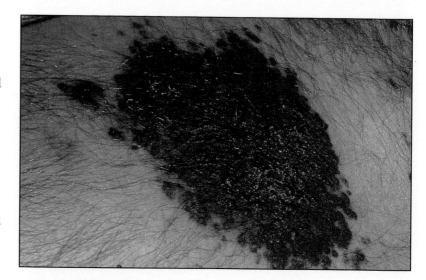

FIGURE 13-29. Epidemic Kaposi's sarcoma (KS). The nose is very frequently involved in HIV-associated KS. The tip of this patient's nose shows a pink-red macule. A darker purple plaque, located on the ala, represents an older and more advanced lesion. Two nodules of KS are seen on the upper lip. (*Courtesy of* Richard A. Johnson, MD, New England Deaconess Hospital, Boston, MA.)

FIGURE 13-30. Epidemic Kaposi's sarcoma. This photograph shows a more advanced lesion, a large plaque on the skin of an HIV-infected patient. Large lesions such as this one often start as multiple patches or plaques before becoming confluent. Deep involvement of lymphatics and lymph nodes may cause lymphedema. (*Courtesy of* Richard A. Johnson, MD, New England Deaconess Hospital, Boston, MA.)

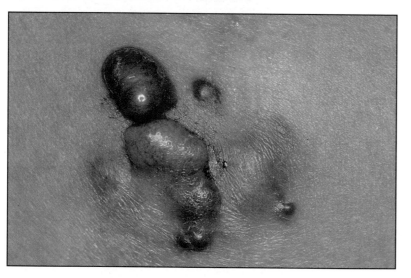

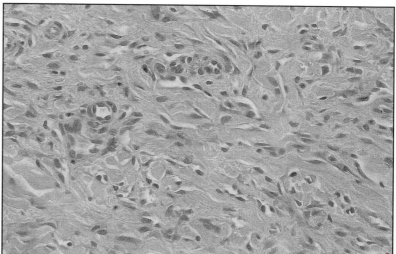

FIGURE 13-31. Epidemic Kaposi's sarcoma (KS). This photograph shows red-purple nodules characteristic of the more advanced nodular stage of KS in this HIV-infected patient. Multiple nodules may enlarge and coalesce to form tumorous masses that may ulcerate and bleed. (*Courtesy of* Richard A. Johnson, MD, New England Deaconess Hospital, Boston, MA.)

FIGURE 13-32. Epidemic Kaposi's sarcoma (KS). This is a typical plaque-stage KS lesion in an HIV-infected patient. In this stage, a diffuse proliferation of spindled cells dissects through dermal collagen and forms characteristic slit-like vascular spaces. Sprinkled throughout the lesion are lymphocytes and plasma cells.

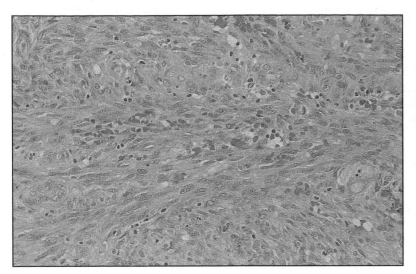

FIGURE 13-33. Epidemic Kaposi's sarcoma (KS). This nodular KS illustrates several fascicles of monomorphic spindled cells that intersect one another at right angles. Slit-like vascular spaces, some of which are filled with red blood cells, are seen. Deposits of hemoglobin and intracellular hyaline globules, which are thought to be erythrocyte breakdown products, may be present. A lymphoplasmacytic infiltrate is seen admixed with tumor cells.

INTERMEDIATE OR BORDERLINE VASCULAR TUMORS

Kaposi's sarcoma
Retiform hemangioendothelioma
Kaposiform hemangioendothelioma
Polymorphous hemangioendothelioma
Malignant endovascular papillary angioendothelioma
  (Dabska tumor)
Composite hemangioendothelioma

FIGURE 13-34. Classification of intermediate or borderline vascular tumors. This class of vascular neoplasm exhibits behavior between the benign vascular tumor and the highly malignant angiosarcoma. Many of the tumors in this class, particularly the hemangioendotheliomas, have been described only recently. The lesions in this family have a tendency to recur locally but have extremely low metastatic potential. While epithelioid hemangioendothelioma was previously considered part of this group, recent discovery of metastatic rates up to 31% has led to the reclassification of this lesion as malignant. Other entities in this group may be reclassified as benign or malignant, as more evidence of their behavior accumulates. The proper classification of these lesions is critical to provide for proper excision to prevent local recurrence while avoiding the more radical treatments required for malignant neoplasms [8].

RETIFORM HEMANGIOENDOTHELIOMA: CLINICAL SUMMARY

Age:	Young adults
Gender:	Both sexes
Location:	Skin and subcutaneous sites
Clinical:	Cutaneous tumor with indolent growth most commonly found in the extremities, especially the lower limbs; local recurrence is seen; metastasis is extremely rare

FIGURE 13-35. Clinical summary of retiform hemangioendothelioma, including age, gender, location, and clinical presentation. This is a recently described tumor. Histologically, this lesion is reminiscent of the rete testis, as the name implies.

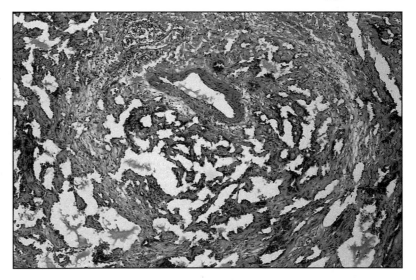

FIGURE 13-36. Retiform hemangioendothelioma. This is a recurrent lesion from the foot of a young adult male and shows arborizing narrow vessels with prominent endothelial nuclei that protrude into the lumen. The absence of endothelial pleomorphism, mitotic activity, and irregular dissection of collagen bundles in the dermis separates this lesion from cutaneous angiosarcoma. In addition, cutaneous angiosarcoma usually presents in a more elderly population (*see* Fig. 13-39). (*Courtesy of* Christopher D. M. Fletcher, MD, FRCPath, Brigham and Women's Hospital, Boston, MA.)

EPITHELIOID HEMANGIOENDOTHELIOMA: CLINICAL SUMMARY

Age:	All age groups, but unusual in childhood
Gender:	Both sexes affected with nearly equal frequency
Location:	Most frequently in soft tissues, subcutis, and muscle; may also occur in the head and neck, liver, lung, and bone
Clinical:	Solitary, sometimes tender mass; 13% of cases recurred and 31% of cases developed metastatic disease in one series

FIGURE 13-37. Clinical summary of epithelioid hemangioendothelioma, including age, gender, location, and clinical presentation. While previously thought to be intermediate or borderline, this tumor has recently been reclassified as malignant. Despite its somewhat better prognosis, this tumor occupies the same class as the highly aggressive angiosarcomas [8].

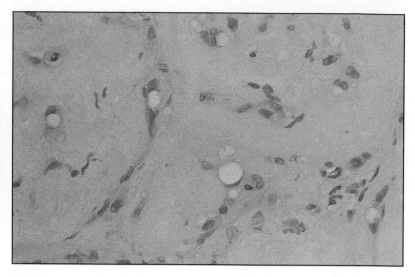

FIGURE 13-38. Epithelioid hemangioendothelioma. This pauci-cellular tumor characteristically has abundant, amorphous, hyaline matrix widely separating clusters of tumor cells. Embedded in the stroma are plump, epithelioid endothelial cells in nests or cords. These neoplastic cells characteristically contain prominent cytoplasmic lumina that recapitulate angiogenesis. Occasional blood cells are seen in these miniature lumina. Well-formed vascular spaces are not readily seen. The endothelial origin of this tumor is supported by ultrastructural studies and immunoperoxidase techniques demonstrating expression of antigens found in endothelial cells [8].

ANGIOSARCOMA: CLINICAL SUMMARY

Idiopathic angiosarcoma	Skin and subcutaneous tissue are the most common locations affected by angiosarcoma; the head and neck region is the most common site with a particular predilection for skin of the scalp on elderly patients, often males; skin lesions present as bluish bruise-like plaques and more superficial red nodules; lesions are prone to ulceration and bleeding
Lymphedema-associated angiosarcoma	An association between angiosarcoma and chronic lymphedema of various etiologies is well recognized; the most common example is Stewart-Treves syndrome (angiosarcoma arising in the setting of post-mastectomy lymphedema); in the past, these tumors have been called lymphangiosarcomas
Post-radiation angiosarcoma	Classically seen in the skin of the breast years after radiation for breast carcinoma, this lesion can be seen in irradiated skin in other locations as well; there is a recent unexplained increase in the incidence of this form of angiosarcoma
Soft tissue angiosarcoma	This lesion is seen in older males, usually in the deep portions of the lower limb and abdomen; while still rare, the discovery that these lesions exhibit epithelioid morphology has led to increased recognition; up to one third of these lesions are associated with syndromes such as neurofibromatosis, Mafucci's syndrome, and Klippel-Trenaunay syndome (*see* Fig. 13-19)

FIGURE 13-39. Clinical summary of angiosarcoma. Angiosarcomas are rare, highly malignant tumors derived from endothelial cells and are seen in many different organs in characteristic clinical settings. In all settings, the neoplasm has a highly aggressive course with dismal 5-year survival rates. Angiosarcomas can adopt a range of histologic appearances from vascular to spindle cell to epithelioid morphologies [1,8].

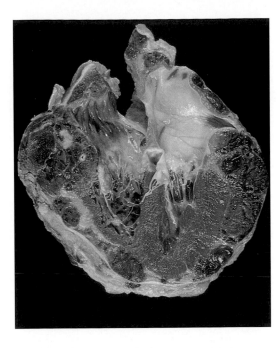

FIGURE 13-40. Angiosarcoma of the heart. This example of a rare angiosarcoma of the heart can be seen involving the atria and both ventricles. The tumor is a dark brown, spongy, and markedly hemorrhagic mass involving all chambers. The variegated nature of this tumor is attributed to the presence of clotted blood of varying ages. Angiosarcoma, although rare, is the most common primary malignant tumor of the heart [9]. (*From* Schoen [9]; with permission.)

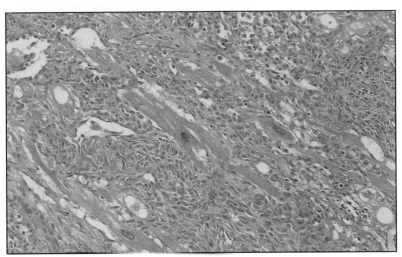

FIGURE 13-41. Angiosarcoma of the heart. This micrograph shows several residual myocytes surrounded by an infiltrating angiosarcoma. The majority of tumor cells are spindled and the vascular origin of this tumor is not always readily apparent on routine histologic examination. Immunophenotyping is often necessary in such cases to make a definitive diagnosis.

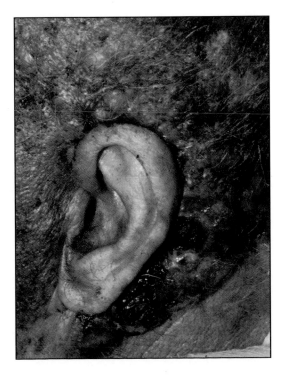

FIGURE 13-42. Cutaneous angiosarcoma. This lesion is very aggressive and locally destructive. Most of these lesions initially present as bruise-like areas with an indurated edge. As the lesion advances, it becomes raised and nodular and may ulcerate. Cutaneous angiosarcoma is difficult to treat because many of the lesions are multifocal at presentation. Metastasis to lymph nodes and lung is common. (*Courtesy of* Phillip H. McKee, MD, FRCPath, Brigham and Women's Hospital, Boston, MA.)

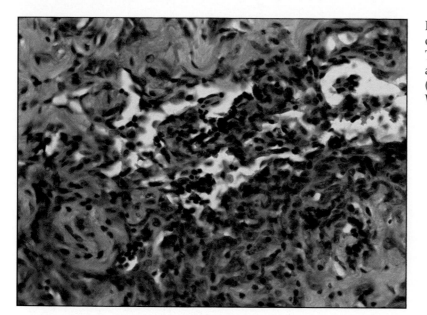

FIGURE 13-43. Cutaneous angiosarcoma. This lesion is composed of pleomorphic cells in multiple layers lining the vascular spaces. The infiltrating tumor cells form irregular anastomotic spaces as they dissect through the collagen bundles of the dermis. (*Courtesy of* Phillip H. McKee, MD, FRCPath, Brigham and Women's Hospital, Boston, MA.)

REFERENCES

1. Fletcher CDM: *Diagnostic Histopathology of Tumors*, 2nd ed. London: Churchill Livingston; 2000:45–86.

2. Weiss SW, Goldblum JR: *Enzinger and Weiss's Soft Tissue Tumors*, 4th ed. St. Louis: Mosby; 2001:985–996.

3. Warner T, Wilson-Jones E: Pyogenic granuloma recurring with multiple satellites: a report of eleven cases. *Br J Dermatol* 1968, 80:218–227.

4. Tappero JW, Mohle-Boetani J, Koehler JE, *et al.*: The epidemiology of bacillary angiomatosis and bacillary peliosis. *JAMA* 1993, 269:770–775.

5. Olsen TG, Helwig ED: Angiolymphoid hyperplasia with eosinophilia: a clinicopathologic study of 116 patients. *J Am Acad Dermatol* 1985, 12:781–796.

6. Mircea I, Kaelin WG, Jr: The von Hippel-Lindau tumor suppressor protein. *Cur Opin Gen Dev* 2001, 11:27–34.

7. Antman K, Chang Y: Medical progress: Kaposi's sarcoma. *N Engl J Med* 2000, 342(14):1027–1038.

8. Kempson RL, Fletcher CDM, Evens HL, *et al.*: *Tumors of the Soft Tissues, Atlas of Tumor Pathology*, fasicle 30, series 3. Washington, DC: Armed Forces Institute of Pathology; 2001:307–370.

9. Schoen FJ: *Interventional and Surgical Cardiovascular Pathology: Clinical Correlations and Basic Principles*. Philadelphia: WB Saunders; 1989: 209–210.

Lymphoscintigraphy
  of bilateral lymphedema, 248
  normal, 243

M

M-mode echocardiography, 220
Macromolecular tracer, lymphatic transport
    of, 243
Maffucci's syndrome, 261
Magnetic resonance angiography
  for carotid stenosis and stroke, 131
  of carotid stenosis and stroke, 133
  for chronic mesenteric arterial insufficiency,
    111–112
  for renal artery stenosis, 90, 97, 98
  sensitivity of, 98
  of vertebrobasilar circulation, 143
Magnetic resonance imaging
  accuracy of, 37
  advantages and disadvantages of, 37
  in aortic aneurysm diagnosis, 7
  for aortic dissection, 25, 36–37
    diagnostic performance of, 40
  black-blood technique in, 36
  for cerebrovascular disease, 129
  for cortical infarct, 134
  for stroke, 131
Magnetic resonance venography, 212
Malon-dialdehyde, 177
Marfan syndrome, 2, 4
  aorta in, 6
  in aortic dissection, 26
  cystic medial necrosis in, 27
Masson's tumor, 260
Mastectomy
  lymphedema associated with, 249
  lymphedema of arm after, 247
    therapy for, 251
Meandering artery, 113
Mechanical thrombectomy, 221
Media, 1
Medical Research Council European Carotid
    Surgery Trial, 139
Mesenteric arterial beds, 113
Mesenteric arterial insufficiency, chronic, 122
Mesenteric artery, 112
  colonic branches of, 113
  mycotic aneurysm of, 20
  occlusion of
    atrial fibrillation with, 119
    bowel injury patterns with, 117
    patterns of, 116
  small intestinal branches of, 112
  stenosis of, 123
  superior
    occlusion of, 124
      bowel injury patterns with, 117
      patterns of, 116

stenosis of, 123, 126
vasospasm in, 115
Mesenteric blood flow
  measurement of, 114
  regulation of, 114–115
Mesenteric circulation, 111
  vascular compromise in, 111
Mesenteric insufficiency, chronic, 111–112
  symptom relief with bypass grafting and
    transaortic endarterectomy for, 126
Mesenteric ischemia
  acute
    diagnosis of, 119–120
    pathophysiology of, 116–118
    presentation of, 119
    surgical exploration for, 121
    therapy for, 121
  chronic
    diagnosis of, 122–124
    extent of obstruction in, 122
    signs and symptoms of, 122
    therapy for, 124, 125–126
  comorbidity in, 112
  diagnosis of, 111–112
  nonocclusive, 111
    supportive medical therapy for, 121
  risk factors for, 116
  therapy for, 112
Mesenteric vascular anatomy, 112–114
  redundant, 111
Mesenteric vascular disease, 111–126
Mesenteric veins, 113
  obstruction of, 120
Mesenteric venous occlusion, 111, 112
  therapy for, 121
Mesenteric venous thrombosis
  conditions associated with, 118
  presentation of, 119
  radiologic findings in, 120
Mesh graft, 239
Metatarsal ulceration, 54
Methylprednisolone, 202
Metoprolol, 166
Microarteriolysis, radical, 184
Microscopy, pulmonary, 218
Milroy's disease, 244
Missense mutations, 244
Multi-infarct dementia, 144
Multiple hemispheric lacunes, 144
Mycosis, 6
Mycotic aneurysm, 20
Myeloproliferative disease, 185
  in Raynaud's phenomenon, 177
Myocardial infarction
  antiplatelet drug effects on, 136
  with cerebral embolism, 146
  Kaplan-Meier curves of patients free from, 171
  in Kawasaki disease, 204
  Q-wave, in vascular surgery patients, 155
  risk of in peripheral arterial disease, 59
Myocardial ischemia

atenolol and, 167
heart rate control and, 168
low intraoperative prevalence of, 164
perioperative cardiac outcome and, 166
Myocarditis, 189
Myxedema, 245

N

Nailfold capillary microscopy, 173, 180, 181
National Cholesterol Education Panel (NCEP)
    guidelines, 60
Necrotizing vasculitis, 177
Nephrectomy, 82
Nephrosclerosis, 96
Neurofibromatosis, 85
Neurohumoral mediators, 177
Neurologic disorders
  in chronic venous insufficiency, 229
  in Raynaud's phenomenon, 177
Nevus flammeus, 261
Nicardipine, 182
Nifedipine, 182, 183
Nitrates
  cardiac risk and in vascular surgery
    patients, 166
  predicting outcome of in renal artery
    stenosis, 96
Nitric oxide, 226
Noninvasive cardiac testing, 151
Noninvasive vascular testing, 54–57
North American Symptomatic Carotid
    Endarterectomy Trial (NASCET), 138, 139

O

Obesity, 229, 233
Oncotic pressure, 241
Optic neuropathy, ischemic, 131
Oral contraceptives, 207
Oral hydration, 91
Osler-Weber-Rendu syndrome, 261

P

Pacemakers
  in upper extremity venous thrombosis, 212
  in venous thrombosis, 207
Palma crossover femorofemoral venous
    bypass, 239
Palmaz stents, 67
Parke-Weber syndrome, 261
PARTNERS study, 53
Peau d'orange, 245, 246
Penetrating atherosclerotic ulcer, 44
Pentoxifylline, 62
Percussive injury, 179

a